SURGERY – PROCEDURES, COMPLICATIONS, AND RESULTS

Additional books and e-books in this series can be found
on Nova's website under the Series tab.

SURGERY – PROCEDURES, COMPLICATIONS, AND RESULTS

CASE REPORTS IN SURGERY

SURGERY – PROCEDURES, COMPLICATIONS, AND RESULTS

CASE REPORTS IN SURGERY

AHMAD JABIR RAHYUSSALIM
ISMAIL HADISOEBROTO DILOGO
ACHMAD FAUZI KAMAL
AND
ARYADI KURNIAWAN
EDITORS

nova
Medicine & Health
New York

Library of Congress Cataloging-in-Publication Data

ISBN: 978-1-53616-582-1
Library of Congress Control Number:2019952135

Published by Nova Science Publishers, Inc. † New York

CONTENTS

PREFACE

This book of case reports focuses on a wide variety of surgery cases from the national referral center in Indonesia, Cipto Mangunkusumo Hospital. The thirty-eight reports included in this book range from rare diseases to practices of state-of-the-art surgery methods and materials, all collected in order to answer the needs of fellow clinicians, surgeons and general practitioners alike, who face similar patients and conditions. We believe this book would also be beneficial for the purpose of knowledge sharing and scientific discussions across the medical field.

The reports published in this book were written by handled by surgeons with each respective expertise, ensuring the reliability of the contents. We hope that this publication will continue to be useful and will be followed up by upcoming issues of this case report series.

Chapter 1 - In electrical burn injuries, non vital tissue debridement and adequate defect closure determines the outcome of limb salvage. Clarification of the advantages of groin flap use for soft tissue defect closure is required to assist medical practitioners in deciding if groin flap should be considered as an option for upper limb reconstruction due to electrical burns. Two cases of electrical burn injuries to the extremities with two-stage reconstructive surgery using groin flap were reported. We questioned clinically whether a two-stage surgical method affected the morbidity of patients with electrical burns and investigated the correlation between the type of flap harvesting (delayed and non-delayed groin flap) and flap vitality and did literature search and analysis. We concluded that the use of groin flap as distant pedicle flaps provided an alternative in cases where free flap reconstruction was impossible.

Chapter 2 - Aortic dissection is a condition in which there is a tear in the aorta's tunica intima layer, leading to separation between the tunica intima and the tunica media, forming a false lumen. We report an autopsy of a 60-year-old German man diagnosed with Stanford type B (DeBakey type III) aortic dissection who underwent a debranching aorto-innominate-carotid graft (Y-graft) and TEVAR surgery. The external examination revealed postsurgical scars on the chest and left inguinal region along with injection marks on both upper extremities. The internal examination revealed blood inside the thorax; heart filled with blood and blood clots; cardiac enlargement; a constricted left coronary artery; an aortic wall laceration; separation of the tunica intima from the tunica media and adventitia throughout the ascending, descending, and abdominal aorta, forming a false lumen containing blood clots; atherosclerosis; and signs of damaged internal organs. Histopathological examination revealed an acute myocardial rupture, atherosclerosis in the left coronary artery, dissection of the aorta accompanied with erythrocyte infiltration in the aortic wall, and signs of internal organ congestion.

Chapter 3 - Meningioma is the most common type of benign intracranial tumor. The occurrence of extracranial meningioma is rare, accounting for only 2% of all meningiomas. There are two types of extracranial meningioma: primary and secondary. Primary extracranial meningioma grows extracranially without any connection to intracranial lesions, whereas secondary extracranial meningioma is an intracranial meningioma that extends extracranially. Herein, we report the case of a 45-year-old female patient with secondary extracranial sinonasal meningioma who presented with intermittent headache and unilateral proptosis due to olfactory groove meningioma that expanded to the right ethmoid sinus. Gross tumor resection was achieved in this case.

Chapter 4 - Currently, there has been an increase in the incidence of acute pancreatitis worldwide. Pain control is an important part of supportive management for patients with acute pancreatitis. A 26-year-old woman presented to our emergency department with a distended abdomen and excruciating pain in the upper abdomen. She was diagnosed with acute pancreatitis. She developed acute respiratory distress; thus, she was intubated and admitted to the intensive care unit. Her upper abdominal pain gradually intensified, causing worsening of acute respiratory distress syndrome. Thoracic epidural analgesia at the T7–T8 interspace was considered for pain management. Epidural analgesia is one of the important pain management modalities, and it stops severe acute pancreatitis development by improving splanchnic and pancreatic perfusion, resulting in decreased liver damage and inflammatory responses.

Chapter 5 - ABO-incompatible kidney transplantation (ABOi-KT) is a strategy to overcome the shortage of organ donors. It is considered a high-risk option because of potential antibody-mediated rejection (AMR); however, it results in improved outcomes because of the use of more potent immunosuppressants in combination with splenectomy and therapeutic plasma exchange (TPE). We reported a case of a 54-year-old male O-blood type recipient who received an A-blood type living donor kidney. The desensitization protocol consisted of a combination of three sessions of TPE with immunosuppressants administered prior to transplantation. The anti-A antibody IgM-IgG titers could be reduced and maintained at a range of 1:32–1:4. Additionally, the fibrinogen level was 245 mg/dl prior to transplantation without any fresh frozen plasma(FFP)replacement. There was massive postoperative bleeding due to the low fibrinogen level. The patient received cryoprecipitates and intravenous tranexamic acid and was discharged from the hospital on day-7posttransplantation. Preoperative TPE was the primary therapy for ABOi-KT in this patient. Only three sessions were performed, but it caused hypofibrinogenemia and postoperative bleeding. Coagulation factor monitoring and blood component therapy were essential to prevent these complications.

Chapter 6 - The vulvoperineal region is key to the urinary and reproductive systems and is closely related to the gastrointestinal system. Most vulvar defects result from tumor ablation, but reconstruction after oncological resection remains challenging as the reconstructive target is to restore adequate function with an ideal aesthetic result. Here, we report the case of a 46-year-old female with extramammary Paget's disease of the vulva. She underwent oncological excision for vulvar reconstruction. Keystone perforator island flaps in this patient achieved symmetrical bilateral results of vulva subunits. The patient was satisfied with the vulva appearance and reported no limitations in daily activities. The use of keystone perforator island flaps is a superior option for vulva reconstruction to achieve a symmetrical outcome.

Chapter 7 - Congenital melanocytic nevus (CMN) is a benign proliferation of melanocytes that appears at birth or within weeks of life. The condition occurs in 1%–2% of newborns, with a 2%–42% and 6%–14% risk of transforming into malignancy or developing into multiple myeloma. The occurrence of CMN involving the auricular area is uncommon. Although excision of the nevus is the treatment of choice, this procedure is challenging. A wide area of CMN requires extensive excision coupled with a reconstructive procedure.In this article, we present a case of giant CMN in a 6-year-old female with giant pigmented nevi appearing after birth in all parts of her body, particularly the right facial, auricular, post auricular, mastoid, and neck areas. The diagnosis was reached based on the results of a biopsy revealing the presence of melanocytic nevus. Wide excision of the nevus at the right auricular with cartilage exposure was performed and a split-thickness skin graftwas used for the reconstruction of the auricle. Postoperative follow-up showed good outcome.

Chapter 8 - Parry–Romberg syndrome (PRS) is a rare degenerative disease characterized by unilateral, slow, and progressive atrophy of the facial tissue (including muscle, bones, and skin). Patients with this syndrome often develop a deviated nose. Such condition may lead to various aesthetic and functional issues. Septorhinoplasty plays a central role in the successful management of deviated nose. Here, we discuss the management of deviated nose in a patient with PRS along with evaluation of its characteristics, etiology, and pathophysiology. An 18-year-old female with deviated nose and the angle of her mouth toward the right side of the face underwent septorhinoplasty and labioplasty. Post surgery, functional and aesthetic improvements were observed in the deviated nose and facial asymmetry.

Chapter 9 - The nose is the most prominent structure in the center of the face and plays an important role in the aesthetics of the face. Nasal defects in the dorsum, ala nasi, nostrils, columella, or septum due to trauma, animal bites, and tumor can lead to loss of function and decrease in aesthetic value. Nasolabial and nasal septal flaps are used for the reconstruction of nasal defects after mass extirpation in the lower third of the nose, particularly in cases of ala nasi defects. Here, we report the case of a patient who underwent reconstruction with a combination of nasolabial and nasal septal flaps for an ala nasi defect due to mass extirpation for basal cell carcinoma. We also conducted an evidence-based literature search tailored to the case.

Chapter 10 - Background: Supernumerary nostrils are an extremely rare congenital Purpose: To prepare a standardized procedure for repairing supernumerary nostrils, and to discuss the probable psychological effect on the patient. Patients and Methods: Fistulectomy and cartilage graft from the ear were performed to reconstruct the accessory nostril. Surgery was performed at a young age to prevent further disfiguration and to optimize psychological well-being. Result: The wound showed good healing progress over the lateral side of the nose. Although the symmetry between the two nostrils was not ideal, it was acceptable. Conclusion: The repair aims to create a functioning and normal-appearing nose with minimal deformity. The extra nostril can be excised during fistulectomy. The patient can also be offered social skill training to improve their self-esteem and family acceptance and support are important in the rehabilitation of children with facial disfigurations.

Chapter 11 - Nasal valve, which is the narrowest area in the nasal airway passage, is responsible for about half of the total nasal airway resistance. Functional septorhinoplasty is used to achieve an esthetic shape of the nose while preserving adequate nasal and breathing function. Nasal complaints are subjective; thus, objective measurements obtained through active anterior rhinomanometry are needed to correctly identify nasal valve incompetence. We present reports of two cases where changes in nasal airflow and resistance were objectively assessed before and after functional septorhinoplasty using an alar batten graft. Significant changes were observed postoperatively. Improvement was confirmed by assessment of subjective symptoms of nasal obstruction and rhinomanometry data.

Chapter 12 - Voice therapy is one of the alternative treatments for laryngopharyngeal reflux. To evaluate the effect of voice therapy in addition to medical anti reflux treatment in a patient with laryngopharyngeal reflux with persistent voice-related symptoms with the use of subjective assessment by the Reflux Symptom Index and the Voice Handicap Index and objective evaluation of the vocal cords by laryngovideostroboscopy. A 48-year-old woman with laryngopharyngeal reflux presented with hoarseness and a sensation of lump in her throat for the previous 6 months. Evaluation by subjective and objective assessments showed a significant improvement after the comprehensive treatment strategy. After voice therapy and the use of a proton-pump inhibitor, the Reflux Symptom Index decreased from 19 to 10, and the Voice Handicap Index lowered in functional (from 3 to 0) and physical (from 8 to 6) subscales. The stroboscopic findings showed significant improvement in mucosal wave (from 10% to 60%), amplitude (from 20% to 40%), open–closed phase, phase symmetry, and periodicity.

Chapter 13 - Fibrous dysplasia is frequently managed with open maxillectomy, and the technique employed depends on the location of the lesion. Mid-facial reconstruction after maxillectomy is a complicated and difficult process. Clinicians require expertise and must exercise caution when closing the defect, taking into consideration both aesthetics and function. Post-maxillectomy reconstruction using titanium alloplastic material has various advantages. To present a case of maxillary fibrous dysplasia treated with suprastructure maxillectomy followed by reconstruction to close the defect, we conducted a literature review. From the review we found that reconstruction uses titanium mesh plates and muscle slings, with the facial contour and tissues lost during the suprastructure maxillectomy taken into consideration. Various types of maxillectomy and post-maxillectomy defects have also been classified with the aim of facilitating reconstruction and guiding the clinician through the process. We concluded that the reconstruction of suprastructure maxillectomy using a titanium mesh plate and muscle sling is effective and produces good results in function and aesthetics.

Chapter 14 - Cleft palate is a congenital abnormality of the face, in which the palate does not develop normally during pregnancy. It is caused by failure of the fusion of the lateral palatine procesuss, resulting in the persistence of a slit-like opening between the oral and nasal cavities. Velopharyngeal insufficiency is the inability of the velopharyngeal valve to close owing to a deficit in the velopharyngeal structure, and one of the causes is cleft palate. The activities of swallowing and speaking depend on the ability to achieve adequate closure of the velopharyngeal valve. Here we present a 21-year-old man with cleft palate since birth. He had complaints of nasal sounds (rhinolalia) and water/food coming out from the nose every time he swallowed. He underwent surgery to correct this abnormality. Cleft palate closure was performed using the V-Y pushback technique and a posterior pharyngeal flap as this approach can extend the palate and effectively improve speech function. After the surgery, there were no disruptions in eating and drinking, and the patient spoke more clearly and was satisfied. A good understanding of the anatomy, physiology, and pathophysiology of cleft palate is very important for the appropriate management in order to achieve optimal and comprehensive treatment with regard to all aspects of aesthetics, speech, and swallowing ability.

Chapter 15 - Palatoplasty is a commonly performed procedure in children. A complication of palatoplasty is tongue edema owing to the use of a mouth gag. Tongue edema can compromise the airway and be dangerous for the patient. The objective of this case report was to increase awareness that tongue edema may arise after palatoplasty and to explain how to manage it. We present the case of a 17-month-old female who presented with tongue edema after palatoplasty. Massive tongue swelling developed 2 hours post-surgery. The patient showed signs of upper airway obstruction and was reintubated. The patient was under observation in the intensive care unit for three days until the tongue size returned to the original. A longer observation period in the recovery room after surgery may be required to prevent occurrence of hazardous events after palatoplasty.

Chapter 16 - Facial clefts are extremely rare congenital anomalies. There are various types of clefts, and classifications are required for their description. Nasal anomalies are rare, and currently, there are no standard methods for the management of such defects. The number of operations and types of surgical intervention vary widely according to the pattern and complexity of the deformity. The aim of this case report is to formulate a standardized procedure for the repair of the nasal component of clefts. A nasal dorsum advanced rotational flap was used to close the cleft of ala nasi during the first-stage surgery. Second-stage surgery involved an osteotomy and septoplasty to obtain a better shape for the nasal dorsum. During the third operation, we reconstructed the ala nasi to obtain improved symmetry. The nasal dorsum rotation flap showed good healing over the lateral surface of the nose and in the subciliary region. The closure of the nasal defect was accomplished using a composite downward rotation flap of the ala based on the lateral cleft wall. An advanced rotation-transposition flap was used in the management of a cleft. We also recommend the use of a superiorly based transposition for extensive lateral nasal wall involvement. In the present case, we performed osteotomy and septoplasty to obtain an improved shape for the nasal dorsum. Although the symmetry between the two nostrils was not ideal, it was acceptable.

Chapter 17 - Limb salvage surgery with tumor resection and endoprosthesis insertion is currently the preferred treatment for malignancies of the extremity. However, this procedure is not feasible in many cases and requires expensive implants that may not be available or affordable for many patients, such as in developing countries. We present three cases with distinct malignancies of the knee, osteosarcoma, metastastic bone disease due to lung cancer, and spindle cell carcinoma, treated by resection arthrodesis. After wide excision of the tumor, the combination of plate screws and K-nails with bone cement was used for arthrodesis. Functional outcomes were evaluated using the Lower Extremity Functional Scale (LEFS) score. LEFS scores were 24, 30, and 26out of 80, respectively. These low scores reflected substantial loss of limb immobility. Resection arthrodesis is a viable treatment option for limb salvage in cases of knee tumor for which resection and endoprosthesis insertion are not feasible, but functional outcome is limited.

Chapter 18 - Chordoma is a low-to-intermediate-grade malignant tumor encapsulating the notochord. It is rare, insidious in onset, and frequently diagnosed late. Due to its size, location, and nature, surgical treatment becomes challenging. Here we report a case of sacralchordoma in a 33-year-old woman treated with a combined anterior and posterior approach to remove the tumor en bloc, followed by posterior stabilization using rod–screw system. Total sacrectomy and spinopelvic reconstruction is the treatment of choice for sacral chordoma. We were able to achieve complete resection of the tumor mass with no recurrence after 6 months of follow-up.

Chapter 19 - Dural scarring may develop after laminectomy, resulting in persistent back and leg pain. Laminectomy for decompression exposes the duramater, stimulating the growth of scar tissue on the dural surface. Such scarring can impair nerve conduction and induce chronic pain, localized according to the affected spinal levels. A single case of back pain and pain radiating to the lower limbs is reported 12 months following laminectomy at L4–L5. Magnetic resonance images revealed new soft tissue in the posterior region pressing on the dura. Re-operation was performed for decompression. Intra-operative examination revealed scar tissue around the dural surface at the previous laminectomy site. Decompression and scarectomy were conducted, but the outcome was unsatisfactory because it proved impossible to remove all the scar tissue from the dura without increasing the risk of nerve root damage. As a result, low back pain was mitigated, but the leg pain persisted. We concluded that laminectomy can result in dural scar formation and chronic pain that is intractable to reparative surgery. Thus, it is critical to institute perioperative procedures that reduce the risk of subsequent dural scar formation.

Chapter 20 - Surgical correction for kyphotic deformity in spondilytis tuberculosis is as important as local infection control itself (through debridement and abscess drainage). This report aims to provide information on the clinical and radiological outcomes after two-stage treatment for kyphotic deformity in patients with spondylitis tuberculosis. We present four cases of kyphotic deformity in patients with spondylitis tuberculosis who underwent two-stage surgery at Cipto Mangunkusumo National Hospital, Jakarta, Indonesia. All patients were female, with a mean age of 37.5 years. The mean follow-up period was 45 months. One patient had a lumbar lesion with loss of lordosis (less than 20°lordosis), and the remaining three had thoracic lesions with a kyphotic angle more than 45°. All patients underwent a two-stage surgery involving initial debridement, kyphotic correction, posterior stabilization, and fusion, followed by anterior fusion with a titanium cage and bone graft. The surgical outcomes were evaluated by comparing the preoperative and postoperative Oswestry Disability Index (ODI) scores and kyphotic angles. After surgery, all patients had good outcomes with reductions in the ODI score and kyphotic angle. The mean ODI score reduced from 20 preoperatively to 5 postoperatively. Additionally, the kyphotic angle reduced from 90° preoperatively to 22° postoperatively (after the second stage). Our two-stage procedure for the treatment of spondylitis tuberculosis with kyphotic deformity was associated with good functional and radiological outcomes at long-term follow-up. Thus, we recommend this two-stage procedure as a standard for cases similar to our reported cases.

Chapter 21 - Conus medullaris syndrome is a complex disease entity that is difficult to define because of its location between the spinal cord and nerve roots. The presenting symptoms are not specific and are often missed by primary doctors, making diagnosis challenging. It is even more difficult because the time since onset plays a major role in the outcome. A 47-year-old female displayed neglected conus medullary syndrome due to a compression fracture of L1 that presented as bladder and defecating dysfunctions and leg pain due to lumbar canal stenosis of L4-L5. A decompression surgical procedure involving total laminectomy at the L1 level, posterior stabilization from T11 to L3, and laminotomy, flavectomy, and discectomy at L4 and L5 were performed in this patient. The patient experienced improved motor function after the operation. Her hypoesthesia also improved. However, her bladder and defecating problem were not resolved. Non-full function restoration likely occurred because of the patient's neglected conus medullaris. However, her function still improved; therefore, surgery was a better option.

Chapter 22 - Congenital malformations in bladder and cloacal exstrophy involve the genitourinary tract, musculoskeletal tissue, and occasionally the gastrointestinal tract. We report two cases of a seven-year-old boy and a 12-year old boy who were referred to our pediatric surgery service with the diagnosis of bladder exstrophy. Preoperatively, the pubic diastasis of the two patients was 6 and 9 cm, respectively. Bilateral anterior innominate osteotomy with external fixator placement was executed by the pediatric urological surgical team following bladder closure. Both patients remained hospitalized for two weeks on bed rest. Skin traction was not applied. External fixators were applied for eight weeks. Immediately after surgery, the diastases were reduced to 4 cm in the 7-year-old patient and 6 cm in the 12-year-old patient. No postoperative complications occurred in either patient and both were able to walk with normal gaits. Slight external leg rotation was noted. Urological abnormalities were improved. Despite the technique, it is difficult to achieve perfect closure of the pelvic diastasis in this age group. Pelvic osteotomy remains the most beneficial intervention for corrective exstrophy closure. The bilateral anterior technique is recommended for this procedure and is applicable in neglected cases. Further follow-up is needed to evaluate the effectiveness of this technique.

Chapter 23 - Fracture of the phalanges can be caused by trauma under various circumstances. The common treatment for unstable phalangeal fractures is Kirschner wire (K-wire) fixation using the most commonly used technique of extra-articular cross-pinning. Using this technique, a stable fracture can be fixed and early phalanx mobilization can be facilitated. To achieve these goals, the landmarks and safe portals for the insertion of the K-wire to the fracture site of the phalanges must be identified. Here we present the case of a 48-year-old woman with fracture at the base of the proximal phalanx of the left fourth finger. For 3 weeks, she underwent closed reduction and immobilization using the K-wire via the extra-articular cross-pinning technique.

After 3 weeks of immobilization using the K-wire, no significant events were observed. After removal of the K-wire, we initiated the rehabilitation program. A desirable range of motion (ROM)was achieved at the metacarpophalangeal joint. The safe portals for the insertion of the K-wire for treating proximal phalanx fractures using the cross-pinning technique must be identified to achieve a desirable ROM. Thus, the extra-articular cross-pinning technique along with the safe portals must be used for treating fractures of the proximal phalanges.

Chapter 24 - Bone pain is the most common type of cancer-related pain; it often occurs in cases of advanced cancer that have metastasized to bone, particularly prostate cancer, breast cancer, lung cancer, and multiple myeloma. This type of pain is usually severe, persistent, and hard to manage. Current pain-relieving strategies include the use of strong opioids, bisphosphonates, and radiotherapy. However, these approaches may cause unwanted side effects that affect a patient's quality of life. Acupuncture is an adjuvant therapy for pain relief; it has minimal side effects and may improve a patient's quality of life. This paper discusses a 42-year-old female with cancer-induced bone pain who underwent 12 acupuncture treatments at the LI4 Hegu, SP6 Sanyinjiao, SP9 Yinlingquan, ST36 Zusanli, GB34 Yanglingquan, LR3 Taichong, BL23 Shenshu, and GB30 Huantiao acupoints and experienced improvement in pain.

Chapter 25 - Monomorphic epitheliotropic intestinal T-cell lymphoma (MEITL) is an uncommon subtype of intestinal lymphoma that is usually found in Asian populations. MEITL causes non-specific gastrointestinal-related symptoms; thus, it is often overlooked and misdiagnosed, resulting in complications and improper therapeutic approaches. A 75-year-old Asian female was admitted to the emergency room with signs and symptoms of ileal obstruction. She had no history of celiac disease. Surgical resection was performed; the tumor consisted of small- to medium-sized tumor cells arranged in a monomorphic and diffuse pattern. The tumor was positive for CD3 and CD56 but negative for CD8. She was diagnosed with MEITL. Although most MEITL tumors are positive for CD3, CD56, and CD8, CD8-negative MEITL has been reported in some studies and is thought to originate from double-negative intraepithelial lymphocytes. We described a rare case of MEITL with an unusual negative CD8 expression.

Chapter 26 - Clear cell papillary renal cell carcinoma is an indolent neoplasm composed of clear epithelial cells arranged in tubules and a papillary structure, with predominantly linear nuclear alignment away from the basement membrane. In this paper, we report our experience of diagnosing a rare case of clear cell papillary renal cell carcinoma. A 50-year-old male with a chief complaint of abdominal pain. A computed tomographic abdominal scan revealed a large heterogeneous multicystic mass on the left kidney. On the basis of the macroscopic examination, microscopy, and immunohistochemical staining, we diagnosed the tumor as a clear cell papillary renal cell carcinoma. This tumor is an uncommon variant of a renal cell neoplasm that has distinct histological and immunohistochemical characteristics. Pathologists should be aware of this entity because the biological behavior of this tumor is very different from that of conventional clear cell carcinoma.

Chapter 27 - The actual incidence of adrenocortical adenoma (ACA) remains unknownMyelolipomatous metaplasia is an extremely rare finding in adrenal tumors, particularly in ACA. The pathogenesis of myelolipomatous metaplasia remains unclear. We report the case of a 40-year-old man who presented with a mass in his abdomen which size increased within 4 months of diagnosis. Computed tomography of the abdomen showed a heterogenic mass in the right suprarenal region with fine demarcated outlines, and the result was indicative of an adrenal carcinoma. The patient underwent adrenalectomy. Based on hematoxylin &eosin (H&E) staining and immunohistochemical analysis, the mass was confirmed to be a non-functional ACA with a myelolipomatous metaplasia. ACA is a rare type of tumor. Myelolipomatous metaplasia found within an adenoma of the adrenocortex is an even more uncommon finding. The correlation between clinical, radiological, and pathological examination results must be assessed for a more accurate diagnosis. The combination of H&E staining and immunostaining is helpful in facilitating the diagnosis of adrenocortical tumors and metaplasia within the tumor.

Chapter 28 - Chronic myeloid leukemia (CML) is a myeloproliferative neoplasm of the hematopoietic stem cells, in which granulocytes are the major proliferative component. Approximately 50% of newly diagnosed cases are asymptomatic and discovered when an abnormal white blood cell count is detected. In some cases, the bone marrow shows variable stages of fibrosis, whereas severe reticulin fibrosis is rarely observed. We present a patient with uncommon initial features of CML (i.e., pancytopenia, severe bone marrow fibrosis, and the absence of splenomegaly). Histopathological examination of the bone marrow revealed a hypercellular bone marrow with a normal myeloid to erythroid ratio showing myeloid maturation into segmented neutrophils. The number of megakaryocytes with atypical nuclei was increased, forming a cluster. Reticulin staining showed that fibers were increased diffusely and densely with extensive intersections. This increasing number of megakaryocytes and excessive fibrosis resembles primary myelofibrosis. The presence of theBCR-ABL1 fusion gene confirmed the diagnosis of CML.

Chapter 29 - Clear cell chondrosarcoma is a rare variant of low-grade malignant cartilaginous tumor, representing approximately 2% of all chondrosarcomas. In this article, we report a rare case of clear cell chondrosarcoma in a 21-year-old male. Histopathological findings showed abundant clear cytoplasm or a faintly acidophilic cytoplasm with distinct cytoplasmic borders. The nuclei were round, vesicular, and centrally located, with prominent nucleoli. Mitotic figures are uncommon. Follow-up immunohistochemical staining showed positivity for S-100 protein and negativity for other epithelial markers, supporting the diagnosis of clear cell chondrosarcoma. Clear cell chondrosarcoma mostly involves the epiphyseal long bones, especially in the femur or humerus. Complete surgical excision is the treatment of choice.

Chapter 30 - Hürthle cell carcinoma (HCC) of the thyroid is an unusual and relatively rare type of thyroid cancer. Small series of HCC patients have been reported in the literature, but because of its relative rarity, its pathological and clinical significance have not been well documented. A 55-year-old woman presented with rapid neck mass enlargement and hoarseness. Thorax X-ray imaging suggested intrathoracic struma. Ultrasonographic examination showed struma nodosa in the right lobe. Fine-needle aspiration biopsy results suggested a follicular neoplasm of Hürthle cell type. Grossly, the right thyroid size was6×5×4cm and was brown, firm, and encapsulated. The cut surfaces were brown and lobulated, with no papillary growth or calcification. A histological examination showed large tumor cells in a trabecular arrangement, rounded nuclei, coarse chromatin, some vesicular with prominent nucleoli, and abundant granular eosinophilic cytoplasm. Another section revealed capsular invasion, and a solid area containing scattered bizarre giant cells with irregular nuclei. The histopatological features and imunohistochemical staining results supported a diagnosis of encapsulated angioinvasive HCC with bizarre nuclei. HCC is a rare type of carcinoma that remains controversial and difficult to diagnose. Careful assessment should be performed to look for bizarre nuclei to prevent over diagnosis.

Chapter 31 - Secretory carcinoma is an exceptionally rare type of invasive breast cancer in the special subtype classification of World Health Organization 2012. It occurs in <0.15% of all breast cancers and has a distinct histomorphology, which is characterized by the presence of intracellular and extracellular eosinophilic secretory materials. It generally shows triple negativity for estrogen receptor, progesterone receptor, and human epidermal growth factor 2and shows strong reactivity for S-100 protein. We report the case of a 54-year-old woman with invasive breast carcinoma. The histomorphology mimicked that of secretory carcinoma, with unusual immunohistochemical findings typical of secretory carcinoma. However, secretory carcinoma is associated with a characteristic translocation that creates ETV6–NTRK3 gene fusion, which was not observed in this case. Despite the considerable resemblance with secretory carcinoma, this case was ultimately diagnosed as invasive breast carcinoma of no special type.

Chapter 32 - Langerhans cell histiocytosis (LCH) is a rare clonal proliferative disorder of Langerhans cells with unknown etiology, which occurs predominantly in male children. Histopathology features show polymorphous cells arranged in diffuse sheets. This case study involved the case of a patient who exhibited a nodular pattern that was unusual for LCH. The aim of this case report is to share experience about the unusual histology of LCH. An eleven-month-old boy presented with enlarged neck and inguinal lymph nodes. Ultrasound showed multiple enlargements of the lymph nodes with hypervascularization and a regular and distinct border. The patient underwent open surgical biopsy and the specimen was sent for histopathology analysis. The histopathology showed a nodular pattern with the characteristics of Langerhans cells that have abundant eosinophilic cytoplasm and the presence of nuclear grooves, nuclear folding, and inflammatory cells. The immunostaining was positive for CD1a, Langerin, S100, and CD68. In most cases of LCH, the morphology features showed polymorphous cells arranged in diffuse sheets. There are to our knowledge no published reports to date that show LCH in the nodular pattern. Whether or not there is different pathogenesis or biological behavior in nodular LCH remains unclear.

Chapter 33 - Rhabdomyosarcoma (RMS) is the most common soft tissue malignancy occurring in childhood and adolescence. RMS was previously classified into the following three main subtypes: embryonal, alveolar, and pleomorphic. In the latest classification, a new variant of RMS, spindle/sclerosing RMS, has been included. This variant is rare, occurring in 5%–10% of all cases of RMS. It is characterized by prominent hyaline and sclerosis stroma that mimics an osteoid or chondroid with a pseudovascular, microalveolar, or cord growth pattern. Therefore, it might be easily mistaken during initial evaluation as osteosarcoma, chondrosarcoma, angiosarcoma, infiltrating carcinoma, spindle cell sarcoma, or other RMS types. Awareness of the existence of this entity is important for not only diagnosis but also prognosis and treatment. Here we present the case of a child with sclerosing RMS that was not easily diagnosed. This report aims to discuss the potential diagnostic pitfalls associated with other look-alike sarcomas.

Chapter 34 - Primary malignant giant cell tumor of bone (PMGCTB) refers to a high-grade sarcoma arising from adjacent to benign giant cell tumor located in bone tissue. This time of sarcoma is rare and accounts for approximately 7% of all giant cell tumors. This report shares our experience of diagnosing a rare case. A 53-year-old man presented with a mass on the upper end of his tibia that appeared 6 years before he was admitted to the hospital and had no previous history of radiation therapy or surgery. A radiograph showed an aggressive bone tumor at the metadiaphysis with a suspicious femorotibial joint involvement. Histopathology showed mononuclear cell proliferation, multinucleated giant cells with abundant nuclei, identical with mononuclear cells in the stroma, and a high-grade sarcoma area juxtaposition to the benign giant cell tumor. PMGCTBs arise de novo and are extremely rare. From these findings, we concluded this case as PMGCTB. Malignant giant cell tumor of bone (MGCTB) prognosis is poor with a 5-year survival of 50%, and PMGCTB has a better prognosis than secondary MGCTB.

Chapter 35 - Giant cell tumor of bone (GCTB) is a primary bone neoplasm composed of mononuclear cells proliferating among scattered macrophages and large, osteoclast-like giant cells. Secondary malignant GCTB is a sarcoma arising at a site where a GCTB has been previously documented. This case report is about a 32- year-old female who presented with right knee pain of one year duration. The patient had a history of bone tumor, at the same site, six years ago. Radiographs showed a mass in the epimetaphy seal, extending into the tibiofemoral and patellofemoral junction. Such findings were consistent with a recurrent lesion. Following microscopic investigation, spindle- cell with atypical mitoses and nuclear pleomorphism, admixed with conventional GCTB, were identified. Sarcomatous changes in malignant GCT develop many years, or even decades, following the primary lesion's removal. Radiologic features are represented by large lesions with cortical destruction and prominent invasion into the soft tissue. Microscopically, the conventional GCTB is adjacent to, or intermixed with, the sarcomatous area. Based on such findings, we conclude this case is a secondary malignant GCTB.

Chapter 36 - Segmental absence of intestinal musculature is a distinct histopathological entity with rare occurrence. The condition typically presents in neonates, with the primary manifestation being intestinal obstruction or perforation. Here we present the case of a neonate who initially presented with a high lesion of anal atresia. In the first few days following colostomy, the infant exhibited signs of intestinal obstruction. An exploratory laparotomy revealed ileal stenosis. A resected ileum specimen showed a narrowed segment of the ileum. Histopathological examination showed focal hypoplasia to total absence of muscularis propria with intact mucosal, submucosal, and serosal layers. Histochemical and immunohistochemical studies confirmed the absence and hypoplasia of muscularis propria, presence of ganglion cells, and absence of Cajal cells in the pathological segment. In cases of neonatal intestinal obstruction due to segmental absence of intestinal musculature, the possibility of defects of intestinal musculature should be investigated, particularly in conjunction with other congenital diseases.

Chapter 37 - Most liver hemangiomas are small and asymptomatic, but large, or giant, hemangiomas may be symptomatic and can occur with hemangioma-like vessels (HLVs) distant from the primary tumor. We report three cases of giant cavernous hemangioma of the liver in adults, with the hemangioma recurring in one of the three patients 8 months after surgical resection. All cases had clusters of HLVs located far from the primary tumor and in the resection margin.

Chapter 38 - Ovotesticular disorder of sexual development (OT-DSD) is a rare congenital anomaly characterized by the simultaneous presence of ovarian tissue with mature ovarian follicles and testicular tissue with distinct seminiferous tubules in the same individual. The most common karyotype of OT-DSD is 46, XX. A 12-year-old boy was brought by his parents to our hospital because of a mass in his right groin area that had enlarged over the past 2 weeks. The patient's medical history included multiple surgeries due to hypospadias and unilateral right-side cryptorchidism. Histopathological analysis revealed the presence of ovarian tissue containing multilocular cysts and uterine tissue with an endometrium component, but no testicular component. Hormone analysis showed elevated levels of luteinizing hormone and follicle-stimulating hormone, with normal levels of testosterone and anti-Müllerian hormones. The patient was diagnosed with 46, XX OT-DSD and assigned as a male.

Section 1. General Surgery, Neurosurgery, and Anesthesiology

In: Case Reports in Surgery
Editors: Ahmad Jabir Rahyussalim et al.
ISBN: 978-1-53616-582-1

Chapter 1

THE USE OF GROIN FLAP FOR UPPER EXTREMITY COVERAGE IN ELECTRICAL BURN PATIENTS: EVIDENCE-BASED CASE REPORTS

Nathania Pudya*[*], *Aditya Warhana and Erythrina Permatasari
Division of Plastic Surgery, Department of Surgery, RSUPN Dr. Cipto Mangunkusumo, Universitas Indonesia, Jakarta, Indonesia

ABSTRACT

Electrical burn injuries commonly occur in the extremities, particularly on the wrists, forearms, and hands. In high-voltage burns, the injury extends deeply and damages the underlying tissue, resulting in tissue ischemia and subsequently, a high probability of extensive tissue necrosis. In electrical burn injuries, nonvital tissue debridement and adequate defect closure determines the outcome of limb salvage. Clarification of the advantages of groin flap use for soft tissue defect closure is required to assist medical practitioners in deciding if groin flap should be considered as an option for upper limb reconstruction due to electrical burns. Two cases of electrical burn injuries to the extremities with two-stage reconstructive surgery using groin flap were reported. We questioned clinically whether a two-stage surgical method affected the morbidity of patients with electrical burns and investigated the correlation between the type of flap harvesting (delayed and non-delayed groin flap) and flap vitality. We also performed a literature search for relevant information regarding the use of groin flap in electrical burns injury using PubMed, Clinical Key, and Google and initially identified 56 articles. After screening, the application of inclusion and exclusion criteria, and full-text reading, the three remaining articles were appraised in terms of validity, importance, and applicability. According to the literature, the timing of the reconstruction did not appear to affect flap survival and outcome. Moreover, fasciocutaneous flaps are relatively thin, making them ideal for coverage in regions with exposed tendon and bony structure. One study has

[*] Corresponding Author's E-mail: nathaniapudya@gmail.com.

revealed that the use of fasciocutaneous flaps to cover defects of an acutely burned hand showed a low infection rate comparable with that of muscle flaps, despite the argumentation of a greater susceptibility to infection in comparison to muscle flaps due to a comparatively inferior vascular plexus. No evidence was found from our search of global literature indicating whether the time of flap harvesting affects flap vitality. In conclusion, the use of groin flap as distant pedicle flaps provided an alternative in cases where free flap reconstruction was impossible. The pathophysiology of vascular occlusion causes progressive necrosis of tissue in electrical burn injuries unrelated to the timing of reconstructive surgery. It is critical to debride nonvital soft tissue without jeopardizing the vital structures underlying the burn wound. Although the pliable characteristics that are possessed by groin flap are required to cover small cross-sectional diameter anatomic regions such as the wrist, its bulky appearance requires secondary reconstruction to thin the flap.

Keywords: Electrical injury, groin flap, superficial circumflex iliac artery flap, upper extremity, reconstruction

BACKGROUND

Electrical burn injuries are associated with high morbidity and commonly occur in the upper extremities, particularly the wrists, forearms, and hands. The injury extends deeply into the underlying tissue causing tissue damage, thereby resulting in ischemia and subsequently, a high probability of extensive tissue necrosis.

The passage of an electrical current produces heat, leading to tissue damage. Because the current is transmitted along the path of least resistance through the body, it flows along neurovascular bundles. This causes extensive damage that involves the nerves, blood vessels, muscle, skin, tendon, and fat all the way through to the underlying bone. Bones retain the most body heat and possess the highest electrical resistance, particularly in the periosseous tissue such as that between two bones (e.g., tibia–fibula and radius–ulna). This is a contributing factor to delayed vascular occlusion and progressive tissue necrosis [1].

The cross-sectional diameter area of the involved body part affects its resistance and the magnitude of tissue damage. The wrist is an undersized cross-sectional area with tendon and bony structure areas that are highly resistant to heat and more severe damage. The peripheral nerve in minimal cross-sectional areas is located in close proximity to the bone and fibrous tissue. Therefore, an electrical injury is likely to lead to thrombosis of the perineural region, causing compression syndrome of the peripheral nerves. An experimental study conducted by Jia-ke et al., (2009) has shown irreversible vascular damage post burn injury via optical microscopy that was marked by the necrosis of the vascular walls and thrombosis along the areas of arterial endothelium destruction as well as pyknosis of vascular muscle with the presence of fibrinous exudates. Moreover, muscle viability progressively decreased between 30 min to 72 h after the injury, explaining the appearance of degeneration necrosis in certain muscle cells due to coagulation accompanied by myolysis [2].

Reconstructive surgery of electrical burn injuries is divided into primary and secondary stages. Vogt et al., [4] have described primary reconstruction as the surgical procedures performed in the early phases of the burn injury to decrease infection and improve wound healing. These procedures involve the debridement of devitalized tissue and wound closure using stepladder reconstruction (from skin grafting to free flap). In contrast, secondary reconstruction is performed after the burn wounds have healed to enhance the function and aesthetics of the injured area, such as burn scar contracture release [3].

The timing of debridement remains controversial, with several studies both for and against performing treatment during the acute phase. Some literature suggests that primary reconstructive surgery should be performed within the first 3 weeks following an electrical burn injury because the passage of electric current causes vascular changes similar to ischemia–reperfusion injury, which disturbs the capillary blood flow and results in progressive tissue necrosis. Furthermore, several studies have hypothesized that less secondary reconstruction is required if there is an early coverage of exposed functionally important structures during the acute phase [4], [5].

The use of a distant flap, such as groin flap, may be considered as a substitution for free microvascular tissue transfer for the coverage of raw surfaces and important underlying tissue structures in the wrist. The groin flap is an axial fasciocutaneous flap vascularized by the superficial circumflex iliac artery. The artery is located parallel and approximately 2–3 cm distal to the inguinal ligament, able to cover an area of skin between 5 cm inferior and superior to the artery and approximately 5 cm above the anterior superior iliac spine. In cases of extensive coverage, a flap may be raised based upon the adjacent superficial epigastric artery [6]. We present a case series of electrical burn patients with wrist defects that were treated using an axial groin flap and propose this as an alternative method to free flap reconstruction.

CLINICAL QUESTION

According to a case series of electrical burn patients and evidence-based medicine, we posed the following clinical questions: 1) Does the two-stage surgical method affect the morbidity of electrical burn patients? and 2) Does the time of flap harvesting (delayed and non-delayed groin flap) affect flap vitality?

METHODS

Literature Review

We performed a database search of PubMed, ClinicalKey, and Google on May 30, 2019The databases were searched using the Medical Subject Headings (MeSH) terms "Electric Burn Injuries," "Groin Flap," "Superficial Circumflex Iliac Flap," "Upper Extremities," and "Reconstruction" (Table 1). Inclusion criteria were English literature; adult populations with electrical burn injury in the upper extremities; the provision of preoperative, intraoperative, and follow-up postoperative data; and studies with distant flap intervention. We excluded studies concerning non-burn injury populations, the single intervention of local flap or free microvascular flap surgery, surgical intervention in areas other than the upper extremities, and pediatric populations. Following a full-text reading of the initial screening results, one study of anon-burn injury population was excluded because it was not comparable with the other screened studies (Figure 1).

Table 1. Search strategy used to perform a database search on July 30, 2016

Search Engine	Search Term
PubMed	("electric injuries"[MeSH Terms] OR ("electric"[All Fields] AND "injuries"[All Fields]) OR "electric injuries"[All Fields] OR ("electrical"[All Fields] AND "injury"[All Fields]) OR "electrical injury"[All Fields]) AND ("groin"[MeSH Terms] OR "groin"[All Fields]) AND ("surgical flaps"[MeSH Terms] OR ("surgical"[All Fields] AND "flaps"[All Fields]) OR "surgical flaps"[All Fields] OR "flap"[All Fields]) AND superficial[All Fields] AND "circumflex"[All Fields] AND ("iliac artery"[MeSH Terms] OR ("iliac"[All Fields] AND "artery"[All Fields]) OR "iliac artery"[All Fields]) AND ("surgical flaps"[MeSH Terms] OR ("surgical"[All Fields] AND "flaps"[All Fields]) OR "surgical flaps"[All Fields] OR "flap"[All Fields]) AND ("upper extremity"[MeSH Terms] OR ("upper"[All Fields] AND "extremity"[All Fields]) OR "upper extremity"[All Fields]) AND ("reconstructive surgical procedures"[MeSH Terms] OR ("reconstructive"[All Fields] AND "surgical"[All Fields] AND "procedures"[All Fields]) OR "reconstructive surgical procedures"[All Fields] OR "reconstruction"[All Fields])
ClinicalKey	electrical injury, groin flap, superficial circumflex iliac artery flap, upper extremity, reconstruction
Google	electrical injury, groin flap, superficial circumflex iliac artery flap, upper extremity, reconstruction

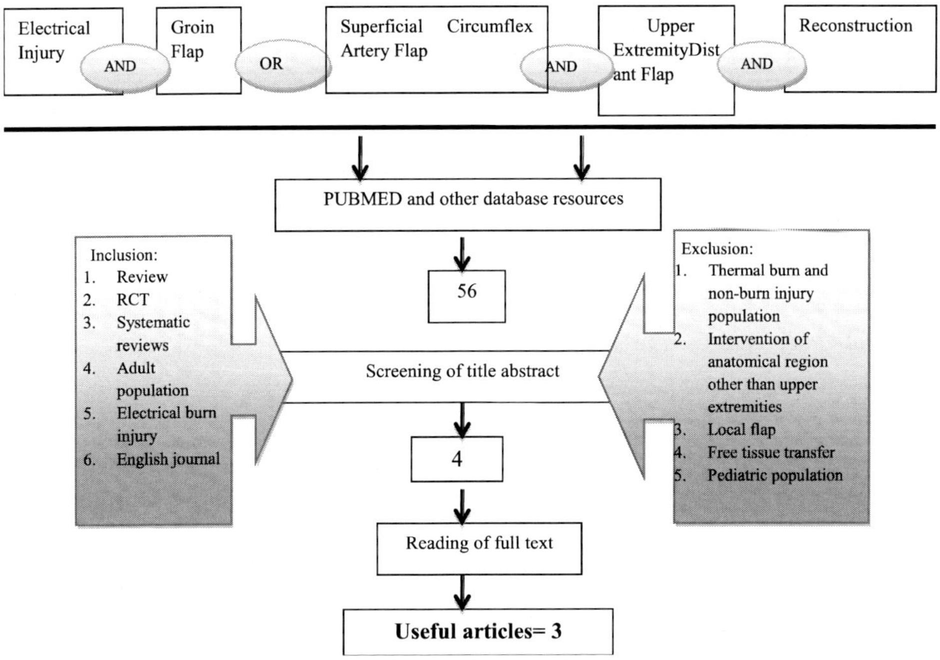

Figure 1. Flow diagram of search strategy of literature performed on July 30, 2016.

Case Studies

We evaluated two case studies of electrical burn injury to the upper extremities with groin flap reconstruction.

RESULTS

Literature Review

The literature search identified three articles meeting our criteria for appraisal. There were one systematic review and two cohort studies, both valued as high-level evidence. Table 1 presents a critical appraisal of the articles. Handschin et al., study [6] included 68 patients with electrical injury, of which 40 suffered from low-voltage electrical burns. Mean burn wound size was 33% ± 22% of the total body surface area, and90% of cases involved the upper extremities. There were three cases wherein the groin flap was used to cover defects in the upper extremities. This study has suggested series debridement for the removal of visible necrotic tissue aggressively followed by immediate reconstruction. Microvascular thrombosis as an indication of flap failure appeared during the first 4 weeks. No information was provided regarding the type of groin flap performed in this study, and there was no history of bleeding reported in the patients undergoing the groin flap reconstruction.

Case 1

A 32-year-old male presented at the emergency room with a chief complaint of electrical burn injury in both wrists and lower extremities that had occurred 2 weeks prior. There was no history of trauma, loss of consciousness, or fever. Fasciotomy and excisional debridement had already been performed twice at another hospital.

A raw surface sized 6.5 × 9.5 cm in the left wrist and 3 × 4.5 cm in first web space were noted. The underlying structure was difficult to identify due to eschar and necrotic tissue appearance in the wrist. The raw surface in the first webspace showed a subdermal wound bed with granulation tissue, and the proximal phalanx of the first digit was visible. The range of movement in the hands was limited due to pain and stiffness (Figure 2).

Radiographic findings revealed bilateral soft tissue swelling in the fascia antebrachii. There was subluxation of metacarpophalangeal digit 1 to the radial side and a closed incomplete fracture of the proximal phalanx digit 1 in the left hand. Destruction of the metadiaphysiscortex of the distal right ulnar bone was detected on the anteromedial side with a lytic lesion in the epidiaphysis. There appeared to be periostitis in the metadiaphysis of the distal radius and ulnar joint (Figure 3).

The patient was diagnosed with a deep dermal electrical burn injury of > 9% of the total burn surface area with 2% raw surface. The debridement of nonvital structures, such as tendons (flexor system), muscle, and fat tissues, was performed 20 days after the burn injury (Figure 4). The ulnar artery was identified as compromised owing to thrombosis; however, adequate vascularization was sourced from the radial artery.

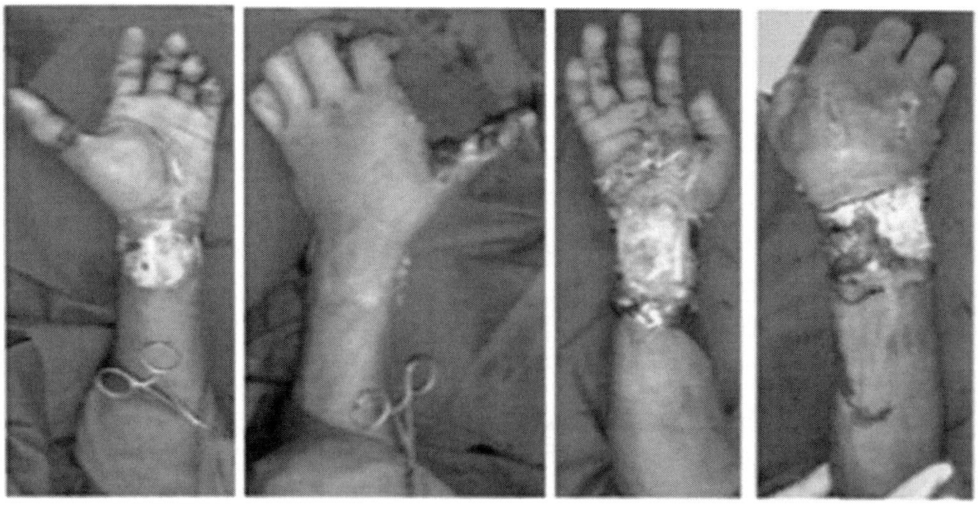

Figure 2. First clinical presentation of a 32-year-old male with bilateral electrical burn injury and raw wrist surfaces.

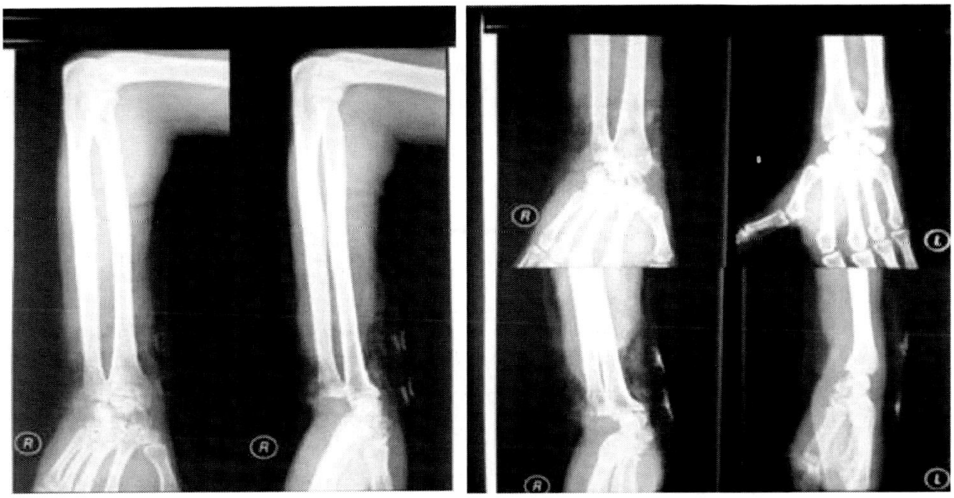

Figure 3. The radiographic findings reveal the appearance of osteomyelitis in the ulnar bone with marked periostitis in the distal region of the right radial bone (left). Subluxation of the left proximal phalange digit 1 to the radial side with an incomplete fracture of the proximal phalange of the left hand (right) is observed.

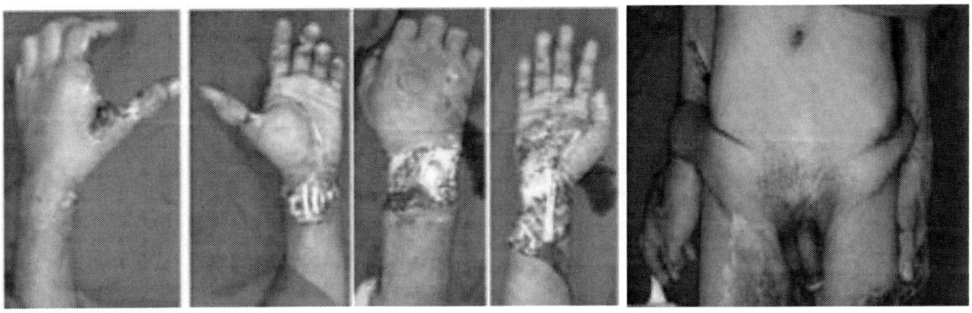

Figure 4. Post debridement (left) and post bilateral groin flap surgery (right).

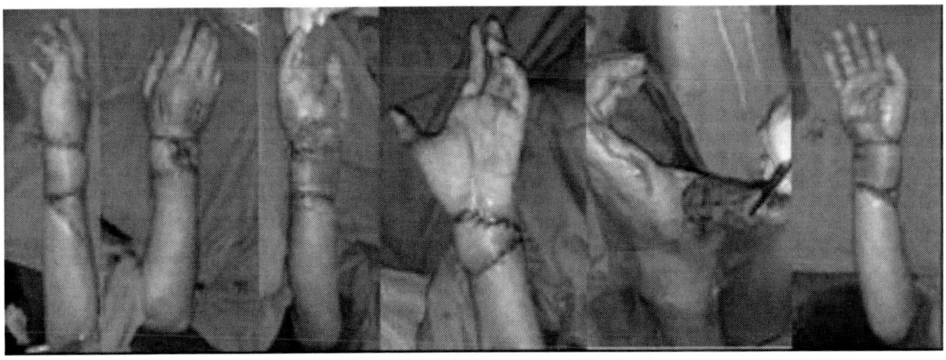

Figure 5. Post groin flap surgery, the remaining raw surface was covered with a split-thickness skin graft.

Groin flap coverage of the bilateral raw surface was performed 5 days after debridement surgery (Figure 5). Due to the extensive circumference of the right wrist, the flap inset was delayed until blood flow to the distal portion was adequate. The right groin flap surgery was performed 10 days after the second procedure. The left side groin flap was separated at 21 days and the right-side groin flap at 11 days post debridement surgery. The evaluation of flap vitality was performed intraoperatively, and good vascularization of both flap pedicles was confirmed. A split-thickness skin graft was performed to achieve closure of the raw surface in the digit 1 of the left hand and the remaining raw surface proximal to the left groin flap. Owing to the instability of the distal radius–ulna joint, a transfixion wire was applied by an orthopedic surgeon.

Case 2

A 25-year-old male was diagnosed with a deep dermal electrical burn injury to his left hand that covered 2% of his total body surface area. The injury occurred 10 days prior to hospital admission. There was no history of trauma or loss of consciousness. A raw surface (8 × 4 cm) in the central palm of the hand extending from the proximal palmar crease to distal of the insertion of the flexor digitorum superficial to digits 2–5 in the left hand was present. Another raw surface covered two-thirds of the circumference of the left wrist region. Exposure of underlying soft tissue (tendons and fascia) with granulation tissue was noted in the digits and wrist (Figure 6). The patient underwent debridement of nonvital structures between flexor zone 1 and 3, including flexor tendons, muscle, and fat tissues. Vascularization was found adequate from the radial artery, because of the non-vitality of the ulnar artery.

A left delayed groin flap closure of the raw wrist surface and a full-thickness skin graft was performed at day 13 post burn injury (Figure 7). An intraoperative evaluation of flap vitality showed good vascularization of the flap pedicle. At day 31, the patient underwent separation of the left delayed groin flap. During the postoperative evaluation, the flap showed no wound dehiscence or infection. However, a skin contraction due to healing of the full-thickness skin graft was observed.

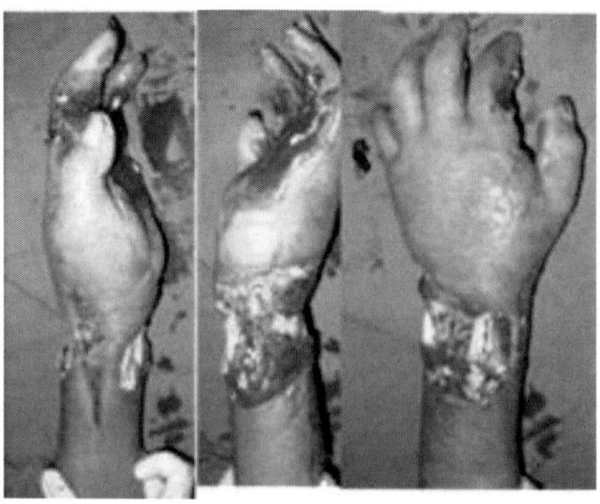

Figure 6. First clinical presentation of a 25-year-old male with electrical burn injury covering two-thirds of the circumference of the left wrist and between the central palm of hand to the site of flexor digitorum superficial insertion.

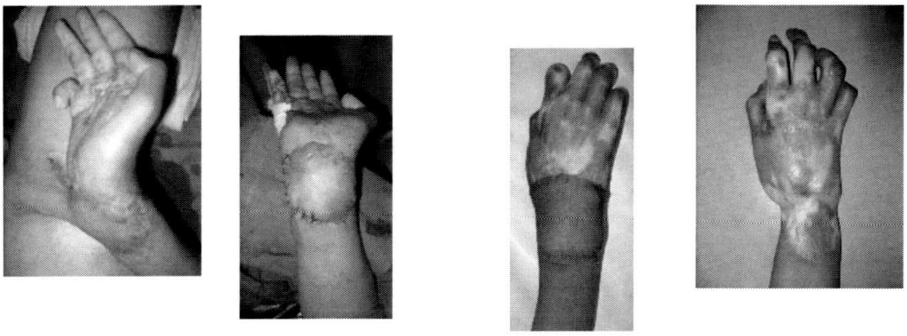

Figure 7. Left delayed groin flap closure at day 13 (left). Post separation of left groin flap (right).

Discussion

Appraised articles are a systematic review and cohort studies, thus it valued as high-level evidences. Figure 2 shows critical appraisal of the articles. Handschin study [5] include 68 patients due to electrical injury and 40 burn patient has low voltage electric burn, with mean size of burn wound 33 +/- 22% of TBSA with commonly involved upper extremities (90%). Total of three groin flap were used to cover defect in upper extremity. This study suggests series debridement for removal visible necrotic tissue aggressively followed by immediate reconstruction. Microvascular thrombosis as failure of flap appeared during the first 4 weeks. No information provided regarding type of groin flap performed in this study, however no history of bleeding reported in the groin flap patient.

Barillo et al., have described six cases of patients with severe hand burns. Three of them underwent primary reconstruction surgery using groin flap to cover the distal regions and fingers. This was followed by liposuction and defatting during the secondary reconstruction procedure at a later stage to decrease the bulkiness of the groin flap. The success rate varied from 50% to 100% flap viability. The Barillo study chose to perform immediate coverage using local, fascial, or fasciocutaneous flaps as well as distant flaps [6].

Jabir et al., have highlighted 12 cases of burn injury that included one patient with electrical burn in whom groin flap reconstruction was performed 4 days post injury. The failure rates were lowest when performed either during the immediate stage (within 5 days of injury) or within the intermediate stage (3 weeks after injury) and were highest when performed during the early stage (15–21 days after injury) [7]. Sabapathy et al., marked secondary reconstruction should be performed in about 6 to 8 weeks after the flap inset consideredema in the flap and induration at the suture line is settled, therefore flap becomes supple and the induration at the suture line reduced [8].

Flap failure was related to inadequate early debridement rather than the timing of reconstruction, and the timing did not appear to affect flap survival and outcome. Fasciocutaneous flaps are relatively thin, making them ideal for coverage in regions with exposed tendon and bony structures. This study revealed that the use of fasciocutaneous flaps to cover acute burn defects of hands demonstrated a low infection rate comparable with that of muscle flaps, despite the argumentation that a greater susceptibility to infection in comparison with muscle flaps would be caused by the comparatively inferior vascular plexus. No global evidence was found in the literature regarding whether the type of flap harvesting affected flap vitality.

Delayed groin flap has disadvantages as multi stage surgery procedure such as immobility of the hand, elbow, and shoulder that will lead to stiffness and edemaformation of the flap and upperextremity as a result of the dependent hand position [9,10]. Graf et al., study highlight decrased mobility of joint in arm, increased with patient'sage [11], furthermore patient aged younger than 50 years hadless likely develop permaent problem with shoulder or elbow mobility. Evaluation post separation flap in mobility of shoulder and elbow joints compared to non injured side in both of patients showed no limitation in movement. Both patient were able to lift hand over 90 degrees and no complained to do daily activities.

Table 2. Evidence-based case report review

	Barillo (2001)	Handschin (2009)	Jabir (2014)
Design	Case series	Case series	Systematic review
Location	America	Zurich	Essex
Population	14-64 years adult population	A 53 yo male, chinese	A 52 yo female, chinese
Anatomical region	Upper extremities injury Lower extremities injury	Upper extremity	Upper extremity Head and neck Lower extremity
Intervention	Groin flap as primary reconstruction	Groin flap as primary reconstruction procedure	Groin flap with immediate (<5 days), early (5-22 days) and intermediate (23 days-6 weeks) post injury
Outcome	Two stage reconstruction surgery	Multiple stage surgery with serial debridement	Two stage reconstruction, primary reconstruction less than 5 days

Conclusion

The use of groin flap as distant pedicle flaps in cases of electrical burn injury provides an alternative when free flap reconstruction cannot be performed. In electrical burn injury, flap compromise is unrelated to the timing of the reconstruction surgery and caused by the pathophysiology of vascular occlusion and progressive tissue necrosis.

The ability to debride nonvital soft tissue without jeopardizing vital structures underlying the burn wound is critical. Pliable characteristics, such as those of groin flap, are required when covering small cross-sectional diameter anatomic regions such as the wrist. However, due to its bulky appearance, secondary reconstruction will be required to thin the groin flap.

REFERENCES

[1] Hunt, J.L., McManus, W.F., Haney, W.P., Pruitt, B.A., Vascular lesions in acute electric injuries. *J. Trauma*, 1974; 14, 461-473.

[2] Jia-ke, C., Li-gen, L., Quan-wen, G., Xiao-peng, S., Hai-jun, Z., Zhi-yong, S., Zhi-qiang, W., Cai, Z. Establishment of soft-tissue-injury model of high-voltage electrical burn and observation of its pathological changes. *Burns,* 2009; 35, 1158-1164.

[3] Arnoldo, B.D., Hunt, J.L., Sterling, J.P., Purdue, G.F. Chapter 38: Electrical Injuries. In: Herndon, D.N.(Ed.),*Total Burn Care.* Saunders; 2012; 433-439.

[4] Vogt, P.M., Niederbichler, A.D., Jokuszies, D. Electrical injury: Reconstructive problems. In: Herndon, D.N. (Ed.),*Total Burn Care.* Saunders; 2012; 441-448.

[5] Handschin, A.E., Vetter, S., Jung, F.J., Guggenheim, M., Künzi, W., Giovanoli, P. A case-matched controlled study on high-voltage electrical injuries vs thermal burns. *J. Burn Care Res.,* 2009; 30, 400-407.

[6] Barillo, D.J., Arabitg, R., Cancio, L.C., Goodwin, C.W. Distant pedicle flaps for soft tissue coverage of severely burned hands : an old idea revisited. *Burns*, 2001;27:613-619.

[7] Jabir, S., Frew, Q., El-Muttardi, N., Dziewulski, P. A systematic review of the applications of free tissue transfer in burns. *Burns*, 2014; 40, 1059-1070.

[8] Strauch, B.,Vasconez, L.O., Hall-Findley, E.J.(Eds.). *Grabb's Encyclopedia of Flaps, Volume II: Upper Extremities.* Boston: Little Brown; 1990.

[9] Arner M, Moller. Morbidity of the pedicled groin flap. A retrospective study of 44 cases. *Scand J Plast Reconstr Surg Hand Surg.*, 1994; 28(2): 143-146.

[10] Goertz, O., Kapalschinski, N., Daigeler, A., et al. The effectiveness of pedicled groinflaps in the treatment of hand defects: Results of 49 patients. *J Hand Surg Am.*, 2012;37(10):2088-2094.

[11] Graf, P., Biemer, E. Morbidity of the groin flap transfer: are we gettingsomething for nothing. *Plast Reconstr Surg.*, 1992;45:86-88.

In: Case Reports in Surgery
Editors: Ahmad Jabir Rahyussalim et al.
ISBN: 978-1-53616-582-1

Chapter 2

AUTOPSY OF AORTIC DISSECTION AFTER TEVAR INSTALLATION: A CASE REPORT

Yuli Budiningsih and Insil Pendri Hariyani*
Department of Forensic Medicine and Medicolegal Studies
Cipto Mangunkusumo National Hospital,
Universitas Indonesia, Jakarta, Indonesia

ABSTRACT

Aortic dissection is a condition in which there is a tear in the aorta's tunica intima layer, leading to separation between the tunica intima and the tunica media, forming a false lumen. The incidence of aortic dissection is reportedly 5–30 cases per 1 million people per year. Thoracic endovascular aortic repair (TEVAR) is a recommended first-line therapy for patients with type B aortic dissection. The reported 30-day mortality rate and major complication rate with TEVAR are 5%–7% and 8%–10%, respectively. We report an autopsy of a 60-year-old German man diagnosed with Stanford type B (DeBakey type III) aortic dissection who underwent a debranching aorto-innominate-carotid graft (Y-graft) and TEVAR surgery. The external examination revealed postsurgical scars on the chest and left inguinal region along with injection marks on both upper extremities. The internal examination revealed blood inside the thorax; heart filled with blood and blood clots; cardiac enlargement; a constricted left coronary artery; an aortic wall laceration; separation of the tunica intima from the tunica media and adventitia throughout the ascending, descending, and abdominal aorta, forming a false lumen containing blood clots; atherosclerosis; and signs of damaged internal organs. There were some vascular Y-graft anastomoses from the ascending aorta to the end of the brachiocephalic artery and just before the branching of the left common carotid and left subclavian arteries. There was also an endovascular graft in the aortic lumen from the aortic arch to the thoracic aorta. Histopathological examination revealed an acute myocardial rupture, atherosclerosis in the

* Corresponding Author's E-mail: insil.pendri@yahoo.com.

left coronary artery, dissection of the aorta accompanied with erythrocyte infiltration in the aortic wall, and signs of internal organ congestion.

Keywords: Aortic Dissection; Acute Myocardial Infarction; Thoracic Endovascular Aortic Repair.

INTRODUCTION

Acute aortic dissection is an age-related cardiovascular disease that has high morbidity and mortality due to complications. Autopsy studies confirm that acute aortic dissection is a life-threatening pathological state [1].

In recent years, 5–30 cases of aortic dissection per 1 million people have been reported annually [2,3]. Population-based studies have confirmed approximately three cases of aortic dissection per 100,000 people per year [1,4]. There are at least 7,000 cases per year in the United States [2].

Thoracic endovascular aortic repair (TEVAR) has recently emerged as the first-line approach for patients with type B aortic dissection. A 30-day mortality rate of 5%–17% and a major complication rate of 8%–10% after installation of TEVAR, have been reported [5].

CASE REPORT

On May 15th, 2017, the Department of Medical Forensic and Medicolegal Studies CMNH received a request from the German Embassy to perform a clinical autopsy on the body of a 60-year-old German man who had died after hospitalized at another hospital.

According to the medical resume, the man was diagnosed with Stanford type B (DeBakey type III) aortic dissection and had been treated for 15 days. His general physical examination revealed that his blood pressure was 190/96 mmHg, his pulse rate was 106 beats/minute, and his respiratory rate was 18 times/minute. The patient had undergone a Y-graft and TEVAR procedures.

The external examination took place on May 15th, 2017, at 16.45 Western Indonesian Time, while the body was still frozen. There were postoperative incision scars on the chest and left inguinal region, along with some needle tracks on both upper extremities.

An internal examination took place on May 15th, 2017, at 18.55 Western Indonesian Time. The examination revealed: 670 and 200 ml of blood inside the right and left thorax, respectively; an opened pericardial sac containing 130 ml of blood and 250 g of blood clots; heart enlargement; constriction of up to 75%–85% of the left coronary artery lumen; two irregular lacerations in the aortic arch (1 cm) and the descending aorta (2 cm), surrounded by infiltrated blood; separation of the tunica intima from the tunica media and adventitia throughout the ascending, descending, and abdominal aorta, forming a false lumen containing blood clots; atherosclerosis along the aortic arch to the abdominal aorta; and some signs of organ damage, such as pulmonary edema and aneurysms in the brain, digestive tract, liver, kidneys, and bladder. There were some vascular Y-graft anastomoses from the ascending aorta to the end of the brachiocephalic artery and just before the branching of the left common carotid and the left subclavian artery. There was also an endovascular graft in the aortic lumen from the aortic arch to the thoracic aorta.

Histopathological examination revealed an acute myocardial rupture, erythrocyte infiltration, aortic dissection, atherosclerosis in the left coronary artery, and damage to the brain, lungs, liver, and lymph nodes.

DISCUSSION

Aortic dissection is a condition in which the tunica intima and the tunica media of the aorta separate and form a false lumen due to a laceration in the tunica intima. The International Registry of Acute Aortic Dissection reported the incidence of aortic dissection was highest during the sixth and seventh decades and mostly involved 62-year-old men. The incidence was more than twice as high in men than in women (68% vs. 32%). Likely, younger patients were also susceptible; the average age of male and female patients was 60 and 67 years, respectively. Seventy-five percent of patients, including the patient in our study, had a history of hypertension [4,6].

Three main systems are used to classify aortic dissection: DeBakey types I, II, and III; Stanford types A and B; and proximal and distal aortic dissection. The classifications are based on where the laceration in the tunica intima of the aortic wall and the false lumen are located. DeBakey type I is an aortic dissection in which the laceration is located in the ascending aorta and the false lumen is found along the aortic arch. In DeBakey type II, only the ascending aorta is involved. In DeBakey type III, the laceration is in the tunica intima in the descending aorta without involvement of the aortic arch and the ascending aorta. DeBakey type III has two subtypes. In subtype IIIa, the laceration is located only in the thoracic aorta; in subtype IIIb, the laceration also involves the abdominal aorta [1,7].

Stanford type A aortic dissection is located in the ascending aorta (DeBakey types I and II); Stanford type B aortic dissection is located in the descending aorta (DeBakey type III) [1,7].

A recent classification divides aortic dissections into five types, as shown in Figure 1.

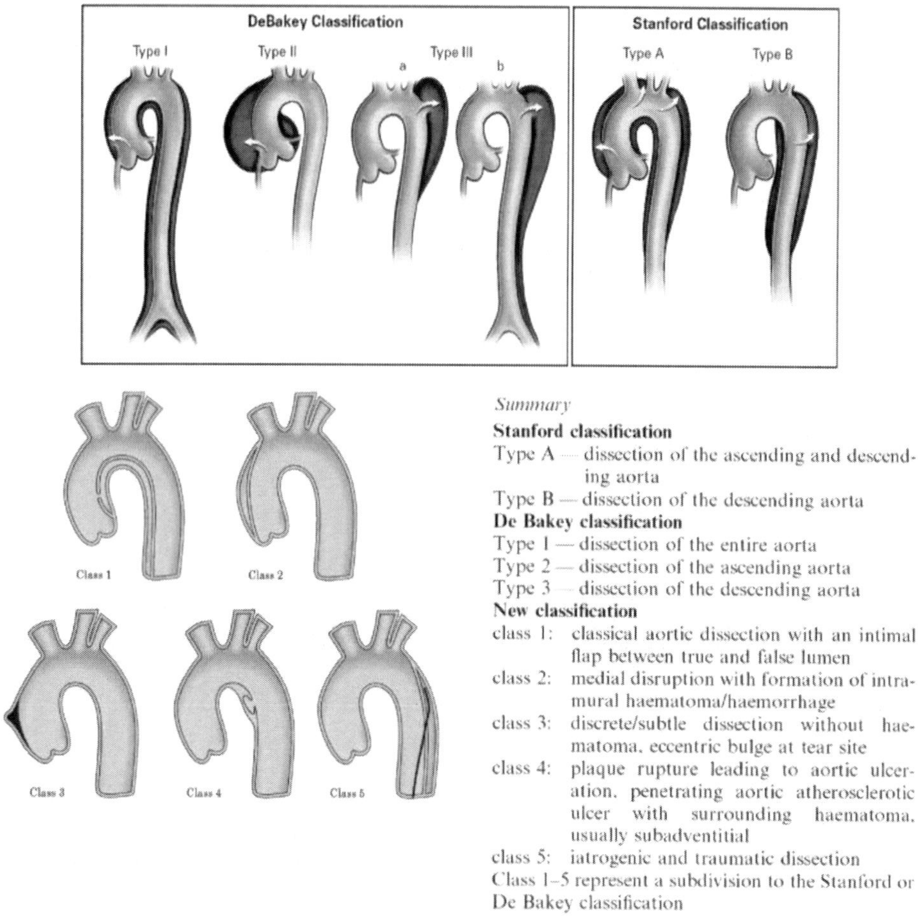

Figure 1. A recent classification of aortic dissections.

The aortic wall is composed of three layers: the innermost tunica intima, the middle tunica media, and the outermost tunica adventitia. Acute aortic dissection occurs from the stress of systemic hypertension, which damages the aortic wall. Generally, this condition begins with a tear in the tunica intima, which then spreads to the tunica media along the aortic wall by pressure from the blood, resulting in a false lumen. The dissection can extend distally, proximally, and, eventually, throughout the aorta. In 90% of cases, a secondary tear in the intimomedia layer forms as the dissection extends, allowing blood to flow back into the true aortic lumen. While the primary laceration is often located in the thoracic aorta, the secondary tear is likely to appear below the descending aorta or in the abdominal aorta [8].

A cohort study by Bailey et al. [9] of 369 autopsies of aortic dissection cases over 16 years (1993–2008) suggested that atherosclerosis was a risk factor in 73% of fatal aortic dissections. The ulcerated atherosclerotic plaque might cause more damage to the tunica intima and lead to aortic dissection [9].

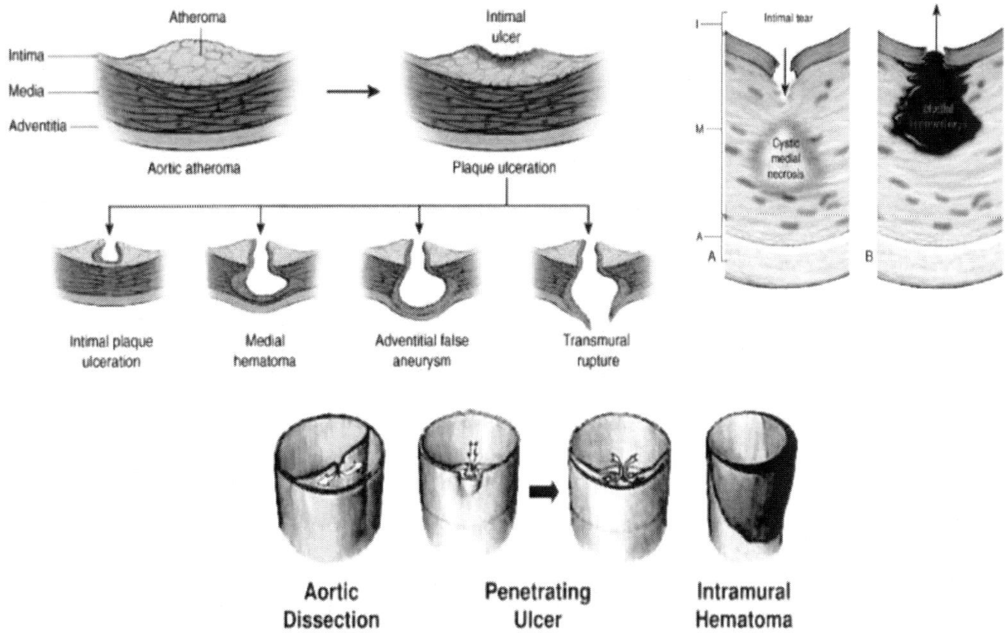

Figure 2. Dissection of the aortic wall.

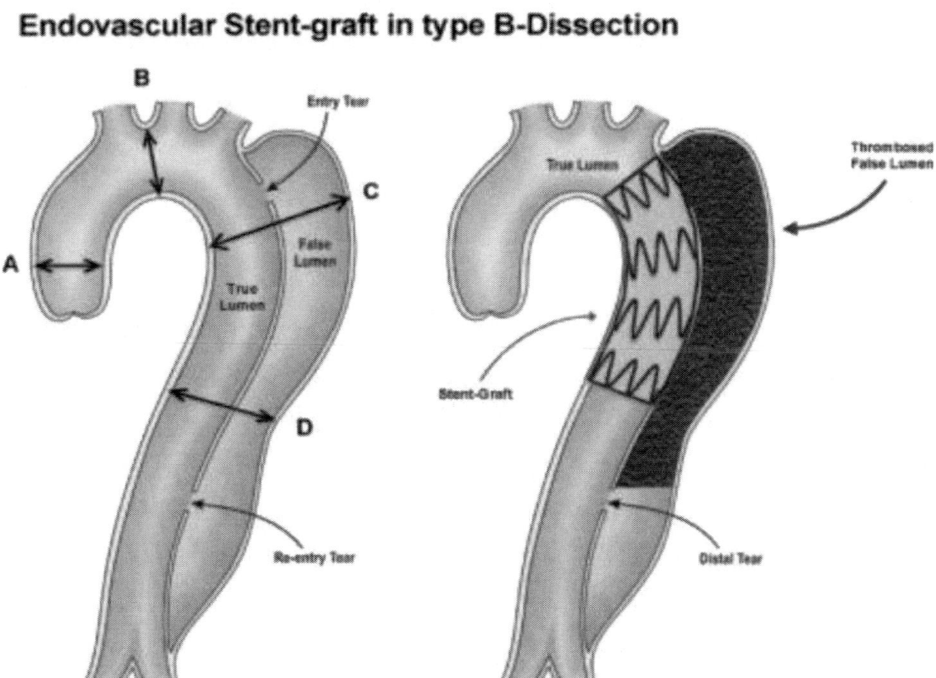

Figure 3. Location of installation of TEVAR for Stanford type B [10] aortic dissection.

The recent INSTEAD-XL studies indicated that TEVAR could prolong the lives of aortic dissection patients by five years and delay progression of the Stanford type B aortic dissection, which often occurs as a complication of diseases such as uncontrolled hypertension, ruptured aorta, and end-organ ischemia. However, TEVAR's effectiveness for treating chronic complications of Stanford type B aortic dissection remains controversial [5].

Our autopsy results showed that the frailty of the aortic wall due to atherosclerosis led to laceration in the ascending aorta, which resulted in blood flowing out to the cardiac and thorax. Blood inside the cardiac could promote pericardial tamponade and disrupt cardiac movements. We also found a laceration in the tunica intima of the descending aorta and dissection along the descending aorta to the bifurcation of the iliac arteries. We detected a TEVAR graft in the aorta and blood clots inside the false lumen.

Our autopsy also revealed a lumen constriction of up to 75%–85% due to a thickened left coronary artery and an acute myocardial infarction image in the myocardium.

Atherosclerosis of the coronary arteries is a potentially fatal disease. This disease reportedly causes at least 25%–40% of deaths. One interesting finding of our autopsy is that atherosclerotic constriction of the left coronary artery occurred in more than 75% of the lumen. This finding is contrary to most atherosclerotic constriction cases where the constriction occurred in less than 75% of the lumen. Necrotic myocardium may occur if the lumen is constricted by 20% or less, followed by ischemia in the artery distribution area [6, 11].

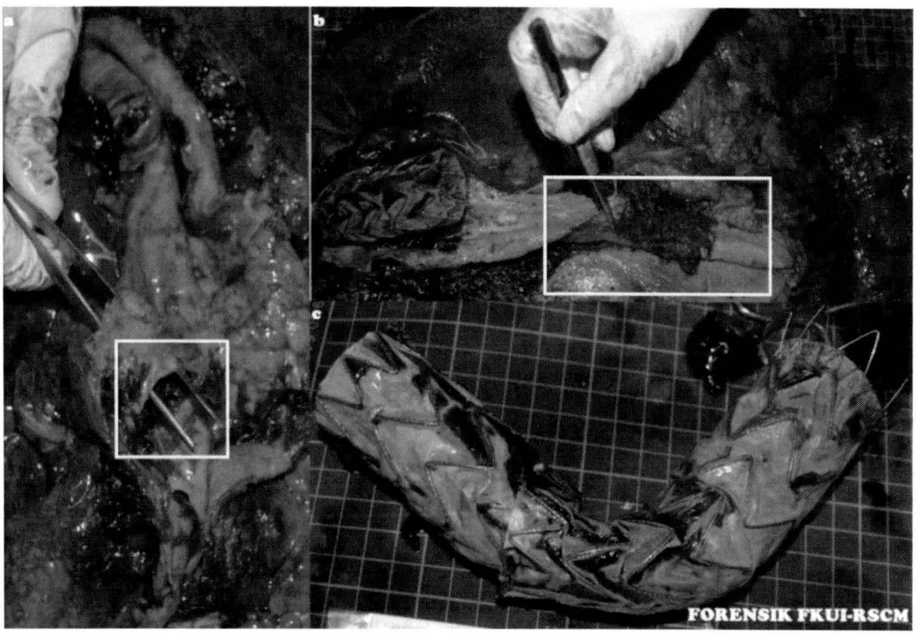

Figure 4. (a) Laceration in the ascending aorta; (b) aortic dissection; (c) TEVAR graft.

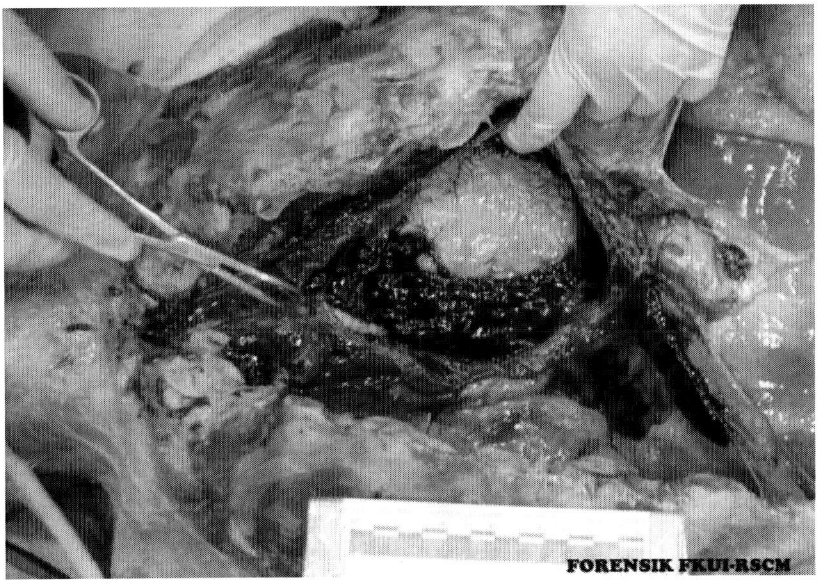

Figure 5. Blood and blood clots inside the pericardium.

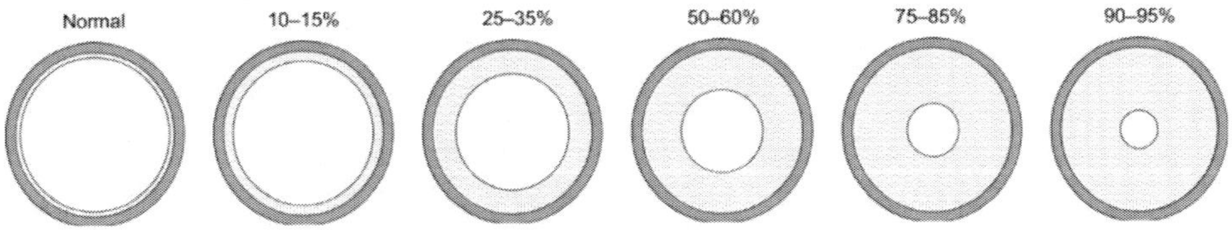

Figure 6. Anatomical cross sections of constriction in atherosclerotic arteries.

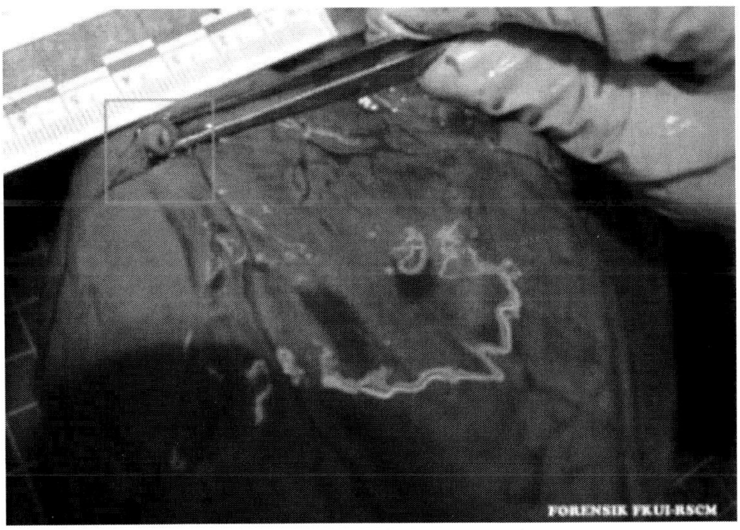

Figure 7. Narrowing of the left coronary artery lumen opening.

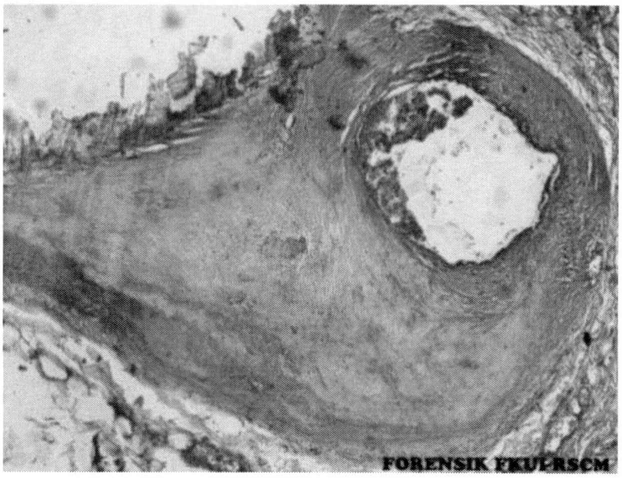

Figure 8. Histopathological image of the left coronary artery.

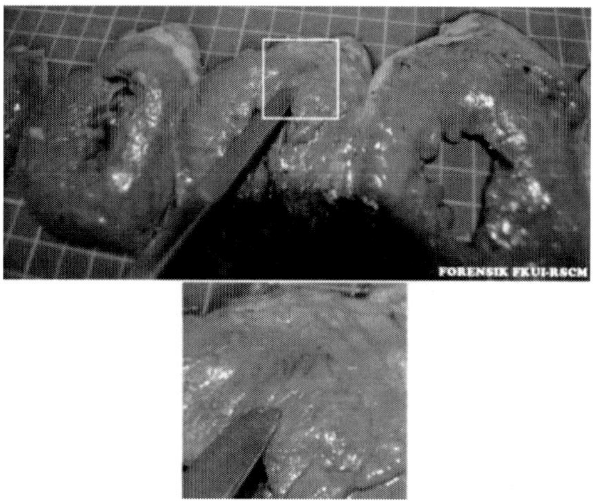

Figure 10. Myocardial infarction.

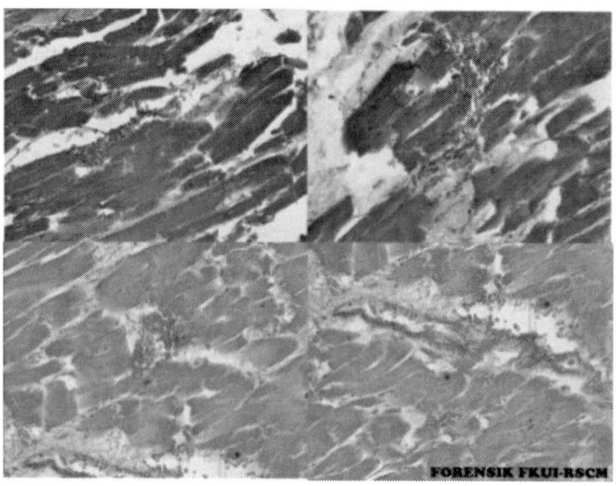

Figure 11. Histopathological image of the myocardium showing myocardial rupture.

This 60-year-old German man appeared to die from natural causes. The external examination revealed several postoperative wounds and signs of damage. The internal examination revealed a TEVAR-corrected Stanford type B (DeBakey type III) aortic dissection. The autopsy also revealed a laceration in the ascending aorta that caused bleeding in the thorax and cardiac. The autopsy confirmed constriction of the left coronary artery lumen by 75%–85% due to atherosclerosis and myocardial infarction. We observed blood and blood clots inside the cardiac that caused cardiac tamponade. The histopathological images confirmed our internal examination findings of myocardial infarction, left coronary artery atherosclerosis, aortic dissection with erythrocyte infiltration, and signs of damage to the brain, lungs, and liver. In this case, cardiac tamponade caused myocardial infarction, which disrupted cardiac movements and led to death.

REFERENCES

[1] Ayala, I., Chen, Y.F. Acute aortic dissection: an update. *Kaohsiung Journal of Medical Sciences*, 2012 28, 299-305.

[2] Isselbacher, E.M. Epidemiology of thoracic aortic aneurysms; aortic dissection; intramural hematoma and penetrating atherosclerotic ulcers. In: Eagle, K.A., Baliga, R.R., Isselbacher, E.M., Nienaber, C.A., editors. *Aortic dissection and related syndromes. Developments in cardiovascular medicine*. Boston: Springer; 2007.

[3] Demengiu, S., Ceausu, M., Hostiuc, S., Curca, G.C., Demengiu, D., Turculet, C. Spontaneous aortic dissection due to cystic medial degeneration report of a sudden death case and literature review. *Romanian Journal of Legal Medicine,* 2009 17, 89-96.

[4] Tai, H.C.H., Chen, W.L. Acute aortic dissection mimicking as ureteral calculus. *Journal of Acute Medicine,* 2016 6, 61-3.

[5] Miyazaki, Y., Furuyama, T., Matsubara, Y., Yoshiya, K., Yoshiga, R., Inoue, K., et al. Thoracic endovascular aortic repair for complicated chronic type B aortic dissection in a patient on hemodialysis with recurrent ischemic colitis. *Surgical Case Reports*, 2016 2, 38.

[6] Saukko, P., Knight, B. Knights Forensic Pathology. Fourth Edition. London: CRC Press; 2016.

[7] Tran, T.P., Khoynezhad, A. Current management of type B aortic dissection. *Vascular Health and Risk Management*, 2009 5, 53.

[8] Wahyudi, D., Dakota, I., Kaligis, R.W.M., Sunu, I. Laporan kasus endovaskular stent graft pada diseksi aorta tipe B. 2007.

[9] Bailey, K., Duflou, J., Puranik, R. Fatal cases of aortic dissection: an autopsy study. *International Journal of Cardiology*, 2012 158, 148-9.

[10] Nienaber, C.A., Rousseau, H., Eggebrecht, H. Randomized comparison of strategies for type b aortic dissection—the Investigation of Stent Grafts in Aortic Dissection (INSTEAD) Trial. *Journal of Vascular Surgery*, 2010 51, 1321-29.

[11] Dolinak, D., Matshes, EW., Lew, E.O. Forensic Pathology Principles and Practice. London: Elsevier Academic Press; 2005.

In: Case Reports in Surgery
Editors: Ahmad Jabir Rahyussalim et al.
ISBN: 978-1-53616-582-1

Chapter 3

RARE OCCURRENCE OF SECONDARY EXTRACRANIAL SINONASAL MENINGIOMA: A CASE REPORT

Renindra Ananda Aman**, Adhitya Syahada, Aryandhito Widhi Nugroho, David Tandian, Samsul Ashari, Syaiful Ichwan, and Setyo Widi Nugroho
Department of Neurosurgery, Faculty of Medicine,
RSUPN Dr. Cipto Mangunkusumo,
Universitas Indonesia, Jakarta, Indonesia

ABSTRACT

Meningioma is the most common type of benign intracranial tumor. The occurrence of extracranial meningioma is rare, accounting for only 2% of all meningiomas. There are two types of extracranial meningioma: primary and secondary. Primary extracranial meningioma grows extracranially without any connection to intracranial lesions, whereas secondary extracranial meningioma is an intracranial meningioma that extends extracranially. Herein, we report the case of a 45-year-old female patient with secondary extracranial sinonasal meningioma who presented with intermittent headache and unilateral proptosis due to olfactory groove meningioma that expanded to the right ethmoid sinus. Gross tumor resection was achieved in this case.

Keywords: extracranial meningioma, sinonasal meningioma, secondary extracranial meningioma, transitional meningioma

* Corresponding Author's E-mail: renindra03@yahoo.com.

INTRODUCTION

Meningiomas are originated from meningeal coverings and arachnoid cap cells found in the arachnoid villi at cranial vault and base, as well as in the spinal region [1]. Hitherto, various registries from countries worldwide have shown an increase in meningioma incidence [2-5]. Although studies on meningiomas in general are abound, particular studies on extracranial meningiomas are lacking.

Extracranial, or ectopic, meningioma accounts for approximately 2% of all meningiomas [6-8]. There are two types of extracranial meningioma: primary and secondary.

While the former has no connection to intracranial lesions, the latter is a direct extension of intracranial lesions to extracranial sites [6-8]. Due to the rare occurrence of secondary extracranial meningioma, its diagnosis and management requires a thorough and cautious approach. In this report, we present the rare case of a secondary extracranial meningioma in the sinonasal area that originated from the olfactory groove area.

CASE REPORT

A 45-year-old female patient presented with a history of progressive intermittent headache since 3 years, followed by progressive protrusion of the right eye since 2 years ago (see Figure 1). The patient had no complains of blurred vision, visual field deficit, double vision, epistaxis, nasal obstruction, rhinorrhea, and smell disorder. Upon neurologic examination, proptosis was identified with a slight decrease in visual acuity in the right eye (6/8.5 on the Snellen chart), unilateral ophthalmoparesis, unilateral anosmia, and bilateral papilledema. No other abnormalities were found. Contrast-enhanced brain computed tomography (CT) revealed a homogenous hyperdense lesion in the bilateral frontal bone with expansion to the right ethmoidal sinus (see Figure 2). Further imaging with contrast-enhanced T1-weighted magnetic resonance imaging (MRI) revealed homogenous hyper-intense enhancement of the lesion (see Figure 3). The patient underwent craniotomy for removal of the tumor, which had areddish-white macroscopic appearance, firm consistency, and could easily bleed (see Figure 4). Histopathologic examinations revealed a grade 1 meningioma (mixed meningioma, also referred to as transitional meningioma) based on the World Health Organization (WHO) classification (9). The case was uneventful, and the patient was discharged 1 week after surgery. Post-operative CT exhibited gross total tumor removal (see Figure 5).

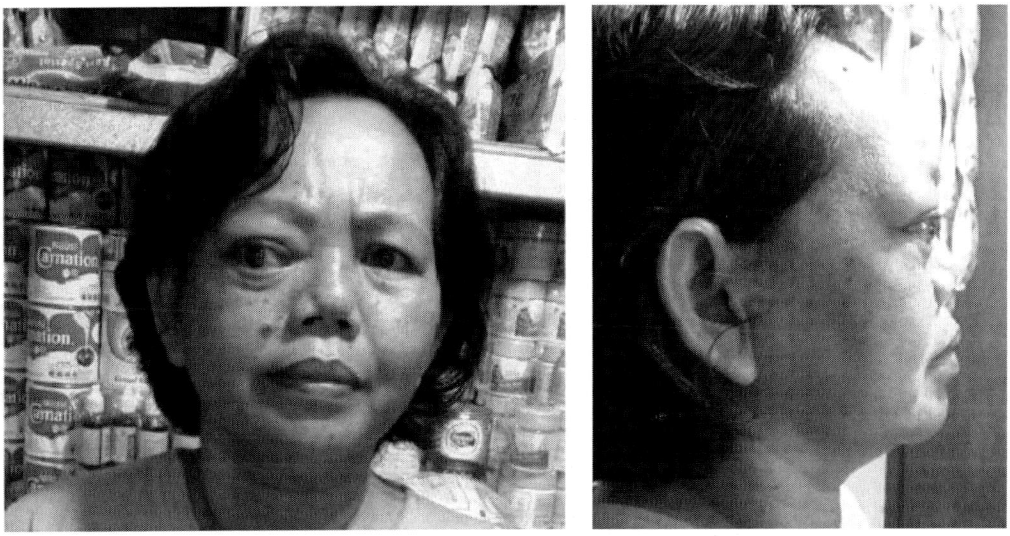

Figure 1. Anterior and lateral view of the patient's face showing obvious protrusion in the right eye.

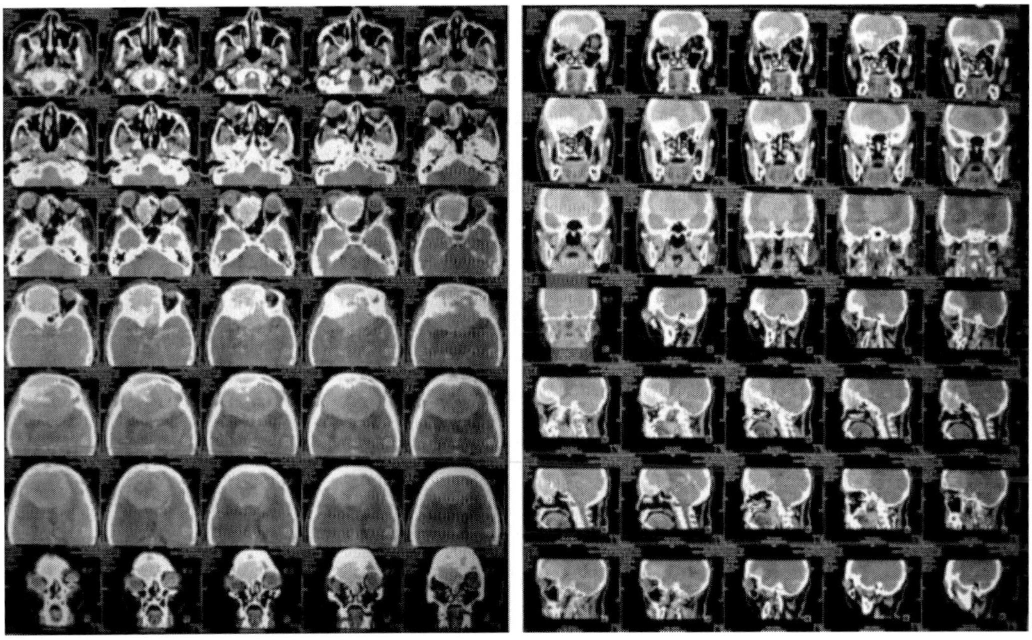

Figure 2. Axial, coronal, and sagittal views of contrast-enhanced computed tomography scan revealed a bilateral frontal mass that expands to the right ethmoidal sinus.

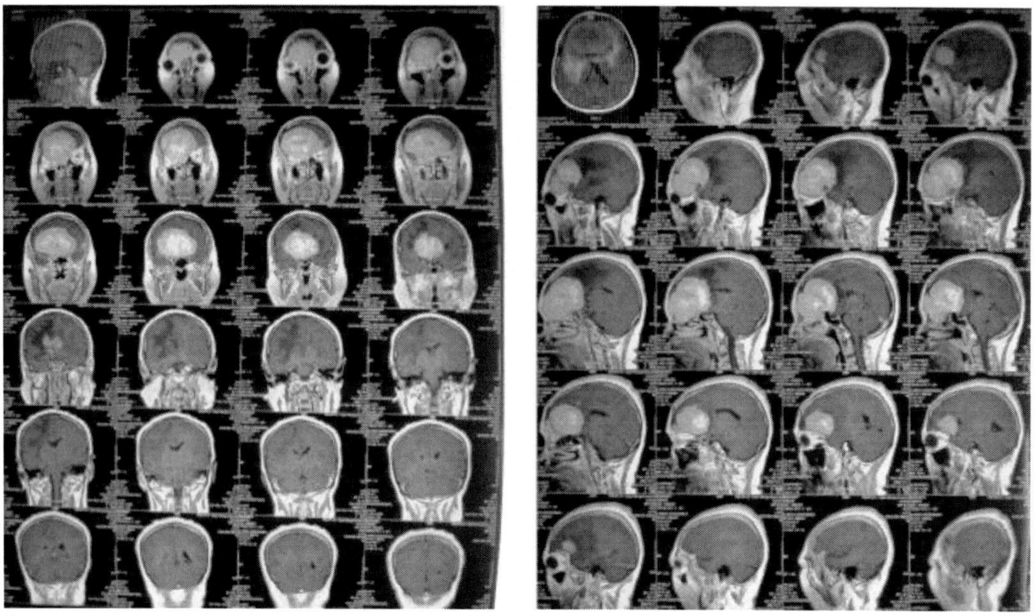

Figure 3. Contrast-enhanced T1-weightedmagnetic resonance imaging revealed a homogenous hyper-intense lesion in the bilateral frontal lobes extending to the right ethmoidal sinus.

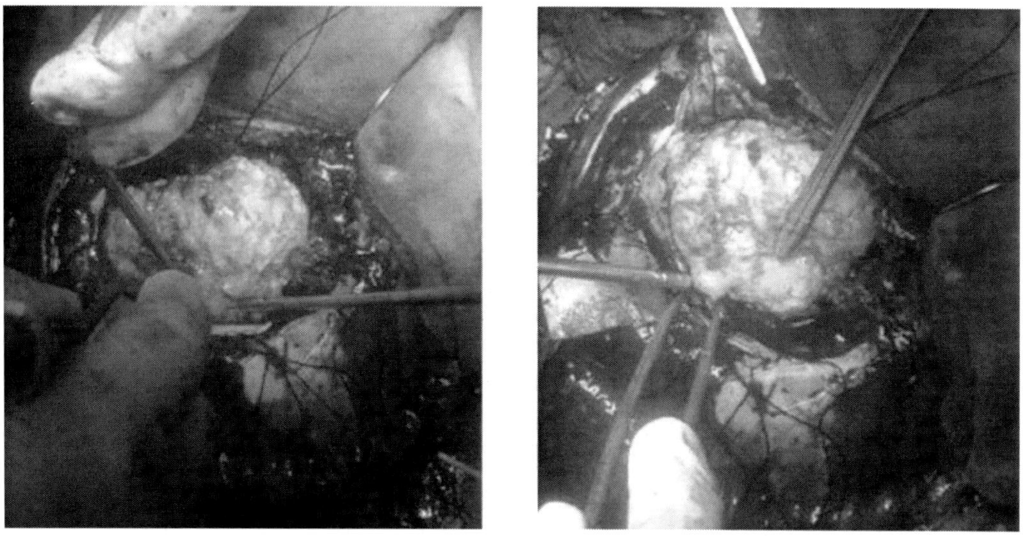

Figure 4. Intraoperative macroscopic view of the lesion: reddish-white appearance, firm, and bleeds easily.

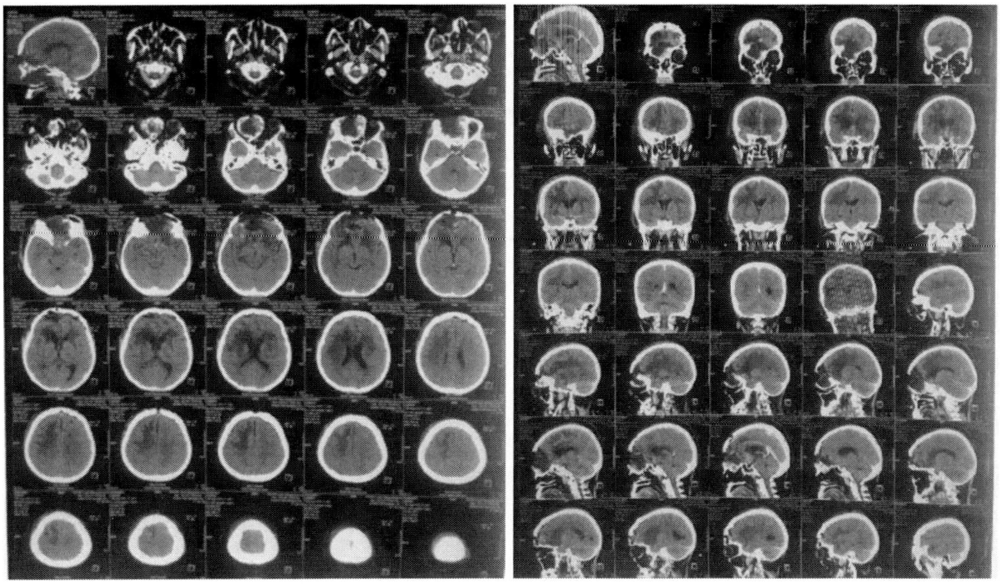

Figure 5. Postoperative axial, coronal, and sagittal computed tomography scan images.

Discussion

Meningioma is the most common benign intracranial tumor, which accounts for 13% – 30% of primary intracranial tumors [6, 7]. Genetic factors, such as neurofibromatosis type-2 and multiple endocrine neoplasia type-1, increase the likelihood of meningiomas [11, 12]. Other risk factors for meningioma are ionized radiation exposure, hormonal exposure, brain trauma, and history of breast cancer. Although there is no evidence that hormonal exposure increases the risk of developing meningioma significantly, its incidence is more prevalent in women than in men (2:1), particularly for grade I meningioma. Meanwhile, for grade II and III meningiomas, the incidence is higher in men than in women (1.2:1) [10-12].

There are two types of meningioma: intracranial and extracranial. Intracranial meningioma is covered by dura mater, whereas extracranial meningioma is not covered by dura mater. The extracranial subtype accounts for approximately 2% of all meningiomas [6-9]. Extracranial meningioma can be classified into two types: primary and secondary. Meningiomas that arise extracranially without any association with an intracranial mass are referred to as primary extracranial meningiomas. Secondary extracranial meningiomas are extentions from intracranial disease. The tumor may enter the orbit and nasal cavity through preformed bony pathways, surgical defects, or foramina of the skull base [6-8]. Hoye (1960) has developed a classification system of extracranial meningiomas (Table 1) [14]. Another classification system was established by Atherio et al., which divided extracranial meningioma into four groups [15]:

(i) primary extracranial meningiomas extending from the skull,
(ii) extracranial meningioma arising from the arachnoid cell rests of cranial nerve sheaths,
(iii) meningiomas with no obvious connection with the foramina or cranial nerves, and
(iv) metastasis of malignant intracranial meningiomas.

Table 1. Hoye classification of extracranial meningiomas [14]

Primary	Secondary
Extracranial extension of a meningioma arising from the neural foramina	Extracranial extension of the meningioma from the intracranial meningioma
Ectopic, without any connection to the neural foramina or intracranial structure	Extracranial extension from metastasis of intracranial meningioma

Several theories regarding the mechanism of primary extracranial meningioma have been proposed, which were as follows: extradural entrapment of arachnoid cells during embryogenesis, ectopic migration of arachnoid cells in the development of peripheral nerves, and metaplasia of mature peripheral nerve sheath or progenitor cells [8]. The most common site for extending intracranial meningioma is the orbit, and other sites include the nasopharyx, scalp, sinuses (frontal sinus, maxillary sinuses, ethmoidale sinus, and sphenoid sinuses), parapharyngeal region, and parotid gland [8]. Although meningiomas have the capability to expand extracranially, they rarely invade the brain [8].

Cautious and systematic anamnesis; physical examinations;and imaging histopathological, and immunohistochemical studies must be conducted to diagnose meningiomasaccurately. Anamnesis and physical examinationscan help identify signs and symptoms with regard to tumor location. In our patient, intermittent progressive headache, unilateral proptosis, and anosmia were identified. Non-contrast-enhanced CT can reveal hyper- or isodense lesion (15% – 20% cases can present with reveal calcification), which enhances homogenously.

T1-weighted MRI can reveal iso- to hypo-intense lesions, which are homogenously enhanced with the administration of gadolinium, whereas T2-weighted MRI usually reveal iso- to hyper-intense lesions. Peritumoural edema is observed in 60% of cases [13]. Histopathology studies aim to classify meningiomas according to WHO grading and to determine the most appropriate treatment. Immunohistochemical studies have used vimentin and epithelial membrane antigens for the diagnosis of meningiomas [16]. However, both were not examined in this study.

Gross total resection remains the standard treatment for all meningiomas [13], although this may not be the case for the management of skull base meningiomas. Nevertheless, surgeons should aim to achieve Simpson grade I resection during the first surgery.

Conclusion

This study reported a case of secondary extracranial sinonasal meningioma. Physical examinations; cautious and systematic anamnesis; and imaging, histopathological, and immunohistochemical studies must be performed to diagnose this rare type of meningioma accurately. Gross total resection of the tumor, dural attachment, and abnormal bone should be performed to achieve low recurrence, although tumor location may be used as basis for the extent of resection.

References

[1] Baldi, I., Engelhardt, J., Bonnet, C., Bauchet, L., Berteaud, E., Grüber, A. & Loiseau, H. (2018). Epidemiology of meningiomas. *Neurochirurgie*, *64*, 5-14.

[2] Ostrom, Q. T., Gittleman, H., Farah, P., Ondracek, A., Chen, Y., Wolinsky, Y., Stroup, N. E., Kruchko, C. & Barnholtz-Sloan, J. S. (2013). CBTRUS Statistical Report: primary brain and central nervous system tumors diagnosed in the United States in 2006–2010. *Neuro-Oncology*, *15*, 1-56.

[3] Radhakrishnan, K., Mokri, B., Parisi, J. E., O'Fallon, M., Sunku, J. & Kurland, L. T (1995). The trends in incidence of primary brain tumors in the population of Rochester, Minnesota. *Annals of Neurology*, *37*, 67–73.

[4] Nakamura, H., Makino, K., Yano, S., Kuratsu, J. & Kumamoto Brain Research Group. (2011). Epidemiological study of primary intracranial tumors: a regional survey in Kumamoto prefecture in southern Japan – 20-year study. *International Journal of Clinical Oncology*, *16*, 314–21.

[5] Surawicz, T. S., McCarthy, B. J., Kupelian, V., Jukich, P. J., Bruner, J. M. & David, F. G. (1999). Descriptive epidemiology of primary brain and CNS tumors: results from the Central Brain Tumor Registry of the United States, 1990–1994. *Neuro-Oncology*, *1*, 14–25.

[6] Counsell, C. E., Collie, D. A. & Grant, R. (1996). Incidence of intracranial tumours in the Lothian region of Scotland, 1989–90. *Journal of Neurology, Neurosurgery, and Psychiatry*, *61*, 143–50

[7] Albu, S., Florian, I. Æ. & Bãciuå, G. (2014). Secondary extracranial meningiomas extending into the paranasal sinuses. *Chirurgia*, *109*, 858-861.

[8] Iaconetta, G., Santella, A., Friscia, M., Abbate, V. & Califano, L. (2012). Extracranial primary and secondary meningiomas. *International Journal of Oral and Maxillofacial Surgery*, *41*, 211-217.

[9] Louis, D. N., Perry, A., Reifenberger, G., von Deimling, A., Figarella-Branger, D., Cavenee, W. K., Ohgaki, K., Wiestler, O. D., Kleihues, P. & Ellison, D. W. (2016).

The 2016 World Health Organization Classification of Tumors of the Central Nervous System: a summary. *Acta Neuropathologica*, *131*, 803-20

[10] Rogers, L., Barani, I., Chamberlain, M., Kaley, T. J., McDermott, M., Raizer, J., Schiff, D., Weber, D. C., Wen, P. Y. & Vogelbaum, M. A. (2015). Meningiomas: knowledge base, treatment outcomes, and uncertainties. A RANO review. *Journal of Neurosurgery*, *122*, 4-23.

[11] Wiemels, J., Wrensch, M. & Claus, E. B. (2010). Epidemiology and etiology of meningioma. *Journal of Neurooncology*, *99*, 307-314.

[12] Barnholtz-Sloan, J. S. & Kruchko, C. (2007). Meningiomas: causes and risk factors. *Neurosurgical Focus*, *23*, 1-8.

[13] Fogh, S. E., Johnson, D. R., Barker, F. G., Brastianos, P. K., Clarke, J. L., Kaufmann, T. J., Oberndorfer, S., Preusser, M., Raghunathan, A., Santagata, S. & Theodosopoulos, P. V. (2016). Case based review: meningioma. *Neuro-Oncology Practice*, *3*, 120-134.

[14] Sharma, J. K., Pippal, S. K. & Sethi, Y. (2006). A rare case of primary nasoethmoidal meningioma. *Indian Journal of Otolaryngology and Head and Neck Surgery*, *58*, 101-103.

[15] Atherino, C. C. T., Garcia, R. & Lopes, L. J. (1985). Ectopic meningioma of the nose and paranasal sinuses (report of a case). *The Journal of Laryngology & Otology*, *99*, 1161-1166.

[16] Thompson, L. D. & Gyure, K. A. (2000). Extracranial sinonasal tract meningiomas. *The American Journal of Surgical Pathology*, *24*, 640-650.

In: Case Reports in Surgery
Editors: Ahmad Jabir Rahyussalim et al.
ISBN: 978-1-53616-582-1

Chapter 4

THORACIC EPIDURAL ANALGESIA IN A CRITICALLY ILL PATIENT WITH ACUTE PANCREATITIS

Dita Aditianingsih, Raden Besthadi Sukmono**[*]**,
Oryza Eureka, Willy Yant Kartolo and Erika Sasha Adiwongso
Department of Anesthesiology and Intensive Care,
Faculty of Medicine, Universitas Indonesia, Jakarta, Indonesia

ABSTRACT

Currently, there has been an increase in the incidence of acute pancreatitis worldwide. Despite the improvements in access to care, imaging, and interventional techniques, acute pancreatitis continues to be associated with significant morbidity and mortality. Pain control is an important part of supportive management for patients with acute pancreatitis. A 26-year-old woman presented to our emergency department with a distended abdomen and excruciating pain in the upper abdomen. She was diagnosed with acute pancreatitis. She developed acute respiratory distress; thus, she was intubated and admitted to the intensive care unit. Her upper abdominal pain gradually intensified, causing worsening of acute respiratory distress syndrome. Opioids did not considerably relieve her pain; moreover, their side effects worsened acute pancreatitis. Moreover, thoracic epidural analgesia at the T7–T8 interspace was considered for pain management. After the administration of epidural analgesia, pain substantially improved, abdominal distention markedly reduced, amylase and lipase levels gradually returned to normal, and she was eventually weaned off the ventilator. Epidural analgesia is one of the important pain management modalities, and it stops severe acute pancreatitis development by improving splanchnic and pancreatic perfusion, resulting in decreased liver damage and inflammatory responses.

[*] Corresponding Author's E-mail: besth25@gmail.com.

Keywords: thoracic epidural analgesia, acute pancreatitis, ARDS

INTRODUCTION

The most severe forms of acute pancreatitis (AP) are associated with high morbidity and mortality. AP has an overall mortality rate of approximately 5%, and most patients with severe AP require intubation and mechanical ventilation [1, 2]. Although the pathophysiologic cascade of its development and progress is poorly understood, microcirculatory disturbances are considered important factors [3]. Different therapeutic interventions for improving pancreatic microcirculation have been evaluated in recent years. The current treatment for AP involves supportive medical therapy, which is sometimes associated with endoscopic procedures and/or surgical interventions. Therapeutic efforts are aimed at saving injured tissue from infarction and necrosis by improving microcirculatory perfusion and oxygen supply [2, 3].

Pain control is an important part of supportive management in patients with AP. Therefore, in the absence of any patient-specific contraindications, a multimodal analgesic regimen is recommended, including narcotics, nonsteroidal anti-inflammatory drugs (NSAIDs), and acetaminophen [4, 5]. The optimal recommendation is adherence to the most current acute pain management guidelines in the perioperative setting. However, all patients with AP should receive some form of analgesia in the first 24 hours of hospitalization to avoid compromise of quality of life [6, 7, 8]. Recently, increasing evidence from preclinical and clinical studies has supported the beneficial effects of thoracic epidural analgesia (TEA) in AP, such as improved gut barrier function and splanchnic, pancreatic, and renal perfusion; decreased liver damage and inflammatory responses; and reduced mortality [1]. Here, we present a report on a critically ill patient with AP who was successfully treated with TEA.

CASE REPORT

A 26-year-old woman was referred to our emergency department with excruciating pain in the upper abdomen and a distended abdomen. Her clinical findings supported a diagnosis of AP. She developed acute respiratory distress syndrome (ARDS) and was intubated. She was then admitted to the intensive care unit (ICU) for further management.

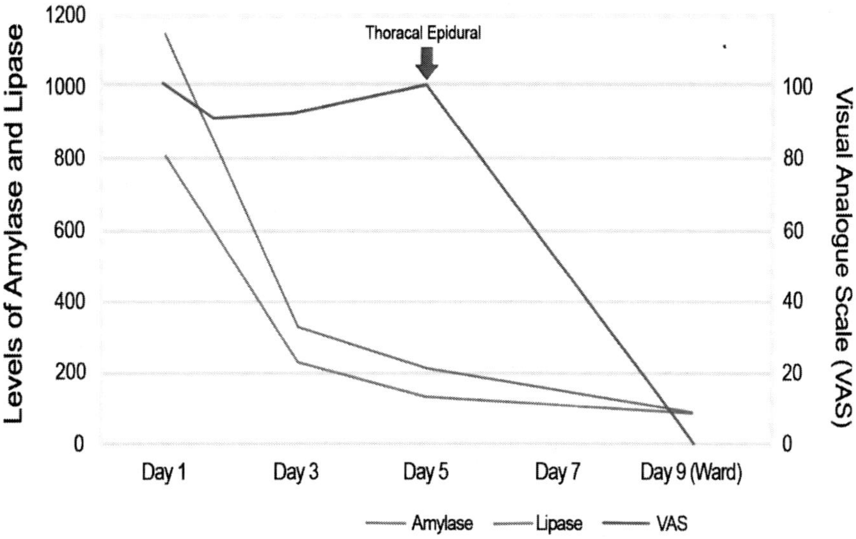

Figure 1. Amylase and lipase levels and pain intensity according to the visual analogue scale during treatment before and after thoracic epidural analgesia in our patient.

Her upper abdominal pain gradually intensified, causing worsening of ARDS and ventilator-patient asynchrony, and therefore, difficulty in ventilator weaning. Several AP laboratory markers, such as amylase and lipase, increased (Figure 1).

Opioids did not significantly relieve her pain; moreover, the side effects worsened her AP. TEA was then considered for pain management, in addition to the prevention of the development of severe AP owing to redistribution of splanchnic blood flow to non-perfused pancreatic regions.

DISCUSSION

The most common and significant complain associated with the diagnosis of AP is pain, and therefore, adequate analgesia represents an important part of the treatment approach [2]. Sensory information from the pancreas is transmitted to the central nervous system via both vagal and spinal pathways. Cell bodies of the spinal afferent pancreatic neurons are located in the T6–L2 dorsal root ganglia, and their axons traverse the splanchnic nerves and celiac plexus before they enter the pancreas [9]. Sensory nerves are responsible for the regulation of pancreatic blood flow, and stimulation of the sensory nerves could produce hyperemia in the pancreatic microcirculation. Previous studies have shown that the protective effects of the sensory nerves on necrotizing pancreatitis are manifested by decreases in plasma amylase and lipase activities, a reduction in the plasma IL-1 level, and an increase in pancreatic DNA synthesis [10, 11].

AP treatment depends mainly on the severity of progression, but almost all cases will require supportive treatments, such as analgesics. Effective treatments of pain in AP range from the administration of simple analgesic drugs, which might be sufficient for patients with mild AP, to the administration of potent opioids, administration of high doses of antibiotics for infected pancreatic necrosis, and even surgical or interventional procedures for cases of severe AP. The World Health Organization analgesic ladder (Figure 2), which includes the use of NSAIDs or their combination with highly potent opioid analgesics in an escalating regime, for the management of abdominal pain mentions the use of interventional strategies depending on the occurrence of AP-related complications [12]. Opioids, such as morphine and its derivatives, are commonly used; however, there is no concrete evidence for their effectiveness and safety. They might hide disease resolution and might increase pain by causing spasms [13]. Besides parenteral pain control, epidural analgesia can be used as an alternative treatment. A previous experimental prospective study assessed the effects of sympathetic block by thoracic epidural anesthesia and found enhanced microcirculatory perfusion and end-organ perfusion and improved survival compared with controls in animal experiments [3]. However, these positive experimental results cannot be automatically transposed to humans since the investigation on regarding the sphlanic perfursion in human have not been cleared [2, 14]. Nevertheless, as the risk of significant morbidity with severe AP is high, it might be reasonable to accept a low rate of TEA complications if a major reduction in mortality is confirmed [14].

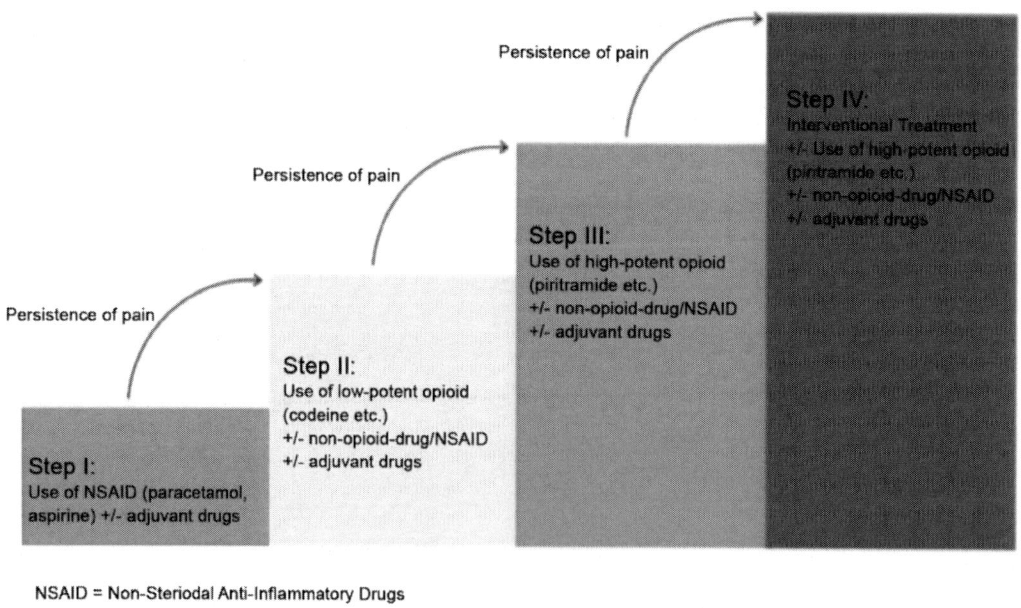

Figure 2. The modified World Health Organization analgesia ladder according to Vargas-Schaffer [12].

TEA can be considered for patients with severe and critical AP who require high doses of opioids for an extended period. Although it has been reported that analgesics could be administered transdermally or rectally, no RCTs have compared the different routes of administration of the same analgesic in patients with AP [15]. The use of TEA in the acute clinical setting of severe AP and sepsis remains a fascinating area of research. Reliable non-invasive measures of splanchnic perfusion need to be developed for further evaluation of the effects of TEA on basic human physiological parameters and for direct randomized trials in critically ill patients [14].

In the present case, epidural analgesia had benefits for AP. This approach is safe and titratable and has minimum side effects compared to other modalities in such a patient. TEA installation at level T5 to T10 was proven to be appropriate and cover the affected dermatome, this was shown in significant reduce in VAS, thus the patient became more comfortable, marked by synchronized breathing with ventilator. It also prevented further progression of the disease by improving splanchnic and pancreatic perfusion. Shortly after the epidural regimen, abdominal distention markedly reduced, amylase and lipase levels gradually returned to normal, and the patient was successfully weaned off from the ventilator.

Conclusion

Epidural anesthesia has a major role in AP management. It is one of the important pain management modalities, and it stops severe AP development by improving splanchnic and pancreatic perfusion, resulting in decreased liver damage and inflammatory responses.

References

[1] Bulyez, S., Pereira, B., Caumon, E., Imhoff, E., Roszyk, L., Bernard, L., Bühler, L., Heidegger, C., Jaber, S., Lefrant, J. Y. & Chabanne, R. (2017). Epidural analgesia in critically ill patients with acute pancreatitis: the multicentre randomised controlled EPIPAN study protocol. *BMJ Open*, 7: e015280. doi: 10.1136/bmjopen-2016-015280.

[2] Zarnescu, N. O., Barbu, S. T., Zarnescu, E. C., Costea, R. & Neagu, S. (2015). Management of acute pancreatitis in the early stage. *Maedica (Buchar)*, 10: 257-263.

[3] Bachmann, K. A., Trepte, C. J., Tomkötter, L., Hinsch, A., Stork, J., Bergmann, W., Heidelmann, L., Strate, T., Goetz, A. E., Reuter, D. A. & Izbicki, J. R. (2013). Effects of thoracic epidural anesthesia on survival and microcirculation in severe acute pancreatitis: a randomized experimental trial. *Critical Care*, 17: R281. doi: 10.1186/cc13142.

[4] Greenberg, J. A., Hsu, J., Bawazeer, M., Marshall, J., Friedrich, J. O., Nathens, A., Coburn, N., May, G. R., Pearsall, E. & McLeod, R. S. (2016). Clinical practice

guideline: management of acute pancreatitis. *Canadian Journal of Surgery*, 59: 128-140. doi: 10.1503/cjs.015015.

[5] Poma, E. M., Santos, C. L., López, B. G., Arbizu, E. A., Olascoaga, F. Z., Petrov, M. S., Morales, F. A., Garralda, M. A., Villarroya, M. C., Riera, J. S. I. & Camps, V. L. (2012). Clinical pathways for acute pancreatitis: Recommendations for early multidisciplinary management. *Medicina Intensiva (English Edition)*, 36: 351-357. doi: 10.1016/j.medine. 2012.02.008.

[6] Pendharkar, S. A. & Petrov, M. S. (2015). Bringing patient-centered care to the fore in diseases of the pancreas. *Gastroenterology Research and Practice*, 2015: 1-6. doi: 10.1155/2015/459214.

[7] Pendharkar, S. A., Plank, L. D., Windsor, J. A. & Petrov, M. S. (2016). Quality of life in a randomized trial of nasogastric tube feeding in acute pancreatitis. *Journal of Parenteral and Enteral Nutrition*, 40: 693-698. doi: 10.1177/0148607115574290.

[8] Pendharkar, S. A., Salt, K., Plank, L. D., Windsor, J. A. & Petrov, M. S. (2014). Quality of life after acute pancreatitis a systematic review and meta-analysis. *Pancreas*, 43: 1194-1200. doi: 10.1097/MPA.0000000 000000189.

[9] Babic, T. & Travagli, R. A. (2016). Neural control of the pancreas. *Pancreapedia Exocrine Pancreas Knowledge Base*. doi: 10.3998/panc.2016.27.

[10] Li, Q. & Peng, J. (2014). Sensory nerves and pancreatitis. *Gland Surgery*, 3: 284-292. doi: 10.3978/j.issn.2227-684X.2013.10.08.

[11] Bockman, D.E. (2007). Nerves in the pancreas: what are they for? *The American Journal of Surgery*, 194: 61-64. doi: 10.1016/j.amjsurg.2007.05.028.

[12] Schorn, S., Ceyhan, G. O., Tieftrunk, E., Friess, H. & Demir, I. E. (2015). Pain management in acute pancreatitis. *American Pancreatic Association*. doi: 10.3998/panc.2015.15.

[13] Basurto Ona, X., Rigau Comas, D. & Urrutia, G. (2013). Opioids for acute pancreatitis pain. *Cochrane Database of Systematic Reviews*, 7: 79. doi: 10.1002/14651858.CD009179.

[14] Harper, D. & McNaught, C. E. (2014). The role of thoracic epidural anesthesia in severe acute pancreatitis. *Critical Care*, 18: 1-2. doi: 10.1186/cc13718.

[15] Stigliano, S., Sternby, H., de Madaria, E., Capurso, G. & Petrov, M.S. (2017). Early management of acute pancreatitis: A review of the best evidence. *Digestive and Liver Disease*, 9: 585-594. doi: 10.1016/j.dld.2017.01.168.

In: Case Reports in Surgery
Editors: Ahmad Jabir Rahyussalim et al.
ISBN: 978-1-53616-582-1

Chapter 5

PREOPERATIVE THERAPEUTIC PLASMA EXCHANGE WITH HYPOFIBRINOGENEMIA COMPLICATION IN ABO-INCOMPATIBLE LIVING DONOR KIDNEY TRANSPLANTATION

Dita Aditianingsih[1,*], Rudyanto Soedono[1], Endang Susalit[2], Willy Yant Kartolo[1], and Erika Sasha Adiwongso[1]

[1]Department of Anesthesiology and Intensive Care,
Faculty of Medicine, Universitas Indonesia, Jakarta, Indonesia
[2]Department of Internal Medicine,
Division of Nephrology and Hypertension, Faculty of Medicine,
Universitas Indonesia, Jakarta, Indonesia

ABSTRACT

ABO-incompatible kidney transplantation (ABOi-KT) is a strategy to overcome the shortage of organ donors. It is considered a high-risk option because of potential antibody-mediated rejection (AMR); however, it results in improved outcomes because of the use of more potent immunosuppressants in combination with splenectomy and therapeutic plasma exchange (TPE). We reported a case of a 54-year-old male O-blood type recipient who received an A-blood type living donor kidney. The desensitization protocol consisted of a combination of three sessions of TPE with immunosuppressants administered prior to transplantation. The anti-A antibody IgM-IgG titers could be reduced and maintained at a range of 1:32–1:4. Additionally, the fibrinogen level was 245 mg/dl prior to transplantation without any fresh frozen plasma (FFP) replacement. There was massive postoperative bleeding due to the low fibrinogen level. The patient received cryoprecipitates and

* Corresponding Author's E-mail: ditaaditiaa@gmail.com.

intravenous tranexamic acid. The bleeding gradually stopped, and the graft function was good. The patient was discharged from the hospital on day-7 post-transplantation. Preoperative TPE was the primary therapy for ABOi-KT in this patient. Only three sessions were performed, but it caused hypofibrinogenemia and postoperative bleeding. Coagulation factor monitoring and blood component therapy were essential to prevent these complications.

Keywords: ABO-incompatibility, kidney donor, therapeutic plasma exchange, hypofibrinogenemia

INTRODUCTION

Kidney transplantation is the treatment of choice for patients with end-stage renal disease (ESRD); however, there is currently a long waiting list for organ donors. Blood type-incompatible transplantation is one of the alternatives to overcome the shortage of organ donors [1]. ABO-incompatible kidney transplantation (ABOi-KT) is considered a high-risk option because of antibody-mediated rejection (AMR) and declining graft survival. Desensitization protocols for ABOi-KT are designed to improve this outcome. These protocols consist of splenectomy and a combination of immunosuppressants, such as high-dose intravenous immunoglobulin, anti-CD20 monoclonal antibody agents, and therapeutic plasma exchange (TPE) [2]. A splenectomy is performed to remove the major B-cell reservoir and prevent AMR; however, its effect on the immune system is irreversible, and it has a higher risk of infections. In 2004, rituximab, the anti-CD20 monoclonal antibody, was introduced and gradually replaced splenectomy. Rituximab binds to CD20 and produces along-acting B-cell suppression effect by inducing complement cytotoxicity, antibody cytotoxicity, and apoptosis on immature and mature B-cells, except for memory B-cells and plasma cells [3]. Preoperative antibody removal is achieved by plasma exchange or plasmapheresis as a part of desensitization for ABOi-KT. TPE removes high-molecular-weight antibodies from the plasma by using an automated blood cell separator to filter the plasma and separate the immunoglobulins to be discarded. TPE can remove 60%–70% of antibodies per session and is more efficient than classic plasmapheresis, which separates immunoglobulins by centrifugation and removes only 40%–50% of antibodies per session. This method requires a femoral, subclavian, or internal jugular double-lumen catheter insertion to ensure adequate blood flow during the procedure. TPE can be performed prior to or post operation, or both. Most cases require three to seven sessions, depending on the initial or elevated antibody titers post transplantation. Each session removes 1–1.5 times the plasma volume (calculated based on hematocrit and predicted body weight), which is replaced by 5% albumin, fresh frozen plasma (FFP), or both. Albumin is a preferable replacement fluid because it has a lower risk of hypersensitivity and infection transmission compared with FFP. However, TPE has a higher risk of bleeding due to the removal of coagulation factors; therefore, FFP is usually reserved to correct coagulation factor and bleeding complications [4].

CASE REPORT

A 54-year-old male was scheduled to undergo a living donor kidney transplant. His blood type was O rhesus +, and the donor blood type was A rhesus +. The recipient had hypertension since 2008. He was diagnosed with end-stage chronic kidney disease in 2015 and underwent hemodialysis for four months prior to transplantation. A physical examination revealed a good general appearance, with a body mass index (BMI) of 24.9 kg/m2 and grade I hypertension (BP 140 – 150/70 – 80 mmHg), which was treated with amlodipine 1 × 10 mg, clonidine 4 × 0.15 mg, bisoprolol 1 × 5 mg, and valsartan 1 × 160 mg. The donor-recipient complement-dependent cytotoxicity crossmatching result showed 10% – 20% lysis (negative result). A desensitization protocol was initiated eight days prior to transplantation. The protocol consisted of immunosuppressants (tacrolimus 10 mg/day PO, rituximab 500 mg/m2 IV, mycophenolate mofetil 1,000 mg/day PO, and methylprednisolone 24 mg PO), and TPE was performed with the Prismaflex system (Gambro, Sweden), only three times every other day, five days prior to transplantation. The hemoglobin level of the patient was 6.1 g/dl, and he received a transfusion of leucodepleted packed red cells (PRCs) before the first TPE was conducted. One and a half times the plasma volume was removed, and 5% albumin with anticoagulant heparin was used as the replacement in every session. A timeline of the protocol is explained in Figure 1.

INVESTIGATIONS

The initial anti-A antibody IgM-IgG titers were 1:256 – 1:4, which were reduced to 1:64 – 1:4 and 1:32 – 1:4 in response to three sessions of TPE. The prothrombin time (PT), activated prothrombin time (APTT), and fibrinogen levels were within normal limits without any replacement of fresh frozen plasma (FFP) or cryoprecipitate during the TPE sessions prior to surgery. Basiliximab (20 mg) was administered in the morning prior to transplantation. The transplantation procedure took 3 hours and 45 minutes to complete, with a primary warm ischemic time of 2 minutes and 27 seconds, a cold ischemic time of 23 minutes and 12 seconds, and a secondary warm ischemic time of 30 minutes and 24 seconds. The recipient's urine was produced on the 40th minute after reperfusion. During the surgical procedure, the patient received 1,250 cc of IV solution; conversely, the total output was 850 cc, with 250 cc coming from blood loss during the procedure and 600 cc from urine output. The patient had significant bleeding from the wound and 450 cc drainage production of serous hemorrhage within one hour postoperatively. The hemoglobin level decreased to 6.1 gr/dl, and the fibrinogen level was low (30.2 mg/dl). The graph of antibody titers, creatinine level and fibrinogen level dynamics before, during and after TPE, and after transplantation procedure was explained in Figure 2.

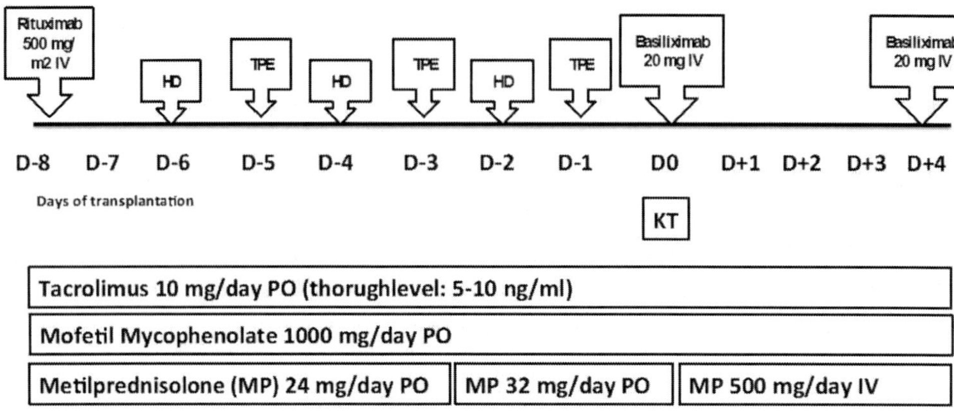

Figure 1. The ABOi-KT desensitization protocol used for this patient. TPE, therapeutic plasma exchange; HD, hemodialysis; KT, kidney transplantation.

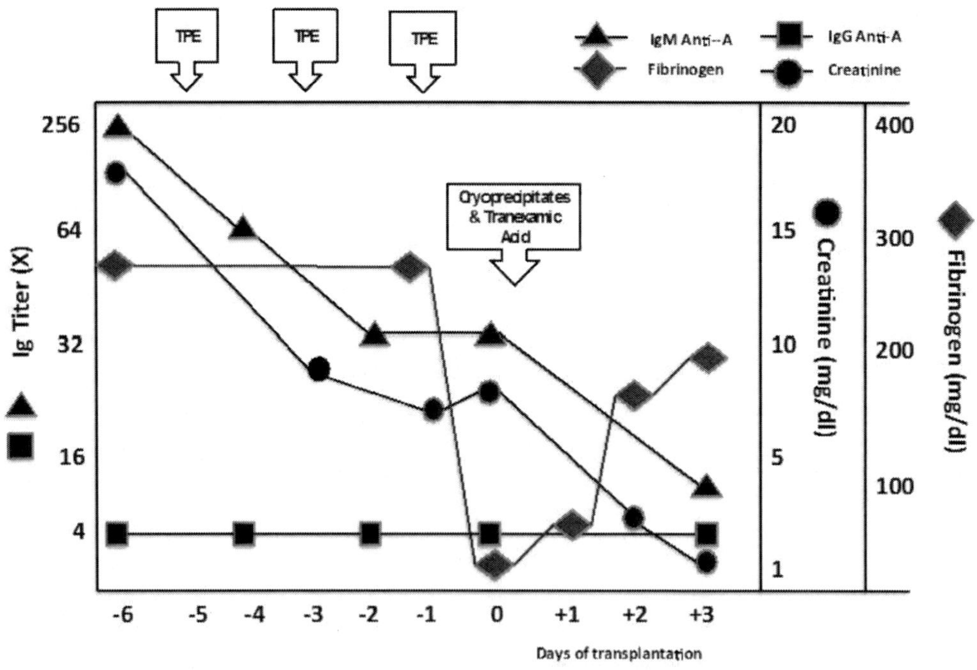

Figure 2. ABO-IgM-IgG antibody titers, creatinine level, and fibrinogen level before and after TPE, during TPE, and after transplantation. TPE, therapeutic plasma exchange; IgM-G, immunoglobulin M-G.

TREATMENT

The patient had significant bleeding from the wound and a drainage production of 450 cc serous hemorrhage within one hour post transplantation. His hemoglobin level decreased to 6.1 gr/dl, and his fibrinogen level was low (30.2 mg/dl). Therefore, 500 ml of leucodepleted PRCs and 10 units of cryoprecipitate were administered along with tranexamic acid, which was given as a1 gram bolus followed by the infusion of 3 grams over 24-hour. The total blood loss after the operation was approximately 840 ml in 17 hours, and drainage production decreased over the next 24 hours. His fibrinogen level increased to 190 mg/dl, and his hemoglobin level was 7.3 gr/dl. The general condition of the patient was stable.

OUTCOME AND FOLLOW-UP

The patient was followed up for seven days post transplantation, and the general condition of the patient was stable. His fibrinogen level increased to 173 mg/dl on postoperation day-1 and to 190 mg/dl on postoperation day-2. His urine output was greater than 1 ml/kgBW/h with serum creatinine level and estimated glomerular rate (eGFR) showed improvement postoperatively. There was no sign of rejection or transfusion-related complications, and the patient was discharged from the hospital on the 8th day post-transplantation.

DISCUSSION

The principle of the immunosuppressive strategy in ABOi-KT is a desensitization strategy that consists of antibody removal or depletion, induction, and maintenance of immunosuppression agents. Alexandre et al. successfully attenuated the immunologic reaction and prevented hyperacute rejection by initiating a desensitization protocol that involves preoperative splenectomy and plasmapheresis. However, since 2004, splenectomy has rarely been performed because of the elimination effect on the immune system and the increased risk of infection [5]. Rituximab has become an alternative to splenectomy because it reduces B-cell production and attenuates the T-cell response within 1 to 3 days after induction; these responses persist for up to two years [6]. TPE is performed prior to transplantation to maintain the anti-A antibody titer between 1:4 and 1:32 in the beginning of transplantation. Several studies have shown that if the titer is less than 1:32, AMR is unlikely to occur [7]. Two studies also reported that the level of anti-ABO IgG antibodies was a more significant independent risk factor of AMR than IgM [8, 9]. After receiving only three sessions of TPE prior to the operation, this patient reached the following preoperative levels: IgM anti-A 1:32 and IgG anti-A 1:4. Since the prognostic value of the baseline anti-ABO titer is not yet established, it was considered safe to proceed with the transplantation for this patient.

TPE with one plasma volume can remove 40% – 50% of the antibodies per session because of the movement of extravascular constituents to the intravascular compartment and the resynthesizing of antibodies [10]. We performed TPE with 1.5 plasma volumes to increase the efficiency of antibody removal per session, which is calculated by the following formula:

$$(100 - \text{Hematocrit})\% \times (\text{KgBW} \times 70) \times 1.5 \text{ ml}$$

TPE removes anti-ABO antibodies along with plasma proteins, such as albumin, coagulation factors, and important immunoglobulins. It is replaced by 5% albumin solution or ABO group FFP during the sessions. Albumin is preferred to FFP because it has a lower risk of infection, hypersensitivity reaction, and reduced risk of ABO-related rejection. However, TPE increases the risk of bleeding, particularly during and after operation because of depleted coagulation factors other than antibodies. We replaced the 1.5 plasma volumes with only 5% albumin in each TPE session. PT, APTT, and fibrinogen levels were measured after each TPE session. FFP or cryoprecipitate were not used during TPE because the PT and APTT results were normal and the fibrinogen level was always above 100 mg/dl until two days prior to the operation. The patient suffered from bleeding complications after the operation. The fibrinogen level was very low, whereas the PT and APTT levels were still within normal limits. After administering 10 units of cryoprecipitate and tranexamic acid infusions, the bleeding gradually stopped, and the fibrinogen level increased. We closely monitored the bleeding events for 72 hours since the effects of hypofibrinogenemia may persist for up to three days, although the fibrinogen biosynthesis rate may increase two- to four-fold per day during the acute phase. TPE may reduce fibrinogen levels by 64% – 80% depending on the individual's condition and extensive rate of TPE. Immunoadsorption is another technique that selectively removes immunoglobulins from separated plasma through high-affinity absorbers and only reduces the fibrinogen level by 20% – 35%. However, our center had no experience using this technique. The incidence of bleeding after the TPE was relatively low (0.06% – 2.3%). Hypofibrinogenemia contributes to bleeding complications in patients using anticoagulants who undergo invasive procedures or surgery [11].

Using FFP in addition to 5% albumin as a replacement during TPE can decrease the reduction in fibrinogen levels. However, the prevention of hypofibrinogenemia by FFP administration during TPE is currently not recommended. The FFP replacement is reserved for patients who are already hemostatically compromised or have a high risk of bleeding. This is because of the risk of adverse events, such as hypersensitivity reaction, transfusion-related circulatory overload, and transfusion-related acute lung injury. Cryoprecipitate has similar disadvantages of FFP, but it contains higher concentrations of fibrinogen, factor VIII, and von Willebrand factor with a lower infusion volume. We administered cryoprecipitate combined with a tranexamic acid infusion when the patient presented with significant bleeding and low fibrinogen levels (below 100 mg/dl). Cryoprecipitate and tranexamic acid administration can improve fibrin formation and platelet aggregation. This present combination prevents massive transfusions and is associated with an improved survival rate in trauma-related bleeding [11-13].

Conclusion

TPE reduces the fibrinogen level, and FFP or cryoprecipitate may be administered when there is significant bleeding along with low fibrinogen levels or prolonged APTT to reduce the antibody-related risk of transfusion. Pre- and post-TPE fibrinogen levels should be closely monitored in patients who undergo invasive procedures due to the potentially tremendous decrease in fibrinogen levels, which contributes to bleeding complications. In the present patient, the combination of cryoprecipitate transfusion and tranexamic acid administration replenished the fibrinogen level and overcame the bleeding complications with an acceptable amount of blood products.

References

[1] Wolfe, R. A., Ashby, V. B., Milford, E. L., Ojo, A. O., Ettenger, R. E., Agodoa, L. Y., Held, P. J. and Port, F. K. (1999). Comparison of mortality in all patients on dialysis, patients on dialysis awaiting transplantation, and recipients of a first cadaveric transplant. *N Engl J Med*, 341: 1725–1730.

[2] Lipshutz, G. S., McGuire, S., Zhu, Q., Zimman, A., Davis, R., Goldfinger, D., Reed, E. F., Wilkinson, A. H., Danovitch, G. M. and Pham, P. T. (2011). ABO-blood type-incompatible kidney transplantation and access to organs. *Arch Surg*, 146: 453–458.

[3] Clatworthy, M. R. (2011). Targeting B-cells and antibody intransplantation. *Am J Transplant*, 11: 1359–1367.

[4] Tobian, A. A., Shirey, R. S., Montgomery, R. A., Tisch, D. J., Ness, P. M. and King, K. E. (2009). Therapeutic plasma exchange reduces ABO titers to permit ABO-incompatible renal transplantation. *Transfusion*, 49: 1248–1254.

[5] Alexandre, G. P., Squifflet, J. P., DeBruyere, M., Latinne, D., Reding, R., Gianello, P., Carlier, M. and Pirson, Y. (1987). Present experiences in a series of 26 ABO-incompatible living donor renal allografts. *Transplant Proc*, 19: 4538–4542.

[6] Clatworthy, M. R. (2011). Targeting B cells and antibody in transplantation. *Am J Transplant*, 11: 1359–1367.

[7] Tobian, A. A., Shirley, R. S., Montgomery, R. A., Cai, W., Haas, M., Ness, P. M. and King, K. E. (2010). ABO antibody titer and risk of antibody-mediated rejection in ABO-incompatible renal transplantation. *Am J Transplant*, 10: 1247–1253.

[8] Gloor, J. M., Lager, D. J., Fidler, M. E., Grande, J. P., Moore, S. B., Winters, J. L., Kremers, W. K. and Stegall, M. D. (2005). A Comparison of splenectomy versus intensive posttransplant antidonor blood group antibody monitoring without splenectomy in ABO-incompatible kidney transplantation. *Transplantation*, 80: 1572–1577.

[9] Toki, D., Ishida, H., Setoguchi, K., Shimizu, T., Omoto, K., Shirakawa, H., Iida, S., Horita, S., Furusawa, M., Ishizuka, T., Yamaguchi, Y. and Tanabe, K. (2009). Acute antibody-mediated rejection in living ABO-incompatible kidney transplantation: Long-term impact and risk factors. *Am J Transplant*, 9: 567–577.

[10] Winters, J. L., Gloor, J. M., Pineda, A. A., Stegall, M. D. and Moore, S. B. (2004). Plasma exchange conditioning for ABO-incompatible renal transplantation. *J Clin Apher*, 19: 79–85.

[11] Zöllner, S., Pablik, E., Druml, W., Derfler, K., Rees, A. and Biesenbach, P. (2014). Fibrinogen reduction and bleeding complications in plasma exchange, immunoadsoprtion and a combination of the two. *Blood Purif*, 38: 160–166.

[12] Morrison, J. J., Dubose, J. J., Rasmussen, T. E. and Midwinterm, M. J. (2012). Military application of tranexamic acid in trauma emergency resuscitation (MATTERS) study. *Arch Surg*, 147: 113–119.

[13] Shakur, H., Roberts, I., Bautista, R., Caballero, J., Coats, T., Dewan, Y., El-Sayed, H., Gogichaishvili, T., Gupta, S., Herrera, J., Hunt, B., Iribhogbe, P., Izurieta, M., Khamis, H., Komolafe, E., Marrero, M. A., Mejia-Mantilla, J., Miranda, J., Morales, C., Olaomi, O., Olldashi, F., Perel, P., Peto, R., Ramana, P. V., Ravi, R. R. and Yutthakasemsunt, S. (2010). Effects of tranexamic acid on death, vascular occlusive events, and blood transfusion in trauma patients with significant haemorrhage (CRASH-2): A randomised, placebo-controlled trial. *Lancet*, 376: 23–32.

In: Case Reports in Surgery
Editors: Ahmad Jabir Rahyussalim et al.
ISBN: 978-1-53616-582-1

Chapter 6

SYMMETRICAL BILATERAL KEYSTONE PERFORATOR ISLAND FLAPS FOR VULVAR RECONSTRUCTION AFTER ONCOLOGICAL RESECTION: A CASE REPORT

Indri Aulia*[*]*, Chaula Luthfia Sukasah and Eva Chintia Yessica

External Genitalia Section, Plastic Reconstructive and Aesthetic Surgery Division, Department of Surgery, Universitas Indonesia, Dr. Cipto Mangunkusumo Hospital, Jakarta, Indonesia

ABSTRACT

The vulvoperineal region is key to the urinary and reproductive systems and closely related to the gastrointestinal system. Most vulvar defects are resulted from tumor ablation. Therefore, the reconstruction after oncological resection remains challenging as it aims to restore adequate function with an ideal aesthetic result. We report a case of a 46-year-old female with extramammary Paget's disease of the vulva. She underwent oncological excision for vulvar reconstruction. Keystone perforator island flaps were performed in this patient and it demonstrated a symmetrical bilateral result of vulva subunits. The patient was satisfied with the vulva appearance and no limitations in daily activities was reported. The use of keystone perforator island flaps is a superior option for vulva reconstruction to achieve a symmetrical outcome.

[*] Corresponding Author's E-mail: drindriaulia@gmail.com.

Keywords: Keystone flap, vulvar reconstruction, oncological resection

INTRODUCTION

The vulvoperineal region is key to the urinary, reproductive, and gastrointestinal systems. Most vulvar defects are caused by oncological rescetion [1]. However, the extent of surgery varies from limited resection of pre-cancerous lesions to more extensive, bilateral radical vulvectomy for advanced cancer.

The reconstruction of vulvar defects after oncological resection remains challenging due to the high risk of postoperative infection because the area is easily contaminated and damp [2-4]. Poor wound healing and dehiscence might be also resulted from tension and traction upon movement of the affected region [5, 6]. Therefore, the reconstruction target is to restore adequate function and an ideal aesthetic appearance with minimal postoperative complications.

Various techniques have been developed for the reconstruction of vulvar defects, including the use of pedicled flaps [7-11]. However, this procedure might result in bulky flaps and asymmetrical coverage and could be insufficient for achieving appropriate aesthetic and functional results [12].

CASE

Patients with malignancy, especially vulvar malignancy, are treated with interdisciplinary management. In June 2017, a 46-year-old woman was diagnosed with extramammary Paget's disease of the vulva at the Gynecology Department of Dr. Cipto Mangungkusumo Hospital (Jakarta, Indonesia) and underwent an excision procedure conducted by an oncogynecologist. She was consulted to the Department of Plastic Surgery for further reconstruction of the vulva, which was performed using two keystone perforator island flaps from the lateral sides of the defect.

DISCUSSION

Extramammary Paget's disease is an uncommon skin cancer involving genital, anal and perineum area [13]. It initially manifests as rash, scales and crusts that progresses into a wider and more severe lesion. Thus, a reconstructive surgery is necessary following excision of the primary lesion. In this case, we decided to perform keystone perforator island flaps to close the defect.

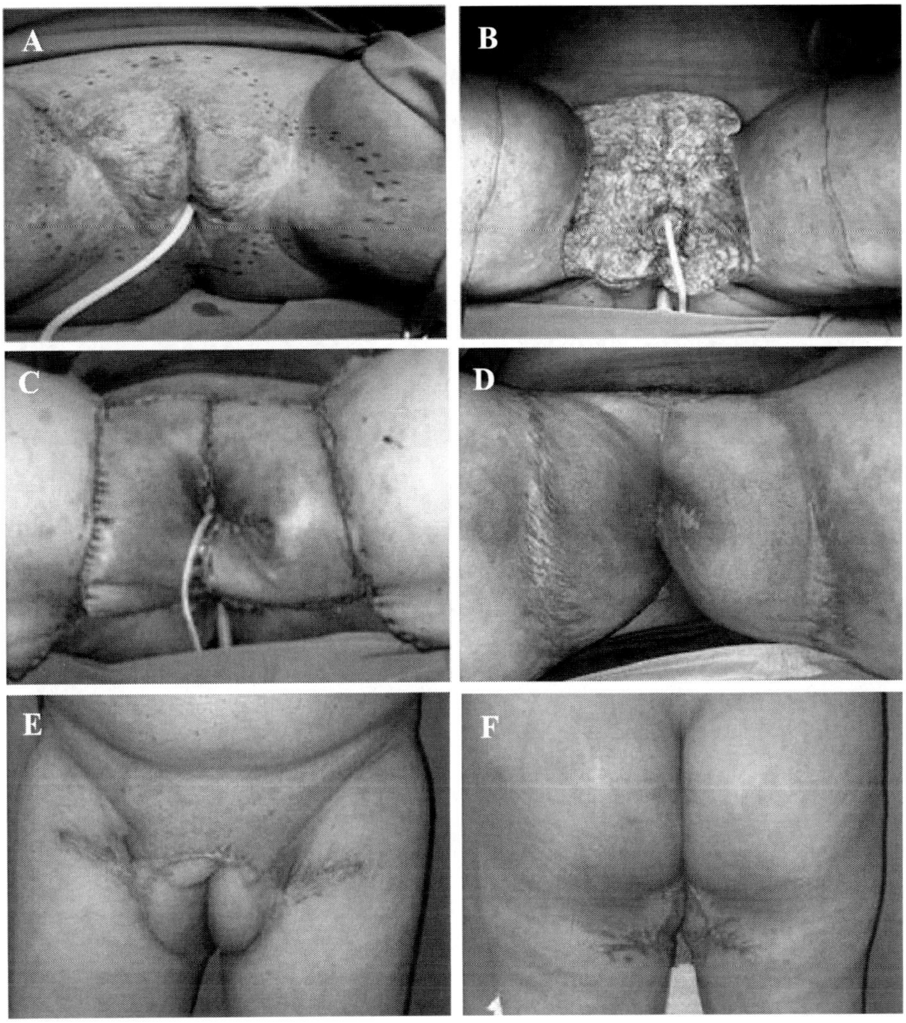

Figure 1. A: Vulvar defects of the patient with extramammary Paget's disease. B: Design of keystone perforator island flap. C: Immediate postoperative appearance. D–F: appearance of the flap 9 months after reconstruction.

The keystone perforator island flaps survived in the patient with no complications of wound dehiscence or postoperative infection. In addition, there was no evidence of recurrence during nine months after the surgery. The vulvar region appeared to be symmetrical. Subjectively, the patient was satisfied with the appearance of the reconstructed vulva and had no complaints with urination, sexual activity, or daily activities. However, after the 9-month follow-up, the patient requested a minor revision to flatten the inferior part of the flap, which was slightly bulky. As with the first reconstruction, there were no complications with the revision procedure.

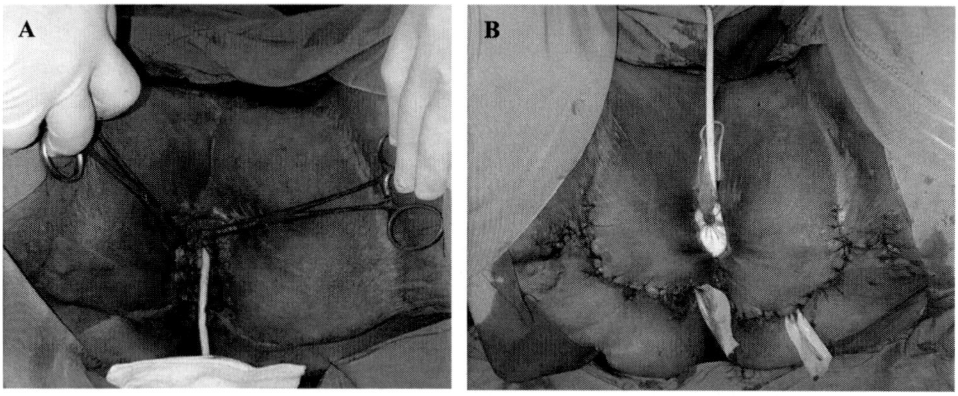

Figure 2. A: Keystone perforator island flap at 9 months after surgery. B: Appearance after revision surgery.

The use of keystone perforator island flaps resulted in symmetrical bilateral outcomes of the vulvar subunits. A 1:1 defect and flap ratio was applied to accurately place the midline. The initial incision and the final sutured lines were placed at the borders of the subunits to create a disguising scar.

Conclusion

Based on our experience, we found that keystone perforator island flaps has a lot of advantages for patients with vulvar defects. It has a simple design, symmetrical vulvar subunits results and it is applicable for defects in any part of the vulva. The appearance of the normal vulva is obtained by resurfacing the defect with tissue alike and applying it tightly as a young women's vulva. Minor revision is an additional procedure based on subjective desires in providing the daily needs and self-confidence. In conclusion, we believe that the use of keystone perforator island flaps is a good alternative for achieving functional and ideal aesthetic results of vulvar reconstruction.

References

[1] Hockel, M; Dornhofer, N. Vulvovaginal reconstruction for neoplastic disease. *Lancet Oncol.*, 2008, 9, 559-568.

[2] Hashimoto, I; Abe, Y; Nakanishi, H. The internal pudendal artery perforator flap: free-style pedicle perforator flaps for vulva, vagina, and buttock reconstruction. *Plast. Reconstr. Surg.*, 2014, 133, 924-933.

[3] Mericli, AF; Martin, JP; Campbell, CA. An algorithmic anatomical subunit approach to pelvic wound reconstruction. *Plast. Reconstr. Surg.*, 2016, 137, 1004–1017.

[4] McAllister, E; Wells, K; Chaet, M; Norman, J; Cruse, W. Perineal reconstruction after surgical extirpation of pelvic malignancies using the transpelvic transverse rectus abdominal myocutaneous flap. *Ann. Surg. Oncol.*, 1994, 1, 164–168.

[5] Tan, B; Kang, GC; Tay, EH; Por, YC. Subunit principle of vulvar reconstruction: algorithm and outcomes. *Arch. Plast. Surg.*, 2014, 41, 379-386.

[6] Huang, J; Chang, N; Chou, H; Wu, C; Abdelrahman, M; Chen, HY; Cheng, MH. Pedicle perforator flaps for vulvar reconstruction — new generation of less invasive vulvar reconstruction with favorable results. *Gynecol. Oncol.*, 2015, 137, 66-72.

[7] Elken, JA; Aldeek, NF; Hsu, CC; Chang, NJ; Lin, CH. Algorithmic approach to lower abdominal, perineal, and groin reconstruction using anterolateral thigh flaps. *Microsurgery*, 2016, 36, 104-14.

[8] Negosanti, L; Sgarzani, R; Fabbri, E; Palo, S; Oranges, CM; De Iaco, P; et al. Vulvar reconstruction by perforator flaps: algorithm for flap choice based on the topography of the defect. *Int. J. Gynecol. Cancer*, 2015, 25, 1322-7.

[9] Carramaschi, F; Ramos, ML; Nisida, AC; Ferreira, MC; Pinotti, JA.V-Y flap for perineal reconstruction following modified approach to vulvectomy in vulvar cancer.*Int. J. Gynaecol. Obstet.,* 1999, 65, 157-63.

[10] Salgarello, M; Farallo, E; Barone-Adesi, L; Cervelli, D; Scambia, G; Salerno, G; et al. Flap algorithm in vulvar reconstruction after radical, extensive vulvectomy. *Ann. Plast. Surg.*, 2005, 54, 184-90.

[11] John, HE; Jessop, ZM; Di Candia, M; Simcock, J; Durrani, AJ; Malata, CM. An algorithmic approach to perineal reconstruction after cancer resection: experience from two international centers. *Ann. Plast. Surg.,* 2013, 71, 96–102.

[12] Wallace, CG; Kao, HK; Jeng, SF; Wei, FC. Free-style flaps: a further step forward for perforator flap surgery.*Plast. Reconstr. Surg.*, 2009, 124, 19-26.

[13] Parashurama, R; Nama, V; Hutson, R. Paget's disease of the vulva: a review of 20 years experience. *Int. J. Gynecol. Cancer*, 2017, 27, 791-793.

SECTION 2. OTORHINOLARYNGOROLOGY - HEAD AND NECK

In: Case Reports in Surgery
Editors: Ahmad Jabir Rahyussalim et al.
ISBN: 978-1-53616-582-1

Chapter 7

RECONSTRUCTION OF AURICLE AFTER WIDE EXCISION OF GIANT MULTIPLE CONGENITAL MELANOCYTIC NEVUS OF THE EAR: A RARE CASE REPORT

Dini Widiarni Widodo*[*] *and Ferucha Moulanda
Department of Otorhinolaryngology Head and Neck, Faculty of Medicine,
Universitas Indonesia - CiptoMangunkusumo General Hospital, Jakarta, Indonesia

ABSTRACT

Congenital melanocytic nevus (CMN) is a benign proliferation of melanocytes that appears at birth or within weeks of life. The condition occurs in 1% – 2% of newborns, with a 2% – 42% and 6% – 14% risk of transforming into malignancy or developing into multiple myeloma. The occurrence of CMN involving the auricular area is uncommon. Although excision of the nevus is the treatment of choice, this procedure is challenging. A wide area of CMN requires extensive excision coupled with a reconstructive procedure. In this article, we present a case of giant CMN in a 6-year-old female with giant pigmented nevi appearing after birth in all parts of her body, particularly the right facial, auricular, post auricular, mastoid, and neck areas. The diagnosis was reached based on the results of a biopsy revealing the presence of melanocytic nevus. Wide excision of the nevus at the right auricular with cartilage exposure was performed and a split-thickness skin graft was used for the reconstruction of the auricle. Postoperative follow-up showed a good outcome.

---

[*] Corresponding Author's E-mail: dini_pancho@yahoo.com.

Keywords: auricular reconstruction, congenital melanocytic nevus, melanocyte, split-thickness skin grafts

Introduction

Congenital melanocytic nevus (CMN) is a benign proliferation of nevus cells (melanocytes) located in the epidermis, dermis, and other tissues. It may cause mutation of genes NRAS Q61 and BRAF V600E, andvaries in severity from mild to life-threatening [1-3, 6]. According to Kopf, giant CMN (GCMN) is defined as nevi that will reach a diameter >20 cm in adult life. In addition, the presence and number of accompanying smaller (satellite) nevi should be recorded and classified into: 1) no lesion; 2) 1–20 lesions; 3) > 20 – 50 lesions; and 4) > 50 lesions. GCMN occurs in 1 per 500,000 births, and is associated with a 2% – 42% and 6% – 14% risk of transforming into a malignancy or developing into multiple myeloma, respectively. The available therapeutic modalities for GCMN include surgery and non-surgical, psychological, and/or clinical intervention with particular attention to discoloration, texture, or the surface of lesions [1, 4, 7-10].

GCMN occurring in the auricular area is considered rare. Moreover, reconstruction following large auricular skin defects frequently poses a surgical challenge. Esthetic concerns include symmetrical projection and maintenance of the shell-like shape. Postoperative complications may include contracture interfering with function, seroma, hematoma, infection, dehiscence, and keloid. Full-thickness skin grafts (FTSGs) and split-thickness skin grafts (STSGs) are alternative options for the coverage of large wounds, offering good functional and cosmetic results. Overall patient satisfaction with regards to the esthetic outcome is high (mean, 9.8). In addition, the rating provided by the surgeons is consistent with patient satisfaction [1, 4, 13].

Case Report

A 6-year-old female was admitted to the CiptoMangunkusumo General Hospital following the appearance of black moles throughout the body especially in the ear, behind the ears, neck and right side of the face from birth. The mole grew larger with the advancing age, and the surface of the mole became thicker, hairy, and blackish in the areas of the face, ears and neck. A biopsy conducted by a dermatologist revealed the presence of melanocyticnevus. Hyperpigmentation appeared in the right auricle, preauricular and post auricula, mastoidarea and neck with size > 40 cm, rough surface, and hypertrichosis without tenderness (Figure 1). There were >50 satellite lesions throughout the body. The ear canal, tympanic membrane, and audiometric examinations were normal.

The patient was diagnosed with GCMN. We performed wide excision of the nevus at the right auricular area until the mastoid area, followed by reconstruction using STSGs from the thigh area placed in the preauricular, auricular, post auricular, and mastoid areas to the right area of the coli (Figure 2). Postoperatively, the patient was hospitalized for 5 dayswith daily skincare and administration of antibiotics, and educated regarding wound care.

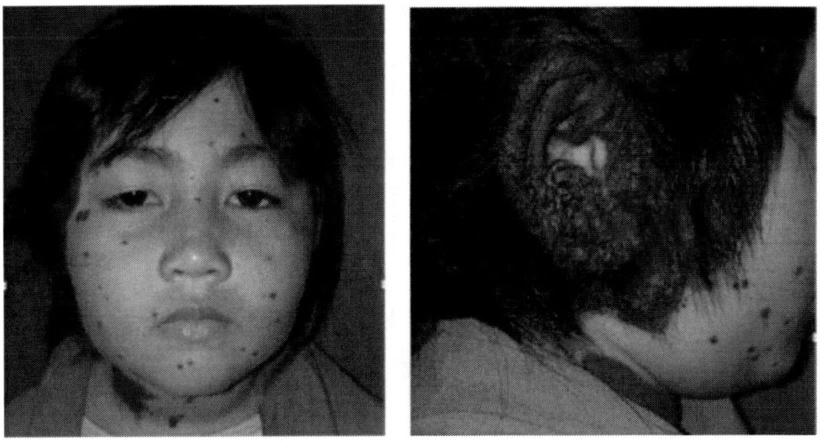

Figure 1. The patient with GCMN. Appearance of satellite nevi on patient's face and neck (left picture) and appearance of GCMN on right auricle, right side of the face and behind the right ear (right picture).

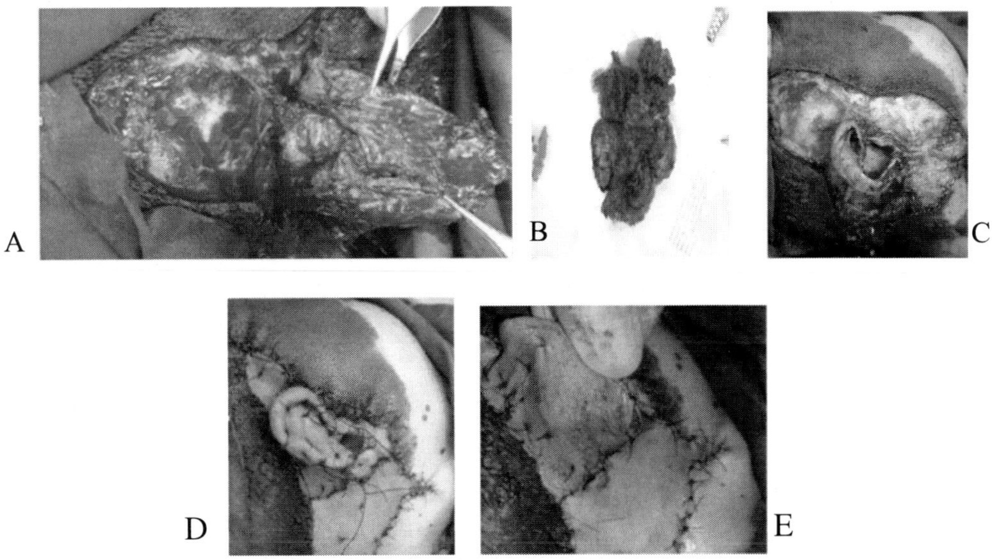

Figure 2. Wide ecision and reconstruction with STSGs. Wide excision procedure of right GCMN (right auricular until mastoid area) with preservation of auricle cartilage (Picture A, B and C). Reconstruction of defect with suturing of STSG (Picture D and E).

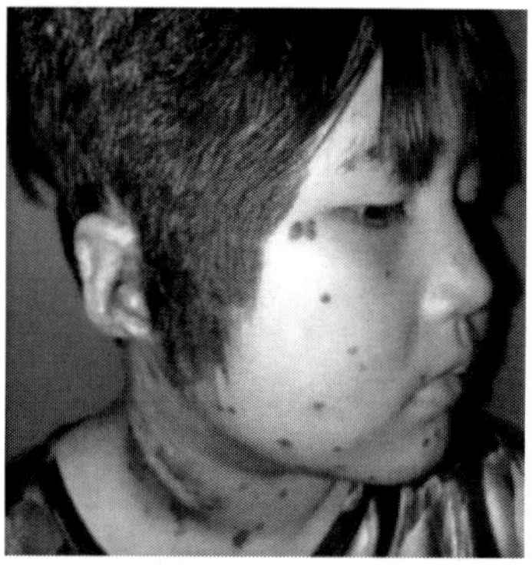

Figure 3. The patient after surgery.

Follow-up was performed in out patient clinic 10 days postoperatively. The tie-over of the graft was removed, the condition of the graft appeared good, and there was no seepage of blood or active bleeding. The stitches were partially removed on day 14. A wet area was observed at the preauricular and neck areas, and treated with amnion.

Follow-up performed 45 days after surgery showed that the wound was dry and the appearance of the epithelium was good (Figure 3). The stitches in the auricular area were the parts removed last to maintain the shape of the cartilage. The patient was subsequently referred to the Dermatology Department for potential laser treatment.

Discussion

GCMN of the ear is a very rare condition. Surgery is currently the treatment of choice for large-sized lesions. It is paramount to note the following in procedures for children: 1) donor skin, 2) grafting technique, 3) early postoperative care. The nevus must be cautiously excised to fully preserve the underlying perichondrium and avoid the presence of residual nevus. For larger nevi, the treatment plan divides the ear into esthetic units as follows: 1) concha, external auditory meatus, and ear canal; 2) antihelix, crura, and scapha; 3) helical rim; 4) lobule; 5) posterior auricular surface; 6) the region of non-hair-bearing skin above and posterior to the ear adjacent to the scalp; and 7) preauricular area (Figure 4) [1, 2, 12].

The reconstruction of large auricular skin defects frequently poses a surgical challenge. Esthetic concerns include symmetrical projection, maintenance of the shell-like shape of the helix, matching the skin color and textures, size discrepancies, presence and symmetry of the tragus as well as the contour of the antihelix, and the concha bowl. In the auricular region, options for the closure of defects typically include second intention healing, posing a risk of cartilage desiccation and webbing of the contoured surface of the ear [13].

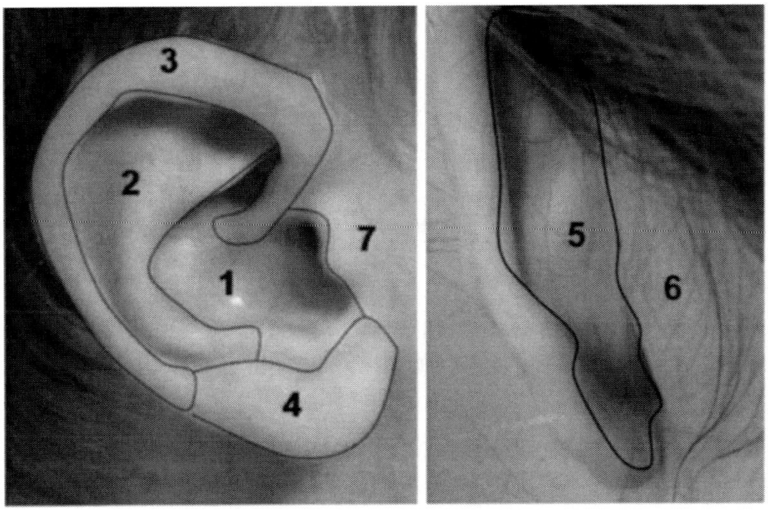

Figure 4. The esthetic units of the ear.

Tailor suturing in the area of auricular is challenging; therefore, it is recommended that the procedure is performed at a sufficiently advanced age (at least at 6 or 7 years of age), for the cartilage to be strong and capable of supporting the graft. The graft can also assist in the evaluation of the risk of recurrence and malignant alterations. FTSGs are an alternative to skin flaps for the auricular region; however, the thickness of FTSGs may be inappropriate for the thin skin of the ear. Failure of FTSGs has been reported in 14% – 30% of reconstruction cases. It has been suggested that STSGs allow rapid coverage of large wounds and offer excellent graft survival. The semitransparent characteristics of STSGs are ideal for covering the wound bed following the excision of an aggressive tumor, as they facilitate the detection of potential recurrence. Notably, thin STSGs match the thin skin of the cartilaginous ear better versus FTSGs, thus offering a distinct advantage [2, 13].

In this case, GCMN of right auricular was treated with wide excision exposing the cartilage, followed by reconstruction of the auricular area using STSGs. Evaluation performed 45 days after surgery showed good outcome.

CONCLUSION

GCMN is a very rare case and require surgical management. Reconstruction of auricle afterwide excision of GCMN is a challenging procedure regarding esthetic, anatomical structure with preservation of auricle cartilage. STSG is the main choice for auricle reconstruction in this case since it allows rapid and match coverage and facilitate detection of potential recurrence [1, 13].

REFERENCES

[1] Viana, A., Gontijo, B. & Bittencourt, F. (2012). Giant congenital melanocytic nevus. *Anais Brasileiros de Dermatologia*, *88*, 863-878.

[2] Adler, N., Margulis, A. & Bauer, B. (2009). Congenital pigmented nevi of the auricle: clinical experience and approach to treatment. *Plastic and Reconstruction Surgery*, *124*, 1932-1939.

[3] Gordon, R. (2013). Skin cancer: an overview of epidemiology and risk factors. *Seminars in Oncology Nursing*, *29*, 160-169.

[4] Salgado, C. M., Basu, D., Nikiforova, M., Bauer, B. S., Johnson, D., Rundell, V., Grunwaldt, L. J. & Reyes-Múgica, M. (2015). BRAF mutations are also associated with neurocutaneousmelanocytosis and large/giant congenital melanocytic nevi. *Pediatric and Developmental Pathology*, *18*, 1-9.

[5] Alikhan, A., Ibrahimi, O. & Eisen, D. (2012). Congenital melanocytic nevi: Where are we now? Part I: Clinical presentation, epidemiology, pathogenesis, histology, malignant transformation and neurocutaneos melanosis. *Journal of the American Academy of Dermatology*, *67*, 1-17.

[6] Scalvenzi, M., Palmisano, F., Cacciapuoti, S., Migliaro, F., Siano, M. & Staibano, S. (2013). Giant congenital melanocytic Naevus with proliferative nodules mimicking congenital malignant melanoma: a case report and review of the literature of congenital melanoma. *Case Reports in Dermatological Medicine*, *1*, 1-6

[7] Nguyen, T., Theos, A., Kelly, D., Busam, K. & Andea, A. (2013). Mitotically active proliferative nodule arising in a giant congenital melanocytic nevus: a diagnostic pitfall. *The American Journal of Dermatopathology*, *35*, 16-21.

[8] Krengeal, S. & Marghoob, A. (2012). Current management approaches for congenital melanocytic nevi. *Dermatologic Clinics*, *30*, 377-387.

[9] Yun, S., Kwon, O., Han, J., Kweon, S., Lee, M., Kim, M., et al. (2012). Clinical characteristic and risk of melanoma development from giant congenital melanocytic nevi in Korea: a nationwide retrospective study. *British Journal of Dermatology*, *166*, 115-123.

[10] Thuile, T., Larcher, L., Gatscher, B., Schwaiger, K., Deluca, J., Fallaha, A., Tappeiner, L., Puviani, M. & Eisendle, K. (2018). Split-thickness skin grafting for reconstruction of auricular skin defects: a statistical analysis. *Deutsche Dermatologische Gesellschaft*, *123*, 1-11.

[11] Depoortere, C., Francois, C., Belkhou, E., Duquennoy-Martinot, V. & Guerreschi, P. (2016). Features of skin graft in pediatric plastic surgery. *Annales de chirurgieplastiqueesthétique*, *7*, 1-10.

In: Case Reports in Surgery
Editors: Ahmad Jabir Rahyussalim et al.

ISBN: 978-1-53616-582-1

Chapter 8

DEVIATED NOSE IN A PATIENT WITH PARRY–ROMBERG SYNDROME: A CASE REPORT

Mirta Hediyati Reksodiputro[1,*], Dewi Puspito Sari[1], Iris Rengganis[2], Endi Novianto[3] and Dini W Widodo[1]

[1]Departement of Otorhinolaringology Head and Neck Surgery, Faculty of Medicine Universitas Indonesia Cipto Mangungkusumo General Hospital, Jakarta, Indonesia

[2]Departement of Internal Medicine, Faculty of Medicine Universitas Indonesia Cipto Mangungkusumo General Hospital, Jakarta, Indonesia

[3]Departement of Dermatology and Venereology, Faculty of Medicine Universitas Indonesia Cipto Mangungkusumo General Hospital, Jakarta, Indonesia

ABSTRACT

Parry–Romberg syndrome (PRS) is a rare degenerative disease characterized by unilateral, slow, and progressive atrophy of the facial tissue (including muscle, bones, and skin). Patients with this syndrome often develop a deviated nose. Such condition may lead to various aesthetic and functional issues. Septorhinoplasty plays a central role in the successful management of deviated nose. Here, we discuss the management of deviated nose in a patient with PRS along with evaluation of its characteristics, etiology, and pathophysiology. An 18-year/old female with deviated nose and the angle of her mouth toward the right side of the face underwent septorhinoplasty and labioplasty. Post surgery, functional and aesthetic improvements were observed in the deviated nose and facial asymmetry.

* Corresponding Author's E-mail: citamirta@yahoo.com.

Keywords: Parry–Romberg Syndrome, deviated nose, septorhinoplasty surgery

Introduction

Hemifacial atrophy or Parry–Romberg Syndrome (PRS) is a rare degenerative disease. It is characterized by slow and progressive unilateral atrophy of the facial tissues, including the skin, subcutaneous fat, muscle, cartilage, and bone. This condition was described for the first time by Parry and Romberg in 1846. The onset of disease occurs during the first decade of life. It slowly progresses for 2–10 years, reaching a stable phase between 18 and 21 years of age [1]. The extension of the atrophy is frequently limited to one side of the face. However, it may occasionally spread to the neck and one side of the body. Occasionally, ocular involvement, deviation of mouth and nose to the affected side as well as unilateral exposure of teeth is also noted. Moreover, patients may present with some neurological complications (e.g., trigeminal neuralgia, facial paresthesia, severe headache, and contralateral epilepsy). Identification of antinuclear antibodies in the serum suggests that the PRS is a kind of localized scleroderma.

Case Report

An 18-year-old girl presented to our hospital with complaints of facial asymmetry and deviation of the nose and angle of mouth to the right side of face. After the age of 7 years old, slow shrinking of the right side of the face was noted by her mother. No symptoms of neurological disturbances or systemic problems were identified. Family history was negative for similar complaints. Additionally, no incidences of trauma or infection were observed to coincide with or precede the onset of the deformity. Clinical examination revealed narrowed right nasal cavity, deviated septum, and eutrophy of the inferior concha. Nasal analysis showed deviation of the nasal axis to the right side ($< 150°$), deviated tip from the basal view, saddle nose below the rhinion axis, and a nasofacial angle of 30° (Figure 1). Rhinomanometry demonstrated higher resistance than normal during inspiration. Additionally, lower air flow in both the right and left nostril at 75 Pa (0.57 Pa/cm3/s and 90.42 Pa/cm3/s, respectively) was noted. The scores of nasal obstruction symptom evaluation and peak nasal inspiratory flowmetry (PNIF) were 35 and 90, respectively. The patient was evaluated by an ophthalmologist and a rheumatologist, and no abnormality was identified. Laboratory examination such as anti-nuclear antibody (ANA) titer in September 2015 was positive, whereas in February 2016, it was negative. Additionally, CRP and ESR were within normal limits. The patient did not receive any medical treatment for immunity disturbance.

In July 2016, the patient underwent septorhinoplasty and labioplasty (Figure 3). Three months after surgery, no nasal congestion was observed, and clinical examination showed a wide right nasal cavity, undeviated septum, and inferior concha eutrophy (Figure 4). An improvement in nasal analysis was observed, with increased angle of nasal axis (174°), no deviated nasal tip, and nasofacial angle post surgery of 40°. Rhinomanometry showed significant changes, with an increased nasal air flow and a lower resistance during inspiration in both the right and left nostrils at 75 Pa (0.41 Pa/cm3/s and 0.37 Pa/cm3/s, respectively) was noted. The scores of nasal obstruction symptom evaluation and PNIF were 10 and 120, respectively.

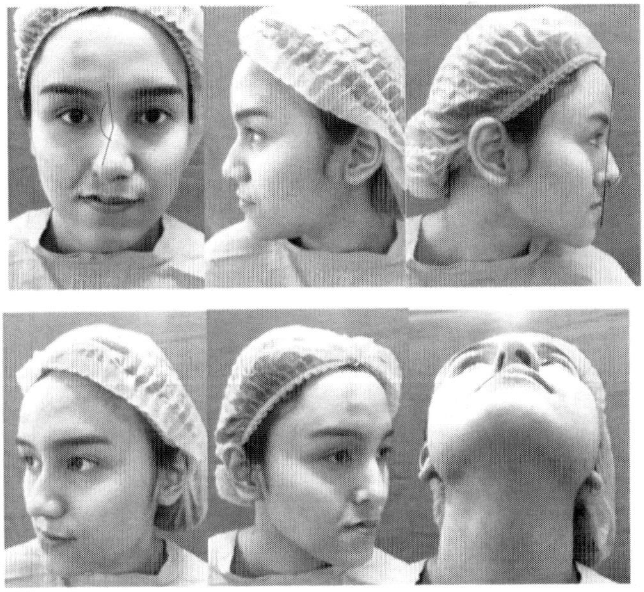

Figure 1. Pre-operative assessment. Nasal analysis showed a nasal axis deviated to the right from the frontal, lateral, and basal view.

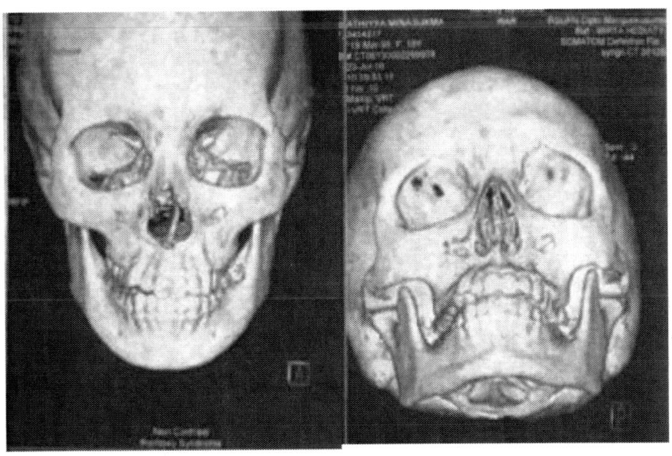

Figure 2. Three-dimensional CT Scan. CT Scan showed no abnormality in the hard tissue, and slight thinning of the soft tissue on the right side of the face, starting from the forehead and buccal cavity.

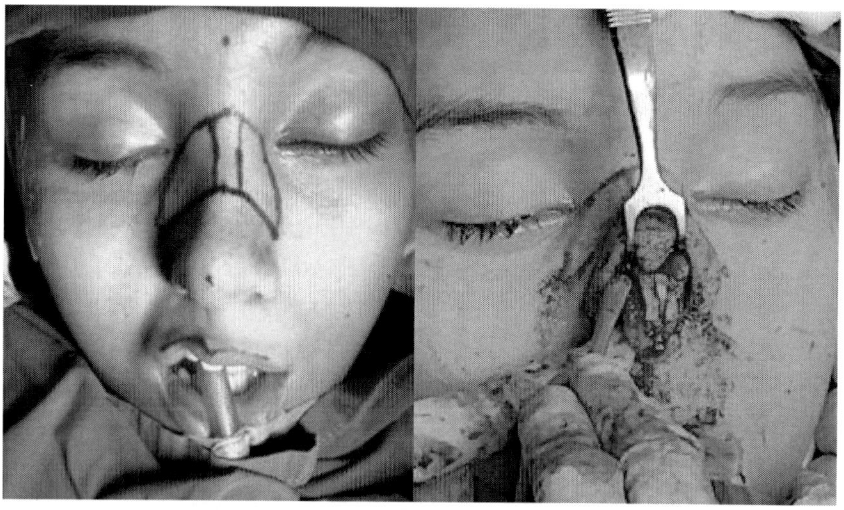

Figure 3. Intraoperative procedure.

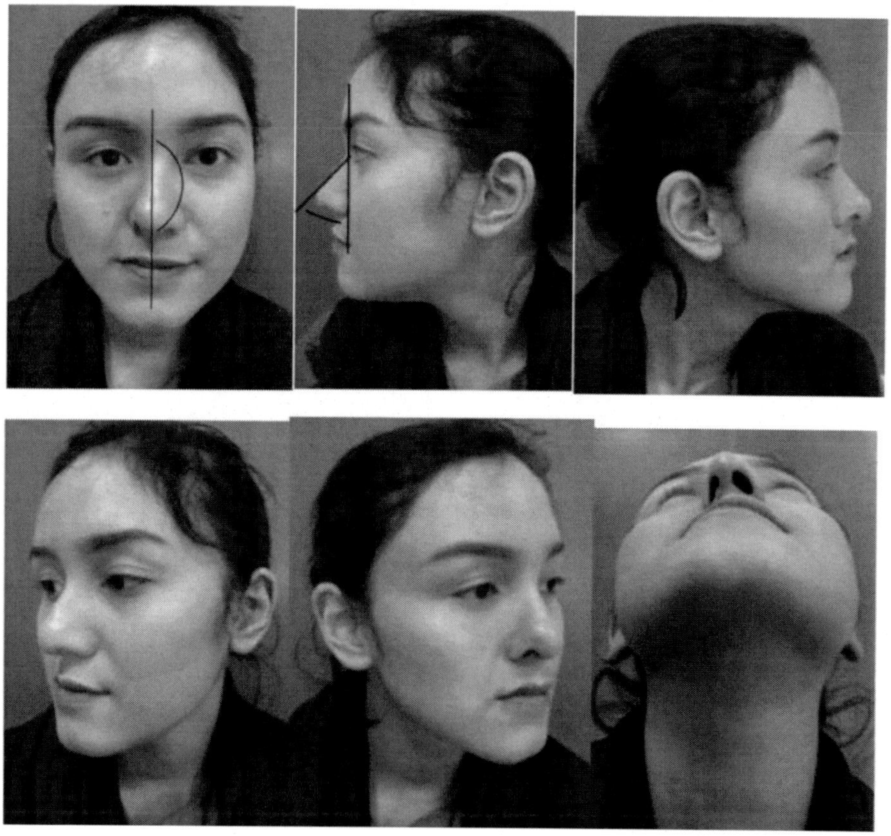

Figure 4. Assessment after three months of surgery.

Nasal analysis showed an improvement in the deviation of the nasal axis from the frontal, lateral, and basal view.

DISCUSSION

In a previous study by Deshingkar et al., it was described that the onset of PRS is insidious. The disease generally manifests itself as an atrophy, with onset during the first decade of life. Prior to becoming quiescent and stabilizing, the syndrome slowly progresses [1]. In this case report, the patient complained of facial asymmetry and deviation of nose and angle of mouth to the right side of face since she was 7 years old. Additionally, 3 years ago, the patient developed nasal congestion. Such findings prove that symptoms slowly develop over the years. In a previous study by Aydin et al., it described that patients with PRS may manifest ophthalmic, and neurological complications. However, the study patient had no symptoms of neurological disturbance and had normal vision [2].

A report by Patel et al. stated that the treatment of PRS should be initiated only after the disease stabilizes [3]. Surgical treatment options depend on the side of atrophy and deformity [3]. The study patient had the deviation of the nose and upper labia to the right side. Consequently, for aesthetic and nasal congestion reasons, the patient underwent plastic reconstruction. Septorhinoplasty and labioplasty were performed after the age of 18 years to ensure that the disease has stabilized and facial growth has slowed down. Of note, performing surgery during facial growth would affect the shape of the nose [2]. Although a deviated nose is one of the greatest challenges in septorhinoplasty, it can be treated with appropriate surgical procedures. Using a precise nasal analysis pre-surgery, the patient was found to have a C-shape deviation. The anterior rhinoscopy showed a deviated right nasal septum and the rhinomanometry showed resistance during nasal inspiration.

To reduce the congestion caused by deviated nose, the septum had to be reinforced and supported in a midline position. The spreader graft was placed following osteotomies, to secure the cartilage in a midline position. The spreader graft was important to smooth the brow-tip aesthetic line and prevent or correct midvault collapse by stenting open the internal nasal valve. As a consequence, medial displacement of the upper lateral cartilages was prevented. The caudal extension graft was used to enhance nasal tip dynamics by controlling the projection, rotation, and strength of the tip. The alar batten graft was used to reinforce the weakness of the lower lateral cartilage, thereby improving nasal patency in correlation with the nasal valve area. Treatment for the atrophy of the cheeks and forehead will be performed by a dermatologist using hyaluronic filling. Four months after surgery, the patient was in good clinical and aesthetic condition.

CONCLUSION

In conclusion, PRS manifests as an atrophy leading to a variety of either or both aesthetic and functional problems. In the study patient, septorhinoplasty was used to successfully manage the deviated nose caused by PRS. The functional septorhinoplasty provided structural support by means of autologous grafts to preserve and augment the nose without compromising aesthetic and functional results.

REFERENCES

[1] Deshingkar, SA; Barpande, SR; Bhavtangkar, JD; Humble, GJ. Progressive hemifacial atrophy. *Contemp. Clin. Dent.* 2012;3(5), S78-81.

[2] Hasan, A; Zeyne, Y; Husamettin, S; Melike, RM. Parry-Romberg syndrome. *Neurosciences.* 2015 Oct; 20(4), 368-371.

[3] Patel, H; Thakkar, C; Patel, K. Parry Romberg syndrome: A rare entity. J. Maxillofac. *Oral Surg.* 2010 Nov 27;9(3), 247-250.

[4] Nasser, IJG et al. Romberg's syndrome: a series of cases. *Rev. Bras. Cir. Plást.* 2013 Jun; 28(2), 201-4.

[5] Reddy, SS; Devaiah, D; Agarwal, K. Parry Romberg syndrome: Report of two cases with rare dental and skeletal findings. *E-Journal of Dentistry.* 2012 Jul;2(3), 68-71.

[6] Sargunar, B; Ebenezer, V; Balakrishnan, R.; Priya, S. Parry Romberg syndrome-A review of treatment options. *Biomed. Pharmacol. J.* 2014;7(1), 207-211.

[7] Prendergast, PM. Anatomy of the face and neck. In: Shiffman MA, Di Giuseppe A, editor. *Cosmetic Surgery: art and techniques.* Berlin: Springer-Verlag Berlin Heidelberg; 2013; 29-45.

[8] Inanli, S; Binnetogl, A. A combined approach to crooked nose deformity. *Aesth. Plast. Surg.* 2016 Jun;40(3), 360-6.

[9] Ahmad, J; Rohrich, RJ; Lee, MR. The crooked nose. *Clin. Plastic. Surg.* 2016 Jan;43(1), 99-113.

[10] Parilla, C; Artuso, A; Gallus, R; Galli, J; Paludetti, G. The role of septal surgery in cosmetic rhinoplasty. *Acta Otorhinolaryngol. Italica.* 2013 Jun;33(3), 146-153.

[11] Teymoortash, A; Fasunla, JA; Sazgar, AA. The value of spreader graft in rhinoplasty: a critical review. *Eur. Atch. Otorhinolaryngology.* 2012 May;296(5), 1411-16.

In: Case Reports in Surgery
Editors: Ahmad Jabir Rahyussalim et al.
ISBN: 978-1-53616-582-1

Chapter 9

USE OF NASOLABIAL AND NASAL SEPTAL FLAPS FOR UNILATERAL LOWER-THIRD NASAL DEFECTS

Mirta H. Reksodiputro, Satria Dipo Putra Asmoro, Dini W. Widodo and Trimartani Koento*
ORL- HNS Department, University of Indonesia, Jakarta, Indonesia

ABSTRACT

The nose is the most prominent structure in the center of the face and plays an important role in the aesthetics of the face. Nasal defects in the dorsum, ala nasi, nostrils, columella, or septum due to trauma, animal bites, and tumor can lead to loss of function and decrease in aesthetic value. Nasolabial and nasal septal flaps are used for the reconstruction of nasal defects after mass extirpation in the lower third of the nose, particularly in cases of ala nasi defects. Here, we report the case of a patient who underwent reconstruction with a combination of nasolabial and nasal septal flaps for an ala nasi defect due to mass extirpation for basal cell carcinoma. We also conducted an evidence-based literature search tailored to the case.

Keywords: Nasal defect, nasal reconstruction, nasolabial flap, nasal septal flap

INTRODUCTION

Nasal soft tissue can be deformed by accidents, surgical trauma, human or animal bites, tumors, and leishmaniasis. Basal cell carcinoma is rather common, with ~80% of the cases

---

* Corresponding Author's E-mail: trimartani@yahoo.com.au.

occurring in the head area, of which 40% occur in the skin of the cheeks and nose. Treatment with surgery in these cases often produces nasal defects [1]. External nose surgery is performed to correct the nasal defects, improve the aesthetic appearance of the nose and breathing, and restore the patient's mental health and self-confidence. However, ala nasi reconstruction for deep or broad defects is rather challenging from an aesthetic as well as a functional perspective. Nasal defects can be reconstructed using many techniques, the best being the use of nasolabial flap, which has a rich blood supply and a suitable texture and color, although it is associated with high donor area morbidity [2]. Nasolabial flap is very useful in ala nasi defect reconstruction [3]. This flap is very well done in elderly patients because it has more flexible skin, and more suitable color evenly. It's difficult to do for patients with hairy skin [4]. Incase with large alae nasi defect, it can be combined with nasal septal flap because it has good blood supply. The septal mucopericondrium can be used for one side in reconstruction [5].

Case Report

A 56-year-old woman underwent wide excision for basal cell carcinoma removal in October 2015 at the Oncology Surgery Division of Dr. Cipto Mangunkusumo Hospital, Jakarta, Indonesia. Reopening of the surgical wound caused a defect on the right side of the lower third of her nose (Figure 1). She did not complain of nasal congestion, recurrent nosebleeds, or pain in the wound. Local examination revealed a 3×1 cm^2 defect in the lateral nasal dorsum toward the right nasal ala nasi, involving the visualizated base of the inferior turbinate mucosa, the right nasal septum, and some of the medial turbinate. The defect edge was hyperemic and dry, with a network of cuffles on the edge of the defect, nasal dorsum, and right nasal collumela. An asymmetrical deflection nasal tip appeared to the right. The trichion, glabella, nasion, rhinion, tip, and subnasal region were not in a straight line. There was no hematoma, edema, laceration, excoriation, or active bleeding.

Reconstruction surgery was perform on November 1, 2016, in the plastic reconstruction division of the otorhinolaryngology outpatient clinic. The island flap surgical technique used a combination of nasolabial and nasal septal flaps. An ear cartilage graft was used as a base support, and the nasal septal mucosa was used to line the nasolabial flap (Figure 2). During follow-up on day 7 postsurgery, the defect was found to be closed, and the nasal septal flap showed growth with no obstruction in the nasal cavity (Figures 3 and 4). During follow-up at 2 months postsurgery, the patient made no complaints of pain, nasal congestion, or runny nose mixed with blood. There was no edema, hematoma, hyperemia, or pus. In addition, there was minimal scar tissue in the surgical wound. Nasoendoscopic examination showed that the surgical wound appeared well; the nasal septal mucosa had formed with good vascularization; the nasal septal flap appeared well; and there was no hematoma, hyperemia, pus, edema, or perforation (Figure 5).

DISCUSSION

The nasolabial flap is very useful in ala nasi defect reconstruction, particularly in the elderly, because of its proximity, suitable color, and ease of use in the nasal recipient area [6]. In addition, the nasolabial flap is rich in blood vessels, including angular arteries (facial artery branches), infraorbital arteries, facial arteries, and infratrochlear arteries, and it is easy to anastomose between the main branches of the blood vessels [9]. Nasolabial flap can combined with nasal septal flaps. Brian, Drisco. defek yang cukup besar pada hidung, dapat digunakan jabir mukoperikondrium septum pada kaudal septum [7]. Jabir ini di suplai darah dari percabangan arteri labialis superior [8].

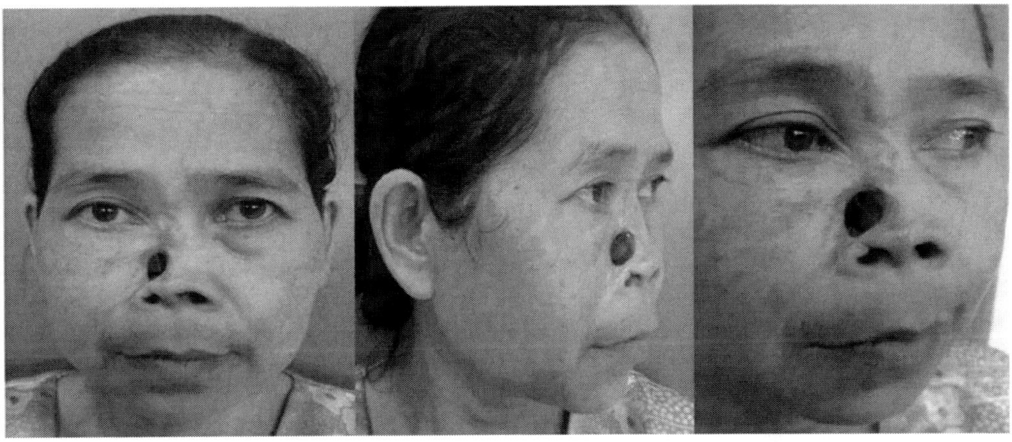

Figure 1. Defect of the right lateral lower third of the nose and ala nasi.

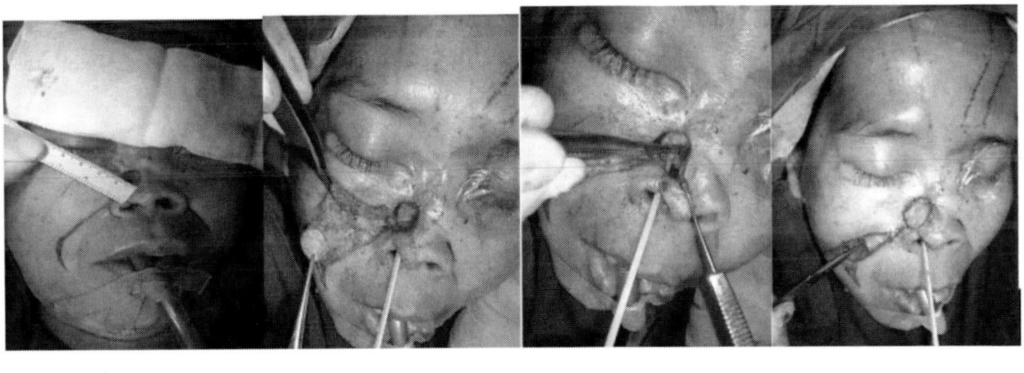

a b c d

Figure 2. (a) Measuring the nasal defect. (b) Island flap technique combining nasolabial flap with nasal septal flap. (c) Nasal septal flap for lining the nasolabial flap. (d) Closing the flap.

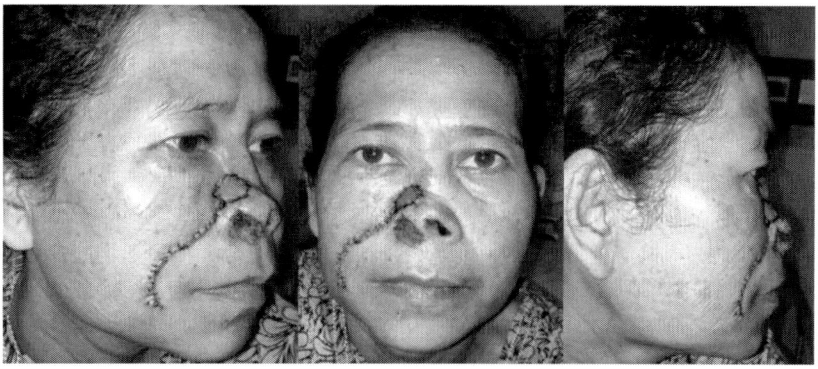

Figure 3. Day 7 postsurgery follow-up.

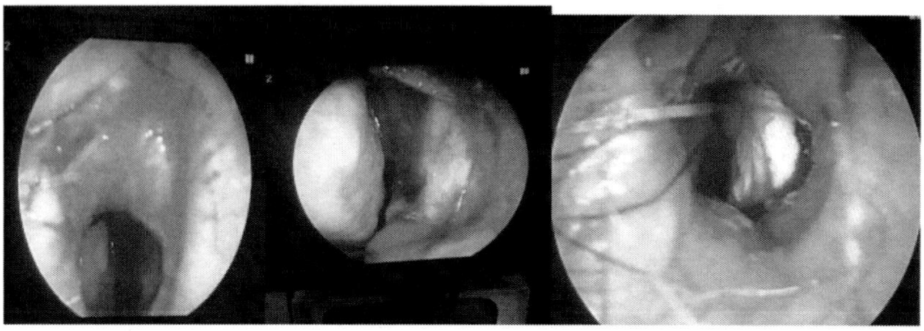

Figure 4. Nasoendoscopic examination on day 7 postdurgery follow-up. Nasal septal flap growth looks good.

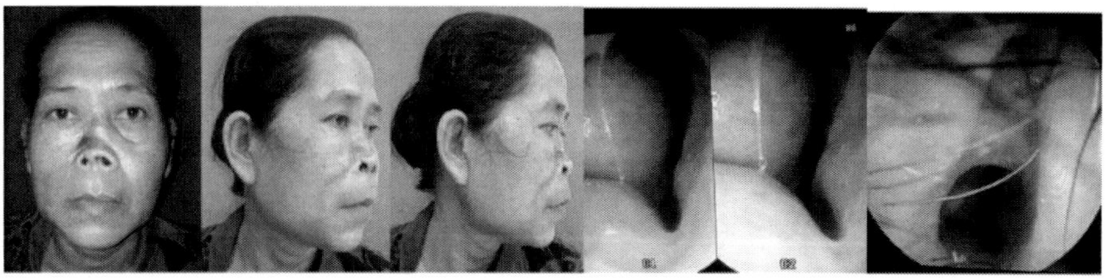

Figure 5. Two-month postsurgery follow-up. The nasal septal flap growth looks good, with no hematoma, hyperemia, pus, edema, or perforation.

In the island flap technique, the nasolabial flap is derived from the cheek area for the reconstruction of nasal defects that are not too large [6]. The nasal septal mocosa is taken as a lining, and an ear cartilage graft is placed above it as support on the contralateral side, making a sandwich [7]. Septal and ear cartilages are used to replace missing parts of the nose and provide good support because of their thin and flexible contours [10].

For a large nasal defect, the mucopericondrium from the nasal septal flap at the caudal septum can be used, which gets blood supply from superior labial artery branches. If needed, most of the one-sided mucopericondrium can be used for reconstruction [2]. The ipsilateral nasal septal flap can be used as a close pediclc, containing superior labial artery branches. This flap is thin and physiological and can be used for defects of the caudal third of the nose [11].

Conclusion

This paper had a case female, 56 years old with right alae nasi defect after tumour extirpation. Reconstruction is performed using nasolabial flap combined with nasal septal flap and ear concha cartilage for base. There was good result for aesthetic and function after two month evaluation. Nasolabial and Nasal Septal Flaps are good option for reconstruction of nasal defect with good and favourable results especially in elderly case.

References

[1] Javaid, M., & Ahmad, N. (2018). Outcome of Nasolabial flap in Reconstruction of the nasal alar defect. *Turkish Journals of Plastic Sugery. Pakistan,* 163-166.

[2] Sand, P. J., & Branham, H. G. (2009). *Skin Grafts and Local Flaps in Facial Plastic Surgery. Nasal Reconstruction. Chapter 41.* New York, NY: Publisher. 660-712.

[3] Werda H. Editor. Coverage of Defects. *Reconstructive Facial Plastic Surgery.* Amsterdam: 2001:12-54.

[4] Rudy J., Triana Jr, Murakami C., Larrabee J. Skin Flap and Local Flaps. In: Papel I., Frodel J., Holt G., Nachlas N., Park S., Toriumi D., et all. Editors. *Facial Plastic Reconstructive Surgery.* 3rd Edition. New York: 2008:41-58.

[5] Brian P., Drisco, Baker S. *Reconstruction of Nasal Alar Defects.* Michigan: 2001:91-100.

[6] Hasan, A. A. (2016). Reconstruction of the nasal defect by nasolabial flaps. *Journal of US-China Medical Science. Iraq,* 64-79.

[7] Alam, M., & Goldberg, L. H. (2019). Oblique advancement flap for defects of the lateral nasal supratip. *Arch, Dermatol.,* 1039-1042.

[8] Larrabee W., Makielski K. Editors. Nose. *Surgical Anatomy of the Face.* United State of America: 2000:153-176.

[9] Martini F. editor. *Fundamental Anatomy and Physiology. The Respiratory System.* 7th Edition. United State of America. 2006:817-819.

[10] Rahpeyma A, Khajehahmadi S. *The place of nasolabial flap in orofacial reconstruction.* Iran: 2016:80-3.

[11] Soetjipto D., Mangunkusumo E., Wardani R. Hidung. In: Soepardi E., Iskandar N., Bashiruddin J., Restuti R. Editor. Buku Ajar Ilmu Kesehatan Telinga Hidung dan Tenggorok. Edisi ketujuh. Indonesia: 2012:96-103.

In: Case Reports in Surgery
Editors: Ahmad Jabir Rahyussalim et al.
ISBN: 978-1-53616-582-1

Chapter 10

Supernumerary Nostril: A Rare Congenital Anomaly

Dini Widiarni Widodo*[*] *and Rindy Yunita Pratamisiwi
Department of Otorhinolaryngology – Head and Neck Surgery,
Faculty of Medicine Universitas Indonesia/Cipto Mangunkusumo General Hospital,
Jakarta, Indonesia

Abstract

Supernumerary nostrils are an extremely rare congenital. The purpose of this study is to prepare a standardized procedure for repairing supernumerary nostrils, and to discuss the probable psychological effect on the patient. Fistulectomy and cartilage graft from the ear were performed to reconstruct the accessory nostril. Surgery was performed at a young age to prevent further disfiguration and to optimize psychological well-being. The result of this study is the wound showed good healing progress over the lateral side of the nose. Although the symmetry between the two nostrils was not ideal, it was acceptable. The repair aims to create a functioning and normal-appearing nose with minimal deformity. The extra nostril can be excised during fistulectomy. The patient can also be offered social skill training to improve their self-esteem and family acceptance and support are important in the rehabilitation of children with facial disfigurations.

Keywords: supernumerary nostril, accessory nostril, psychological effect

[*] Corresponding Author's E-mail: dini_pancho@yahoo.com.

INTRODUCTION

A supernumerary nostril is an extremely rare congenital deformity. Also known as triple nostrils or accessory nostril, supernumerary nostril is defined as an abnormal nostril located above the normal nostril. The specific cause and development of supernumerary nostril are not known. The anomaly seems to develop from a localized abnormality of the lateral nasal process at an early embryonic stage. Various types of the anomaly exist, and different surgery techniques to each are required, but there is still no generally accepted method of repair. The goal of repair is to create a functioning and normal-appearing nose with minimal deformity.

CASE PRESENTATION

A 10-year-old male child, who had a supernumerary nostril located beside his left nostril since birth, was referred to our department. He had no history of nasal obstruction. According to his mother, her pregnancy, the child's birth, and his development were uneventful. The patient had no other congenital abnormalities, and there were no reports of this type of deformity in either parent's family history.

On physical examination, the patient had two nostrils on the left side and the normal ipsilateral nostril was a little smaller than that on the other side. The diameter of the accessory nostril was 2 mm, and there was no discharge from any of the nostrils. We found no inferior and middle turbinate in the accessory nostril and no connective structures to the normal nostril. There was also no upper lateral cartilage in the accessory nostril; thus, the nostril felt soft on palpation. There was fibrous tissue without any columellar structure between the left and accessory nostrils. The nasal mucous lining appeared normal, and the patient was classified with type 3-a supernumerary nostril.

The surgery was performed under general anesthesia. The inner nostril was incised following the accessory nasolabial fold, and a left rim incision was then performed. The tissue between the vestibulum and the accessory nostril was widely undermined. No nasal alar and columellar structures were found during the surgery; therefore, alar reconstruction using ear cartilage was planned.

The left ear concha was marked and dissected. The cartilage was cut into a 0.5 mm × 0.5 mm piece and then inserted in the undermined vestibulum area to form a normal ala. The remaining subcutaneous and skin tissues were then sutured tightly to prevent hematomas.

The nostril size was adjusted with reference to the size of the normal nostril. The incision was sutured using 5-0 Prolene. The new ala was fixated using aluminum foil paper, and a small piece of nasogastric tube was inserted in the nostril as an internal stent, which was then removed after 3 days.

The wound showed good healing progress over the lateral side of the nose. The symmetry between the two nostrils, although not ideal, was acceptable. No hematoma was observed on the left ear, and the incised area showed no sign of infection. The patient and his parents were satisfied with the result, which boosted his confidence.

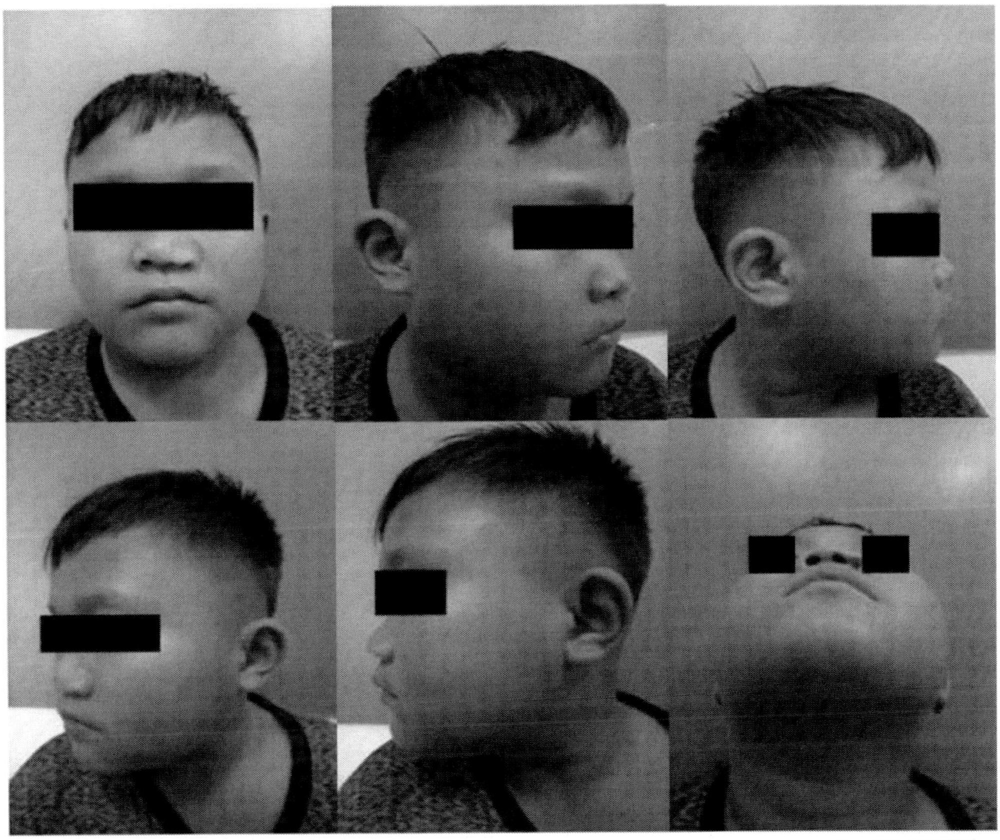

Figure 1. Patient with supernumerary nostril.

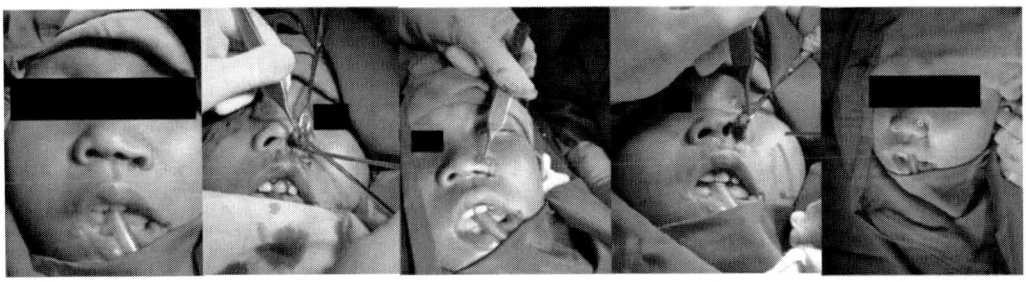

Figure 2. Intraoperative procedure.

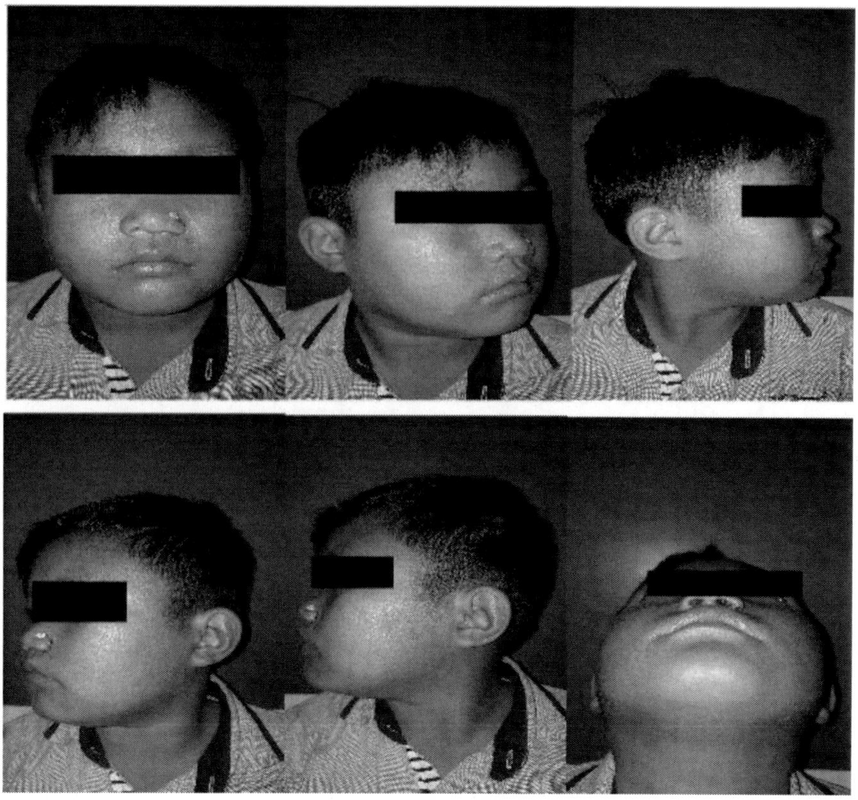

Figure 3. Postoperative result.

DISCUSSION

Supernumerary nostril is an extremely rare type of congenital nasal anomaly with unclear etiology [1]. The first reported case was published in 1906 by Lindsay, who described a patient with bilateral supernumerary nostrils. Most reported cases of supernumerary nostrils have been unilateral, and were associated with other craniofacial malformations, such as a facial cleft [1-3]. A supernumerary nostril may or may not communicate with the ipsilateral normal nasal cavity, depending on the extent of the anomaly's progression. This condition should not be confused with the double nose deformity, which has two septa, four nostrils, four alae, and four nasal cavities [1-3].

Over the past 5 years, four cases of supernumerary nostril have been documented in English. In 2014, Sah et al. [4] reported a case with an accessory nostril located above the left nostril, which was repaired with an elliptical incision and fistulectomy technique. Trimartani and Widayanti in 2015 [5] and Choi et al. [3] in 2016 reported cases with a left accessory nostril treated by fistulectomy. Further, Asadi et al. [6] reported a case with a supernumerary nostril that was treated using an external rhinoplasty approach.

The preoperative workup for supernumerary nostril cases includes a detailed history with special attention to the prenatal course. A comprehensive physical examination is performed to rule out other craniofacial anomalies [7], and the diagnosis is made based on the clinical appearance, physical examination, and histological features of the accessory nostril [2] Consideration of imaging results such as those of computed tomography scans or magnetic resonance imaging to rule out any intracranial communication or skull base defect is balanced with the risk of anesthesia, which is required for imaging [7].

The scarcity and variation of supernumerary nostrils call for innovation during surgical repair. The goal of repair is to create a functioning and normal-appearing nose with minimal deformity. It is vital to resect the entire fistula tract and to preserve the perviousness of the normal nostril. Additionally, the redundant nasal tract should be eliminated, the nasal width reduced, and the alar base repositioned, all the while maintaining the natural alar skin [7].

Most of the above studies advocated that corrective surgery be performed at a young age to prevent any possible alar deformity or deformation of adjacent structures, thereby minimizing related psychological effects [8].

An imperfect appearance may result in overt teasing, bullying, and unwanted questioning. Social responses may also take the form of more subtle modifications in normal patterns of verbal and non-verbal interactions, such as facial expressions. These unfavorable social responses are the result of stigma, where outsiders subconsciously judge an individual negatively because of their imperfect appearance. Individuals affected by supernumerary nostril who are dissatisfied with or who are unrealistic about their appearance need to be identified. These individuals are "at risk" for developing low self-esteem and could be offered some social skills training to improve their self-confidence and increase their self-esteem [8].

The family environment is an important aspect in the rehabilitation of children with facial deformities. The attitudes, expectations, and degree of support shown by parents are likely to have an enormous influence on a child's perception of their impairment. Surgery for disfigurement usually results in increased self-esteem, self-confidence, and satisfaction with appearance, irrespective of whether an objective improvement is detected by independent observers. Unrealistically high expectations for surgical improvement can result in dissatisfaction with post-surgical results; therefore, families should be counseled extensively pre-operatively to identify cases where this may be a problem [8].

CONCLUSION

The documented cases of supernumerary nostril until now are still inadequate. To determinate the embryological implications, anatomic presentations and possible additional anomalies with accessory nose, cases need to be further investigated. We aimed to share this rare congenital anomaly within medical field. In this rare deformity, surgery should be performed at an early age to avoid severe impact on the nasal cartilages because of the fistula, deformation of adjacent structures, and the psychologic effects.

REFERENCES

[1] Mishra, LK. Supernumerary nostril: Report of a rare case and a review of the literature. *Plast. Surg. Case Studies*, 2015;1(3):55-56.

[2] Sun, ZY, Li, H, Zhang, MJ, Zhao, H, Xu, W, Xiao, H, Guo YX, Wen, Z, Yin, GQ. Supernumerary Nostril. *Eur. Surg. Res.*, 2009;42:245-248.

[3] Choi, BE, Ko, SO, Shin HK. Supernumerary nostril: a case report. *Maxillofac. Plast. Reconstr. Surg*, 2016;38(1):43. Published 2016 Nov 5.

[4] Sah, BP, Bhandary, S, Pokharel, A, Shilpakar, SL, Chettri, ST, Paudel, D. A supernumerary nostril associated with dermoid cyst: A rare case report and review of literature. *American Journal of Medical Case Reports*. 2014; 2(3):52-54.

[5] Trimartani, Widayant, N. Rinoplasti pada kelainan hidung kongenital. *Oto Rhino Laryngologica Indonesiana*. 2015;45(1):53-60.

[6] Asadi, M, Tabrizi, AG, Jahanshahi, F. Supernumerary nostril in the twin: case report. *JPRI*, 2017;18(1):1-5.

[7] Shaye, DA, Tibesar, RJ. Repair of supernumerary nostril. *J. Craniofac. Surg*. 2014;25(3): 978-979.

[8] Turner, SR, N, Rumsey, JR, Sandy. Psychological aspects of cleft lip and palate. *Eur. J. Orthod.*, 1998;20(4):407-415.

[9] Saiga, A, Mitsukawa, N. Case of supernumerary nostril. *J. Plast. Reconstr. Aesthet. Surg*. 2013 Jan; 66(1): 126-128. DOI: 10.1016/j. bjps.2012.05.014; PMID: 22687717.

[10] Kawamoto, HK Jr. Rare craniofacial clefts, plastic surgery. Philadelphia, PA: Saunders; 1990. 4:2922-2973.

[11] Losee, JE, Kirschner, RE, Whitaker, LA, Bartlett, SP. Congenital Nasal Anomalies: A Classification Scheme. *Plast. Reconstr. Surg*. 2004. Feb;113(2):676-89.

In: Case Reports in Surgery
Editors: Ahmad Jabir Rahyussalim et al.
ISBN: 978-1-53616-582-1

Chapter 11

OBJECTIVE MEASURES IN FUNCTIONAL SEPTORHINOPLASTY: TWO CASE REPORTS OF NASAL FORM AND NASAL VALVE RECONSTRUCTION

Trimartani Koento[1], Tiara Melati[2] and Mirta H. Reksodiputro[1,*]

[1]Department of Otorhinolaryngology Head and Neck Surgery, Plastic Reconstructive Sub Division, Faculty of Medicine, University Indonesia, Dr. Cipto Mangunkusumo Hospital, Jakarta, Indonesia

[2]Department of Otorhinolaryngology Head and Neck Surgery, Faculty of Medicine, University Indonesia, Dr. Cipto Mangunkusumo Hospital, Jakarta, Indonesia

ABSTRACT

Nasal valve, which is the narrowest area in the nasal airway passage, is responsible for about half of the total nasal airway resistance. Functional septorhinoplasty is used to achieve an esthetic shape of the nose while preserving adequate nasal and breathing function. Nasal complaints are subjective; thus, objective measurements obtained through active anterior rhinomanometry are needed to correctly identify nasal valve incompetence. We present reports of two cases where changes in nasal airflow and resistance were objectively assessed before and after functional septorhinoplasty using an alar batten graft. Significant changes were observed postoperatively. Improvement was confirmed by assessment of subjective symptoms of nasal obstruction and rhinomanometry data.

[*] Corresponding Author's E-mail: citamirta@yahoo.com.

Keywords: rhinomanometry, septorhinoplasty, alar batten graft, nasal valve

Introduction

It is often difficult to objectively quantify the outcomes of functional and esthetic nasal surgery (septoplasty, rhinoplasty, nasal valve surgery, turbinoplasty, and septorhinoplasty) [1], as traditional outcome measures rely on quality-of-life and patient satisfaction. The development and validation of objective measures may allow quantification of surgical outcomes. As nasal form and function are closely intertwined, quantitative assessment can better define this relationship and the effects on these parameters following nasal surgery. Rhinomanometry is an objective measure of nasal airflow and resistance that can be applied to outcome-based research to allow improved comparisons of results across studies. Further development of these objective measures can potentially lead to the identification of clinical predictors for surgical success or the development of standard criteria for surgical decision support. This information is useful not only within academia but also within commercial healthcare, given the mounting external pressure for quantifiable outcomes, particularly in the field of facial plastic surgery, which is increasingly being faced with challenges for insurance approvals and justification of procedures. Thus, the need for objective data will only continue to grow.

Several characteristics of objective assessment techniques, such as nasoendoscopic evaluation and rhinomanometry, are important to achieve accurate reproducible results and to ensure cost-effectiveness. Many available objective measures for functional nasal surgery are lacking in one or more of these characteristics, thereby limiting their routine clinical use. However, advances in computed imaging technologies, such as computed tomography scan (CT scan), have facilitated the development of innovative objective assessment tools for nasal surgery. In this article, we have presented an overview of objective measures in both esthetic and functional nasal surgeries and discussed the assessment of objective outcomes of nasal form and function is discussed.

Case 1

A 24-year-old woman presented with a 5-year history of debilitating nasal obstruction. No other nasal or throat symptoms were noted. On physical examination, there was no nasal deformity or positive sign of Cottle's maneuver (Figure 1). A rigid nasal endoscopic examination showed narrowing of the nasal passages; the internal nasal valves were narrowed, and the inferior turbinates were edematous without septal deviation. The results of anterior active rhinomanometry showed moderate obstruction of right nasal airflow

(Figure 2) with a significant reduction in the flow at rest and maximum respiration (Table 1).

Nasal valve incompetence was addressed through septorhinoplasty, multiple outfracturing of the inferior turbinates, and an alar batten graft. The graft donor site was the cartilage from the left auricular conchal cavity; the site was closed and secured with through-and-through sutures. The patient was discharged the following day. One week postoperatively, the patient had no nasal obstruction. A nasal endoscopic examination revealed a broad nasal passage and widened internal nasal valve areas (Figure 3). A second rhinomanometry examination performed at 2 weeks postoperatively revealed a significant improvement in the right nasal airflow at rest and maximum respiration with enhanced nasal resistance (Figure 4, Table 2).

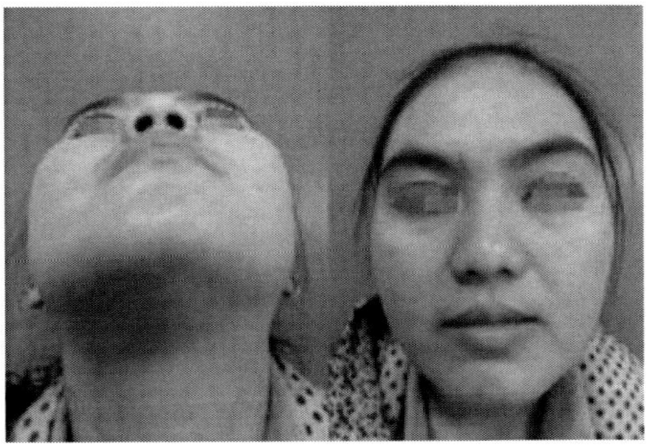

Figure 1. Frontal and basal preoperative views.

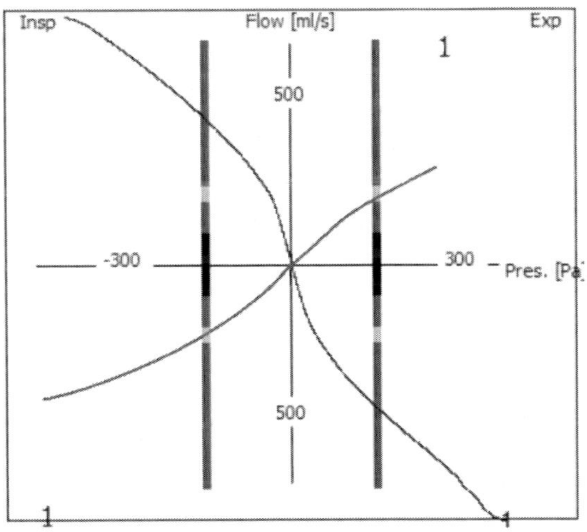

Figure 2. Anterior active rhinomanometry curvature preoperatively.

Table 1. Anterior active rhinomanometry preoperatively data

Pressure	Inspiration			Expiration			Unit
	75 Pa	150 Pa	300 Pa	75 Pa	150 Pa	300 Pa	
Left Airflow	316	456	681	310	452	695	ml/s
Right Airflow	167	257	459	170	235	301	ml/s
Total Airflow	483	716	1140	480	687	996	ml/s
Left Resistance	0.24	0.33	0.44	0.24	0.33	0.43	%
Right Resistance	0.16	0.21	0.26	0.16	0.22	0.3	%

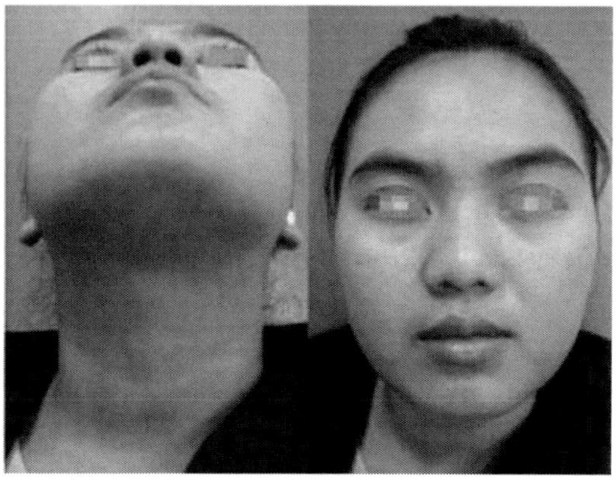

Figure 3. Frontal view before and at 1 week postoperatively.

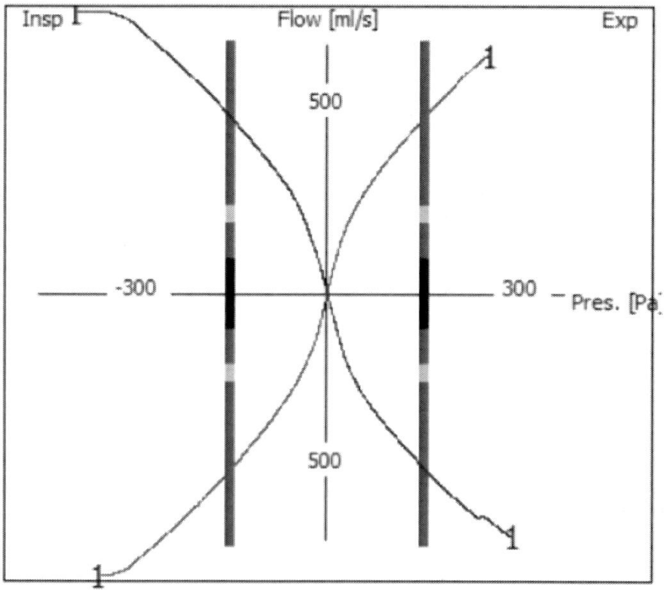

Figure 4. Anterior active rhinomanometry curvature postoperatively.

Table 2. Anterior active rhinomanometry postoperatively data

Pressure	Inspiration			Expiration			Unit
	75 Pa	150 Pa	300 Pa	75 Pa	150 Pa	300 Pa	
Left Airflow	330	493	752	331	485	-	ml/s
Right Airflow	326	496	752	327	489	-	ml/s
Total Airflow	656	989	1540	658	974	-	ml/s
Left Resistance	0.23	0.3	0.4	0.23	0.31	-	%
Right Resistance	0.23	0.3	0.4	0.23	0.31	-	%

CASE 2

A 45-year-old male presented with a chief complaint of nasal obstruction with a history of nasal closed reduction 6 months ago due to an accident (Figure 5). On physical examination, there was no deformity of the nose, with only a scar observed in the right medial canthus. Cottle's maneuver was positive. Nasal endoscopic examination revealed a deviated septum superiorly and collapsed ala nasi during respiration, which reduced the internal nasal valve area. Nasal incompetence in this patient was addressed by septoplasty, and an alar batten graft was placed via the endonasal approach. The patient was discharged the next day, and follow-up examination at 1 week postoperatively was improved, as seen from the nasal endoscopic comparison before and after surgery (Figure 6).

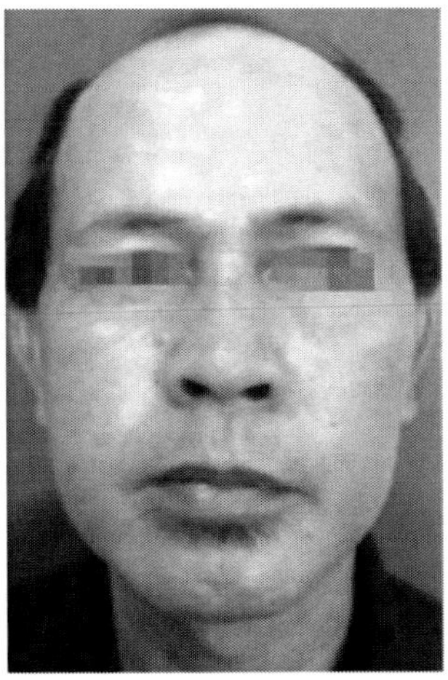

Figure 5. Frontal preoperative view.

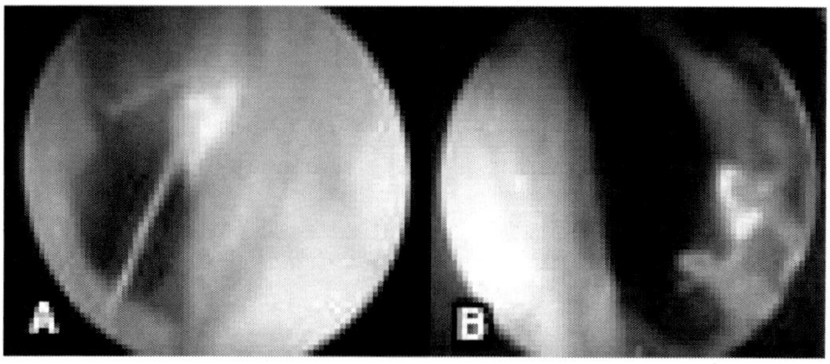

Figure 6. Nasal endoscopic findings: (A) pre- and (B) postoperatively.

DISCUSSION

Objective measurement of nasal obstruction is important to determine a successful surgical outcome. There are many studies that show discrepancy between subjective and objective findings of nasal patency [1]. Therefore objective tools must be reproducible, be able to exclude a mucosal diagnosis, and correctly identify relevant constraints. In the United States, the annual cost of treatment of nasal obstruction exceeds 5 billion USD, with nasal surgery accounting for more than 60 million USD [2]. Rhinomanometry and acoustic rhinometry are expensive, time-consuming, and uncomfortable to the patient [3, 4].

According to Hsu et al. [5], the visual analog scale, the nasal obstruction symptom evaluation questionnaire, and anterior active rhinomanometry are useful tools to assess subjective complaints regarding nasal patency following septoplasty. Rhinomanometry is used to obtain information regarding nasal airflow and resistance. All three of these modalities are helpful in determining the candidacy and success of septoplasty. Bohluli et al. [6] have described the specific equipment and skills required for rhinomanometry, acoustic rhinometry, and computed tomography. The external nasal valve efficacy index by simple photography, which utilizes software to calculate the cross-sectional nostril at rest and respiration, is a relatively simple method that can be routinely performed preoperatively and can be used to document every stage of therapy [6].

Miman et al. [7] identify and classify the shape of the internal nasal valve using nasal endoscopy. In light of the advances in smartphones, Surda et al. [8] perform image analysis to measure the angle and cross-section area of the internal nasal valve. Lee et al. [9] and Moche et al. [10] both studies uses standard CT scan to identify and measure the internal nasal valve.

According to Spielmann et al. [11], identification of the specific underlying cause of nasal valve incompetence is necessary to achieve successful reconstruction. Thus, the most appropriate technique may be to strategically address each cause, and the causes vary across cases. While selecting the technique, long-term advantage to the patient must be considered. Furthermore, Spielmann et al. [11] have recommend routine nasal airflow examination both pre- and postoperatively.

A combination of objective tools such as facial photos, Cottle's maneuver, nasoendoscopic findings, and anterior active rhinomanometry is essential for the diagnosis of nasal obstruction due to incompetence of the nasal valve. Such tools allow specific identification of the area of the lesion and are relatively reproducible. Although rhinomanometry may not be available everywhere and access is limited in many facilities, facial photos, Cottle's maneuver, and nasoendoscopic findings provide integral information, which greatly impacts the selection of the reconstruction technique.

REFERENCES

[1] André, R. F., Vuyk, H. D., Ahmed, A., Graamans, K., Nolst Trenité, G. J., (2009). Correlation between subjective and objective evaluation of the nasal airway. A systematic review of the highest level of evidence. *Clin Otolaryngol.* 34, 518-525.

[2] Chandra, R. K., Patadia, M. O., Raviv, J., (2009). Diagnosis of nasal airway obstruction. *Otolaryngol. Clin. North Am.* 42, 207-225.

[3] Fattahi, T., (2008). Internal nasal valve: significance in nasal air flow. *J. Oral Maxillofac. Surg.* 66, 1921-1926.

[4] Jones, A. S., Viani, L., Phillips, D., Charters, P., (1991). The objective assessment of nasal patency. *Clin. Otolaryngol. Allied Sci.* 16, 206-211.

[5] Hsu, H. C., Tan, C. D., Chang, C. W., Chu, C. W., Chiu, Y. C., Pan, C. J., Huang, H. M., (2017). Evaluation of nasal patency by visual analogue scale/nasal obstruction symptom evaluation questionnaires and anterior active rhinomanometry after septoplasty: retrospective one-year follow-up cohort study. *Clin. Otolaryngol.* 42, 53-59.

[6] Bohluli, B., Varedi, P., Kahali, R., Bagheri, S. C., (2015). External Nasal Valve Efficacy Index: a simple test to evaluate the external nasal valve. *Int. J. Oral Maxillofac. Surg.* 44, 1240-1245.

[7] Miman, M., Deliktas, H., Ozturan, O., Toplu, Y., Akarçay, M., (2006). Internal nasal valve: revisited with objective facts. *Otolaryngol. Head Neck Surg.* 134, 41-47.

[8] Surda, P., Walker, A., Little, S. A., Barnes, M. L., Hassan, D., Toma, A., (2017). Novel outcome measurement tool of the nasal valve surgery image analysis using endoscopic system for smartphones. *Clin. Otolaryngol.* 42, 192-195.

[9] Lee, D. C., Shin, J. H., Kim, S. W., Kim, B. G., Kang, J. M., Cho, J. H., Park, Y. J., (2013). Anatomical analysis of nasal obstruction: nasal cavity of patients complaining of stuffy nose. *Laryngoscope* 123, 1381-1384.

[10] Moche, J. A., Cohen, J. C., Pearlman, S. J., (2013). Axial computed tomography evaluation of the internal nasal vavle correlates with clinical valve narrowing and patient complaint. *Int. Forum Allergy Rhinol.* 3, 592-597.

[11] Spielmann, P. M., White, P. S., Hussai, S. S., (2009). Surgical technique for the treatment of nasal valve collapse: a systematic review. *Laryngoscope* 119, 1281-1290.

In: Case Reports in Surgery
Editors: Ahmad Jabir Rahyussalim et al.
ISBN: 978-1-53616-582-1

Chapter 12

The Role of Voice Therapy in Reducing Voice-Related Symptoms in Laryngopharyngeal Reflux Evaluated by Reflux Symptom Index, Voice Handicap Index, and Laryngovideostroboscopy

Elvie Zulka Kautzia Rachmawati*, Yonian Gentilis[2], Rahmanofa Yunizaf[1], Susyana Tamin[1], Fauziah Fardizza[1] and Luh Karunia Wahyuni[3]

[1]Department of Otorhinolaryngology Head and Neck Surgery,
Faculty of Medicine, Universitas Indonesia,
Jakarta, Indonesia
[2]Otorhinolaryngology Head and Neck Surgery Residency Program,
Faculty of Medicine, Universitas Indonesia,
Jakarta, Indonesia
[3]Department of Physical Medicine and Rehabilitation,
Faculty of Medicine, Universitas Indonesia,
Jakarta, Indonesia

Abstract

Patients with laryngopharyngeal reflux frequently experience refractory voice- related symptoms that are nonresponsive to antireflux therapy. New options, such as voice therapy, are alternative treatments for laryngopharyngeal reflux. To evaluate the effect of voice

* Corresponding Author's E-mail: zulka.elvie@gmail.com.

therapy in addition to medical antireflux treatment in a patient with laryngopharyngeal reflux with persistent voice-related symptoms with the use of subjective assessment by the Reflux Symptom Index and the Voice Handicap Index and objective evaluation of the vocal cords by laryngovideostroboscopy. A 48-year-old woman with laryngopharyngeal reflux presented with hoarseness and a sensation of lump in her throat for the previous 6 months. The patient had taken a proton-pump inhibitor twice a day and undergone lifestyle modification for 6 months, but there was no significant improvement. Voice therapy along with antireflux therapy and lifestyle modification was then conducted. Evaluation by subjective and objective assessments showed a significant improvement after the comprehensive treatment strategy. After voice therapy and the use of a proton-pump inhibitor, the Reflux Symptom Index decreased from 19 to 10, and the Voice Handicap Index lowered in functional (from 3 to 0) and physical (from 8 to 6) subscales. The stroboscopic findings showed significant improvement in mucosal wave (from 10% to 60%), amplitude (from 20% to 40%), open–closed phase, phase symmetry, and periodicity. Voice therapy should be considered as an adjuvant treatment to antireflux therapy and lifestyle modification in patients with laryngopharyngeal reflux presenting with refractory voice-related symptoms.

Keywords: Antireflux therapy, laryngopharyngeal reflux, laryngovide ostroboscopy, RSI, VHI-10, voice therapy

INTRODUCTION

Laryngopharyngeal reflux (LPR) is defined as the backflow of gastric contents into the larynx and pharynx [1]. LPR may be manifested as laryngeal symptoms such as cough, throat clearing, hoarseness, and globus, as well as signs of laryngeal irritation on laryngoscopy [2]. LPR occurs in 4% to 30% of patients who visit otolaryngology departments [3–5]. Up to 71%–79% of the patients with LPR complain of nonspecific symptoms, including hoarseness [6, 7].

Voice problems in LPR patients are best evaluated by subjective and objective approaches. By assessing the patient early both subjectively, using the Reflux Symptoms Index (RSI) and a 10-item Voice Handicap Index (VHI-10), and objectively, using laryngovideostroboscopy, a more efficient model for evaluation and treatment of the patient may be achieved. Vocal fold pathology in LPR is best diagnosed by laryngovideostroboscopy. Among the laryngostroboscopic findings, vocal fold edema has been suggested as the main factor affecting vibration of the vocal folds, leading to hoarseness. In addition, hyperadduction of the true vocal and vestibular folds, the presence of glottal chinks of different lengths, and reduced amplitude and mucosal wave are the main stroboscopic findings [8–11].

Treatment of LPR patients with refractory voice problems is very challenging. Proton-pump inhibitors (PPIs) are still the most effective agents for the treatment of LPR. Belafsky et al., [12] reported that symptom resolution in LPR occurred after 2 months of treatment with PPIs and that the physical findings improved more slowly after at least 6 months of treatment. Refractory voice-related symptoms of LPR that are treated by antireflux therapy have multifactorial causes. The negative loop highlighting the cough and throat clearing secondary to the subsequent accumulation of sticky mucus and globus sensations may be responsible for exacerbation of the tension applied to the mucosa and thus increase vocal microtraumas. Increasing force and subglottal pressure during phonation in the edematous vocal cords may lead to more damage of the mucosal structure. This improper technique of phonation is another factor that prolongs the healing process in injured vocal folds and may cause persistent voice-related symptoms in LPR patients [12–14].

Currently, voice therapy along with medical therapy is the mainstay of treatment for LPR patients with voice problems. The global objective of a program including direct and indirect therapy is the reduction or correction of improper use of the voice. The direct approach aims to correct posture; reduce tension in the laryngeal and cervical muscles; promote respiratory control, efficient glottal closure, and resonant equilibrium; and improve articulation. The indirect methods include raising awareness of healthy vocal habits and their importance. Voice therapy may also help to reverse mucosal changes secondary to acid reflux, inducing rapid resolution of symptoms and shortening the treatment period. Several studies have shown that voice therapy may improve RSI scores in LPR patients when used either with or without a PPI. Furthermore, behavioral voice therapy may result in alleviation of symptoms and reduction in RSI scores that do not occur with antireflux management only [15, 16].

The current study reports a case of LPR with voice disorder that did not respond to antireflux therapy. Voice therapy was conducted in addition to PPI therapy and resulted in many improvements in subjective and objective laryngeal assessment by RSI, VHI-10, and videostroboscopy. The aim of this study is to describe the importance of comprehensive therapy of PPI together with voice therapy in diminishing refractory voice-related symptoms in LPR.

CASE REPORT

A 48-year-old woman with chief complaints of hoarseness and a sensation of lump in her throat for 6 months came to the otorhinolaryngology outpatient clinic of the Ciptomangunkusumo Hospital. The patient had been previously diagnosed with LPR at a private hospital. She had taken a PPI (lansoprazole, 30 mg twice a day) and undergone lifestyle modification for 6 months; however, the symptoms did not diminish. She was then diagnosed with intractable LPR. The VHI-10 questionnaire, which has been validated for the Indonesian language, was used to subjectively evaluate the severity of the patient's dysphonia. At baseline, her VHI-10 score was 13; her RSI score was 19, with the highest scores for voice problems and globus sensation; and her RFS was 10. Neck palpation revealed increased tension of the extrinsic muscles.

The laryngovideostroboscopic evaluation showed an obvious decrease in the mucosal wave of up to 10%/10% and a decreased vibratory amplitude of up to 20%/20%. Supraglottic activity was 20% in the anteroposterior configuration. The periodicity was irregular, with closed phase dominant. There was phase asymmetry with "snake dance" appearance with posterior chink during the closed phase.

Voice therapy along with LPR medication and lifestyle modification was then advised. Voice therapy was tailored to this patient and constituted a combination of indirect and direct approaches. The indirect approaches included patient education, such as discussion of the impact of muscle tension on function, vocal hygiene, and counseling. The direct approaches included physiologic and symptomatic techniques to manipulate subsystems of voicing (respiration, phonation, and resonance). The voice therapy sessions were approximately 50 to 60 minutes in duration and were conducted weekly. All six sessions were completed in one and a half months.

Table 1. Voice Handicap Index (VHI-10) scores in a patient with refractory dysphonia due to laryngopharyngeal reflux before and after voice therapy

VHI-10 (Indonesian version)	Baseline	Follow-up
Functional subscale	3	0
Physical subscale	8	6
Emotional subscale	2	2

Table 2. Reflux Symptoms Index (RSI) scores in a patient with refractory dysphonia due to laryngopharyngeal reflux before and after voice therapy

RSI	Baseline	Follow-up
Voice problem	4	2
Clearing throat	2	0
Postnasal drip	3	3
Difficulty swallowing	3	0
Coughing after eating or lying down	0	0
Breathing difficulty	1	0
Annoying cough	0	0
Sensation of lump in the throat	4	3
Heartburn, chest pain	2	2
Total	19	10

After this comprehensive treatment, the patient was reassessed by RSI, VHI-10, and laryngovideostroboscopy. The VHI-10 showed good results after treatment, especially in the functional and physical subscales (Table 1). The RSI was successfully decreased into

10 with diminishing of voice problems (from 4 to 2 points) (Table 2). In contrast, the globus sensation showed only minimal improvement after treatment (from 4 to 3). Laryngovideostroboscopic examination revealed improvement in the edges of the vocal folds and mucosal wave that reached 60%/60% after therapy (Figure 1 and 2). Amplitude, vibratory portion, supraglottic activity, periodicity, lengthening of the closed phase, and phase symmetry also improved after voice therapy and PPI (Table 3). However, the posterior gap during closed phase was still visualized.

Table 3. Evaluation of the vibratory function of the vocal cords in a patient with refractory dysphonia due to laryngopharyngeal reflux by stroboscopy before and after voice therapy

Stroboscopy parameters	Baseline	Follow-up
Mucosal wave (%)	10/10	60/60
Amplitude (%)	20/20	40/40
Glottic closure	Posterior gap	Posterior gap
Vibratory portion (%)	20/20	60/60
Supraglottic activity (%)		
Lateromedial	0	0
Anteroposterior	20	0
Vocal folds edge	Smooth-convex	Normal
Vertical level	On plane	On plane
Periodicity	Irregular	Regular
Open–closed phase	Closed dominant	Normal
Symmetry	Asymmetry	Symmetry

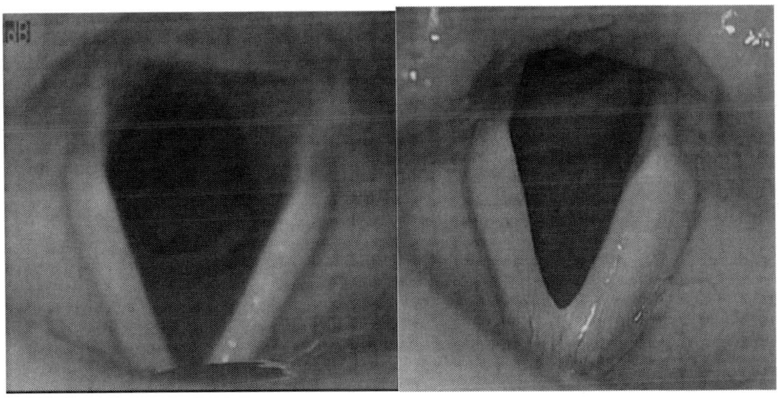

Figure 1. Vocal folds edge improved after voice therapy and proton-pump inhibitor therapy; left, before and right, after therapy.

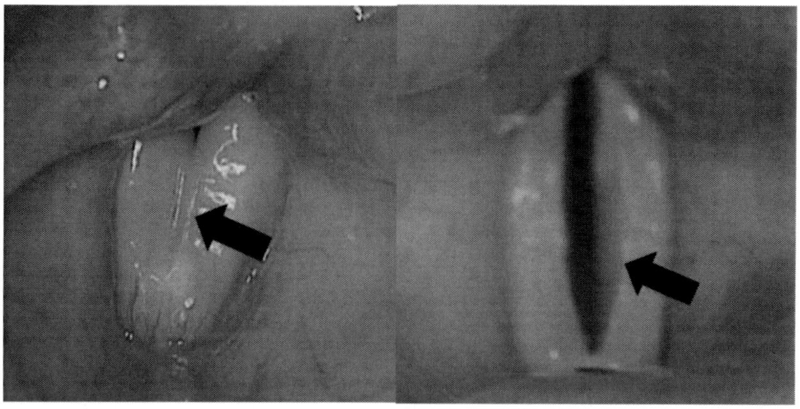

Figure 2. The mucosal wave improved after voice therapy and proton-pump inhibitor therapy; left, before and right, after therapy.

Discussion

According to the Stanford Voice and Swallowing Center Guidelines for LPR Disease, PPIs are the most effective agents for the treatment of LPR [13]. Successful treatment requires high doses for a prolonged period. The PPI should be taken twice daily for at least 6 months, depending on the severity of the LPR changes seen on examination. Improvement of symptoms is expected within 4 to 6 weeks. Usually, the visual signs of improvement according to laryngoscopy lag behind symptomatic relief by several months. Campagnolo et al., [17] recommended that pharmacologic intervention should consist of a minimum of 3 months of treatment with PPIs. Shaw et al., [18] and Pribuisiene et al., [19] analyzed the efficacy of PPIs such as omeprazole and lansoprazole and found a significant response of the laryngeal and voice-related symptoms in 8 weeks. Belafsky et al., [12] reported that symptom resolution occurred after 2 months of therapy with PPIs; however, the physical findings improved more slowly after at least 6 months of treatment. Park et al., [15] reported that 70% of the patients had a good response after 4 months of twice-daily PPI therapy. Thus, twice-daily PPI therapy for at least 4 months is reasonable, and the symptoms should improve by 2 months. However, the patient in this case report was given a PPI for 6 months with no significant subjective improvement.

The persistent voice-related symptoms of LPR treated by antireflux therapy have multifactorial causes. The negative loop highlighting the cough and throat clearing secondary to the subsequent accumulation of sticky mucus and globus sensations may be responsible for exacerbation of the tension applied to the mucosa and thus increase vocal microtraumas [14]. Increasing force and subglottal pressure in edematous vocal cords with abnormalities of vibratory function in reflux laryngitis may lead to more damage to the mucosal structure of the vocal folds. Improper techniques of phonation by LPR patients are another factor that prolongs the healing process in injured vocal folds. The refluxate also causes microtrauma to the lymphoid tissue (lingual tonsils), which may lead to hypertrophy and result in a persistent sensation of lump in the throat. In this condition, the persistent dysphonia caused by ineffective phonation techniques during speaking may induce microtrauma of the vocal folds, which worsens the voice-related symptoms and prolongs the antireflux treatment [14, 20].

Treating persistent vocal problems due to LPR after long-term antireflux therapy is very challenging. Few studies have evaluated the effectiveness of combined medical and voice therapy for this condition. The global objective of voice therapy is the reduction or correction of the improper use of the voice by a program including direct and indirect therapy. The direct approach aims to correct posture; relax the laryngeal and cervical muscles; promote respiratory control, efficient glottal closure, and resonant equilibrium; reduce voice symptoms; improve articulation; and reduce tension in the laryngeal muscles. The indirect methods include raising awareness of healthy vocal habits and their importance. Reposturing of the laryngeal anatomy using laryngeal manipulation, improving the range of motion in the neck and shoulders using manual intervention therapy, and standard physical therapy techniques in conjunction with voice therapy intervention may result in positive changes in outcome measures related to the voice. Lip trills, tongue trills, bilabial fricatives, humming, and phonation into tubes or straws have been used in speech clinics for the treatment of dysphonia. Among these techniques, trill techniques, particularly lip trills, are most commonly used [16].

Voice assessment scales are used to detect the effect of voice therapy in LPR patients. The VHI-10 is a validated voice-related quality of life questionnaire that is used individually to evaluate treatment effectiveness in benign voice disorders. Studies by Rosen et al., [21] and Craig et al., [22] reported that the VHI-10 was applied for the evaluation of treatment efficacy in voice disorders. In this case report, we used the Indonesian version of the VHI-10 that was validated and adapted by Trifani et al., [23]. Voice therapy along with medication resulted in improvement in the functional and physical subscales, but not in the emotional subscale.

Vashani et al., [24] reported that the RSI scores improved in patients who underwent voice therapy. Schneider et al., [16] reported improvements in globus, throat clearing, hoarseness, and postnasal drip after voice therapy in LPR patients, whereas a minority of patients reported improvement in gastroesophageal reflux symptoms (e.g., heartburn). This finding suggests that voice therapy effectively targets voice and laryngeal symptoms in patients with elevated RSI and VHI-10. In this case report, there was improvement in hoarseness and throat clearing, but globus and postnasal drip remained the same. Park et al., [15] showed that the symptom-associated scores (RSI and VHI-10) improved in a clinically significant manner and the time to recovery was shortened by 2 months after voice therapy in LPR patients. The authors also demonstrated that the combination of voice and PPI therapy provided a significantly greater improvement in the RSI and VHI-10 scores than PPI alone in patients diagnosed with dysphonia due to LPR.

In the stroboscopic findings, the vocal folds in patients with LPR often show mucous dehydration, unlike that in individuals with normal phonation. Woo [20] reported that a "salt and pepper" appearance was often found in the vocal folds of patients with LPR due to mucous dehydration. This was followed by reduction of the amplitude and mucosal wave and lengthening of the closed phase during sustained phonation. This finding suggests that a great driving pressure was necessary during the phonatory gesture. In some circumstances, higher driving pressure leads to increased isometric tension on the vocal folds and presses one or both vocal folds inward and reduces the amplitude of vocal fold vibrations. In this case report, the amplitude of the vocal folds was decreased to 20%/20%. Asymmetric inward compression of the vocal folds results in the abnormal vertical level of the midmembranous portion of the vocal cords. This implies that an increased shear force is being applied to the vocal fold margin. It is thought that this high-acceleration vibration is the primary mechanism of phonotrauma that is responsible for the development of benign mucosal lesions such as polyps and nodules in patients with LPR. The possible muscular hyperfunctional effect may also be secondary to a surface inflammatory reaction in LPR. Other minor pathophysiological mechanisms may be involved in voice changes, such as edema of the supraglottic structures. In this case report, the stroboscopic findings revealed that the mucosal wave was decreased to 10%/10%. Woo [20] reported that the normal mucosal wave was about one-half to two-thirds from the visible oscillating vocal folds. A decreasing mucosal wave is a sign of decreased pliability, elasticity, and viscosity in the cordal cover. Leichen et al., [25] reported that reduced hydration of the SLP in LPR may be associated with a reduction of the thickness of the cordal cover, potentiating the stability and the decrease in the mucosal wave, which is highlighted in some clinical studies. The inflammatory process in SLP modifies the biomolecular composition and biomechanical properties of this layer. Thus, the cordal cover could be less compliant, more viscous, and rigid, thus impacting the quality of the mucosal wave of the vocal folds in LPR patients [20, 25, 26].

The increased viscosity also makes it more difficult to start and maintain movement of the vocal folds, and the increased rigidity makes it more difficult to maintain the stability of the pitch; both of these events lead to irregularities in the vibratory process. In this case report, the periodicity of the vibration of the vocal folds was quite irregular [20, 25, 26].

The smooth-convex edges of the vocal folds in this patient show any fluid extravasation process in SLP and edema in the basal membrane that may lead to a "hot-dog" appearance [20]. There was also a posterior gap during the closed phase in this patient. Woo [20] reported that a posterior glottic chink or midfold contact pattern was often found in the vocal folds of LPR patients. These findings lead to an abnormal vibratory process and may lead to lengthening of the closed phase, phase asymmetry, and irregular periodicity that worsens the quality of a patient's voice. "Snake dance appearance" was revealed in this case report as a sign of the asymmetry of the open and closed phases during vibration [20, 25, 26].

Dehqan et al., [27] showed that voice therapy can cause positive changes in the regularity of vibration and suggested that there can be a decrease in excessive action of the laryngeal muscles and hoarseness. Halawa et al., [28] reported that among patients with dysphonia who had alterations in stroboscopic parameters, improvement in glottal closure, mucosal wave, vocal vibration, and asymmetry was found in 33.9%, 50%, 52.27%, and 68.75% of the cases, respectively, after voice therapy. In this case report, there was improvement of approximately 20% in the mucosal wave, amplitude, and anteroposterior supraglottic activity. There was also significant visual improvement in the periodicity, open–closed phase, and phase asymmetry after voice therapy together with PPI. We believe that these changes in the mucosal structure and vibratory function of the vocal cords led to subjective improvement in the RSI and VHI-10 in this patient.

Conclusion

Voice therapy, along with reflux medical treatment and lifestyle changes, is effective in reducing the symptoms in patients with persistent dysphonia due to LPR and should be included in the treatment of patients with LPR that fail to respond to antireflux management. Further research on the effect of voice therapy in LPR patients with dysphonia that do not respond to medical treatment, using subjective assessment tools (VHI-10 and RSI) and objective tools such as stroboscopy and voice acoustic analysis, should be conducted in the future.

References

[1] Vakil N, Zanten, Kahrilas S, Dent P, Jones R. The Montreal definition and classification of gastroesophageal reflux disease: a global evidence-based consensus. *Am. J. Gastroenterol.* 2006;101:1900.

[2] VaeziM, Richter J, Stasney C. Treatment of chronic posterior laryngitis with esomeprazole. *Laryngoscope.* 2006;116:254–60.

[3] Sen P, Georgalas C, Bhattacharyya AK. A systematic review of the roleof proton pump inhibitors for symptoms of laryngopharyngeal reflux. *Clin. Otolaryngol.* 2006;31:20–4.

[4] Jin B, Lee YS, Jeong SW, Jeong JH, Lee SH, Tae K. Change of acoustic parameters before andafter treatment in laryngopharyngeal reflux patients. *Laryngoscope* 2008;118:938–41.

[5] Koufman JA, Amin MR, Panetti M. Prevalence of reflux in 113 consecutive patients with laryngeal and voice disorders. Otolaryngol. *Head Neck Surg.* 2000;123:385–88.

[6] Koufman JA. The otolaryngologic manifestations of gastroesophageal refluxdisease (GERD): a clinical investigation of 225 patients using ambulatory 24-hour pH monitoring and an experimental investigation of the role of acid and pepsin in the development of laryngeal injury. *Laryngoscope* 1991;101:1–78.

[7] Sataloff RT, Castell DO, Katz PO. *Reflux Laryngitis and Related Disorders*. 3rd ed. San Diego, CA: Plural Publishing Inc.; 2006.

[8] Ford CN. Evaluation and management of laryngopharyngeal reflux. *JAMA*. 2005;294:1534–40.

[9] Mesallam TA, Stemple JC, Sobeih TM, Elluru RG. Reflux symptom index versus reflux finding score. *Ann. Otol. Rhinol. Laryngol.* 2007;116:436–40.

[10] Woo P. Stroboscopy. *Intepretation of Laryngeal Stroboscopy*. San Diego, CA: Plural Publishing Inc.; 2010. p. 149−166.

[11] Adhami T, Goldblum JR, Richter JE, Vaezi MF. The role of gastric and duodenal agents in laryngeal injury: an experimental canine model. *Am. J. Gastroenterol.* 2004;99:2098–106.

[12] Belafsky PC, Postma GN, Koufman JA. Validity and reliability of the reflux symptom index (RSI). *J. Voice.* 2002;16:274–7.

[13] Sung CK. Laryngopharyngeal reflux protocol. *Stanford Voice and Swallowing Center Guidelines for LPR Disease.* 2016; 1–4.

[14] Van Lierde KM, Claeys S, De Bodt M. Long-term outcome of hyperfunctional voice disorders based on a multiparameter approach. *J. Voice.* 2007;21:179–88.

[15] Park JO, Shim MR, Hwang YS, Cho KJ, Joo YH, Cho JH, et al., Combination of voice therapy and anti-reflux therapy rapidly recovers voice-related symptoms in laryngopharyngeal reflux patients. *Otolaryngol. Head Neck Surg*. 2011;146:92–7.

[16] Schneider SL, Clary M, Fink DS, Wang SX, Chowdury FN, Yadlapati R, et al., Voice therapy associated with a decrease in the reflux symptoms index in patients with voice complaints. *Laryngoscope* 2018;129:1169–73.

[17] Campagnolo AM, Priston J. Laryngopharyngeal reflux: diagnosis, treatment and latest research. *Int. Arch. Otorhinolaryngol.* 2014;18:184–91.

[18] Shaw G, Searl J. Laryngeal manifestations of gastroesophageal reflux before and after treatment with omeprazole. *South. Med. J.* 1997;90: 1115–22.

[19] Pribuisiene R, Uloza V, Kupcinskas L. Perceptual and acoustic characteristics of voice changes in reflux laryngitis patients. *J. Voice.* 2006;20:128–36.

[20] Woo P. Stroboscopy. *Abnormal Vocal Folds Vibration*. San Diego, CA: Plural Publishing Inc.; 2010. p. 89−104.

[21] Rosen CA, Murry T, Zinn A, Zullo T, Sonbolian M. Voice handicap index change following treatment of voice disorders. *J. Voice.* 2000;14:619–23.

[22] Craig J, Tomlinson C, Stevens K, Kotagal K, Fornadley J, Jacobson B, Garrett CG, Francis DO. Combining voice therapy and physical therapy: A novel approach to treating muscle tension dysphonia. *J. Commun. Disord.* 2015;58:169–78.

[23] Trifani S, Hutauruk S. Uji ValiditasdanReliabilitas Voice Handicap Index-30 Adaptasi Bahasa Indonesia. Tesis Fakultas Kedokteran Universitas Indonesia. 2018.

[24] Vashani K, Murugesh M, Hattiangadi G. Effectiveness of voice therapy in reflux-related voice disorders. *Dis. Esophagus.* 2009;23:27–32.

[25] Lechien JR, Khalife M, Delvaux V. Pathophysiology, assessment andtreatment of laryngopharyngeal reflux. Rev. Laryngol. *Otol. Rhinol.* 2014;135:163–70.

[26] Reichel O, Mayr D, Durst F, Berghaus A. E-cadherin but not beta-catenin expression is decreased in laryngeal biopsies from patients with laryngopharyngeal reflux. *Eur. Arch. Otorhinolaryngol.* 2008; 265:937–42.

[27] Dehqan A, Scherer RC. Positive effects of manual circumlaryngeal therapy in the treatment of muscle tension dysphonia: long term treatment outcomes. *J. Voice.* 2018;35:1–6.

[28] Halawa WE, Munoz IV, Perez SS. Effectiveness of laryngostroboscopy for monitoring the evolution of functional dysphonia after rehabilitator treatment. *Indian J. Otolaryngol.* 2013;65:322–6.

In: Case Reports in Surgery
Editors: Ahmad Jabir Rahyussalim et al.
ISBN: 978-1-53616-582-1

Chapter 13

Maxillary Fibrous Dysplasia Reconstruction after Maxillectomy

Dini Widiarni Widodo*, and Razki Yorivan
Department of Otorhinolaryngology Head and Neck Surgery, Faculty of Medicine
Universitas Indonesia – Dr. Cipto Mangunkusumo General Hospital,
Jakarta, Indonesia

Abstract

Fibrous dysplasia is frequently managed with open maxillectomy, and the technique employed depends on the location of the lesion. Mid-facial reconstruction after maxillectomy is a complicated and difficult process. Clinicians require expertise and must exercise caution when closing the defect, taking into consideration both aesthetics and function. Post-maxillectomy reconstruction using titanium alloplastic material has various advantages. To present a case of maxillary fibrous dysplasia treated with suprastructure maxillectomy followed by reconstruction to close the defect. Reconstruction uses titanium mesh plates and muscle slings, with the facial contour and tissues lost during the suprastructure maxillectomy taken into consideration. Various types of maxillectomy and post-maxillectomy defects have been classified with the aim of facilitating reconstruction and guiding the clinician through the process. The reconstruction of suprastructure maxillectomy using a titanium mesh plate and muscle sling is effective and produces good results in function and aesthetics.

Keywords: fibrous dysplasia, suprastructure maxillectomy, mid-facial reconstruction, titanium mesh plate, muscle sling, aesthetic

* Corresponding Author's E-mail: dini_pancho@yahoo.com.

Introduction

Mid-facial defect reconstruction is an intricate and complicated process and represents a major challenge during head and neck tumor surgery. Available management options are pedicle flap, implant, and free flap, which are often combined with transplantation. The main problem with mid-facial reconstruction is the wide range of defects caused by tumor resection. Corresponding defects not only affect the maxillary bone but also affect the surrounding tissues, facial bone, cranial bone, soft tissue, and orbital bone. An important aspect of maxillary reconstruction is the repair of the maxillary walls. Successful mid-facial reconstruction requires expertise in reconstruction using both implants and a flap to ensure good rehabilitation [1, 2].

Fibrous dysplasia is a fibro-osseous benign lesion with an unknown cause. Fibrous dysplasia lesions in the maxillary area eventually extend to the maxillary sinus, zygomatic bone, sphenoid, and orbital floor. Management of fibrous dysplasia requires taking into consideration the size and location of the lesion. Large lesions require surgical intervention, which may result in significant functional and cosmetic damage to the face and will indirectly affect the quality of life of the patient [3, 4].

This report presents information on a maxillary fibrous dysplasia case treated with suprastructure maxillectomy and subsequently reconstructed with a mesh plate and muscle sling.

Frequency

The frequency of fibrous dysplasia is 1:30,000 individuals, and the disease comprises 2.5% of all bone tumors and 7.5% of all benign bone tumors. The incidence of monostotic fibrous dysplasia is evenly distributed in men and women. This type occurs more often than the polystotic type. The incidence of the polystotic type in men is thrice than that in women. Both types of fibrous dysplasia commonly occur in children and adolescents [5, 6].

Fibrous dysplasia was managed using maxillectomy techniques in 15.2% of 66 cases reported in 2016 in Nigeria. Reports published in 2006 in Malaysia describe the use of maxillectomy for 24 benign maxillary tumor cases, comprising 41% of all cases in the country. The data collected from 2000 to 2009 showed that 26.4% of 65 benign tumor cases were treated with maxillectomy [7–9].

ANATOMY AND PHYSIOLOGY

The mid-facial area includes some of the most prominent structures of the face and separates the oral and orbital cavities. This structure is a polyhedron bounded by skeletal bones. In addition to its structural anatomy, the mid-facial area has functional properties related to breathing, phonation, chewing, swallowing, vision, and smelling. This area has two maxillary bones in the form of polyhedrons separated by the middle part of the face covering the nasal region. The center includes facial features such as the nose, cheeks, and upper lip, whereas the back extends to the anterior skull base. The superoinferior region includes soft tissue and bone from the orbital cavity to the oral cavity, and the middle surface extends towards the temporal bone. This structure includes various tissues surrounded by muscles, skin, and mucosa [10].

An important structure in the mid-facial area is a pair of maxillary bones that join the intermaxilla to form the maxilla. The maxilla contributes to the formation of three cavity walls, namely, the roof of the mouth, the base and lateral wall of the nose, and the medial orbital wall and base. The maxilla attaches to the lateral side of the zygomatic bone. The attachment consists of the base and lateral wall of the orbit, giving the cheek its distinct shape. The maxillary bone is also associated with the frontal and ethmoid bones, nasal bone, lacrimal bone, inferior nasal turbines, palate, and vomer [1]. The orbit is a structure bordering the mid-facial region. The frontal bone is the superior boundary of the orbit, whereas the inferior boundaries of the orbit are the maxilla, palate, and zygomatic bone. The medial boundaries of the orbit are the frontal, lacrimal, and ethmoid bone. The lateral border is the zygomatic bone. The orbit is located inferior to the anterior fossa of the cranial base and superior to the maxillary sinus and is lateral to the nasal cavity. The anterior border of the orbit is the medial fossa of the cranial base and the temporal fossa (Figure 1) [1].

The mid-facial area has a structure called the support wall. This wall functions to maintain the mid-facial area under normal conditions. This support wall is broadly divided into the vertical and horizontal support walls. The vertical support wall is composed of the nasofrontal, pterygomaxillary, and zygomaticomaxillary borders. The three borders serve as the foundation that maintains the mid-facial area in an upright position, forming the anatomy and function of the maxilla. The zygomaticomaxillary border stretches from the maxillary frontal process along the inferior orbital ridge to the zygomatic process of the frontal bone. The pterygomaxillary border extends from the anterior alveolar ridge to the pterygoid plate of the sphenoid bone. The nasomaxillary border extends from the anterior maxillary alveolus along the piriformis aperture to the nasal process of the maxilla (Figure 2) [2, 10].

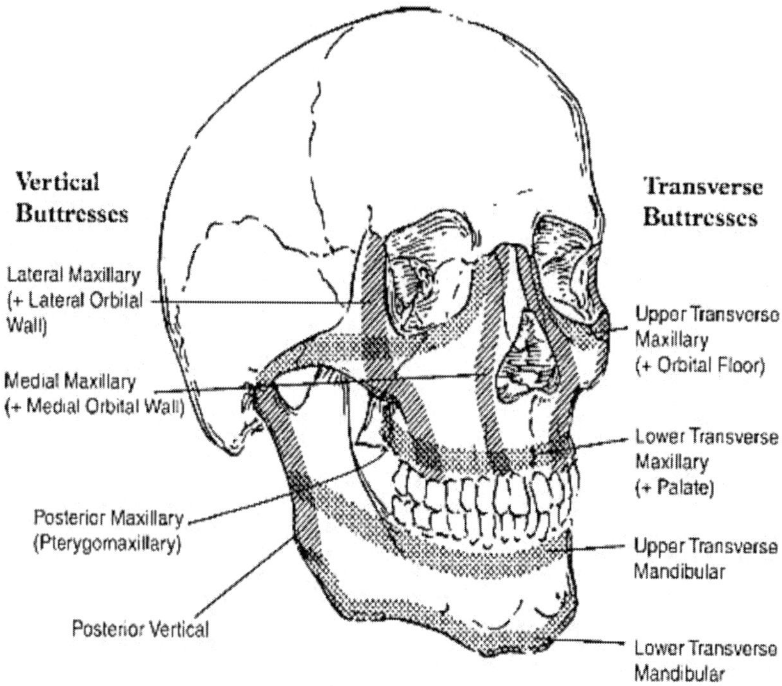

Figure 1. Horizontal and vertical support walls [11].

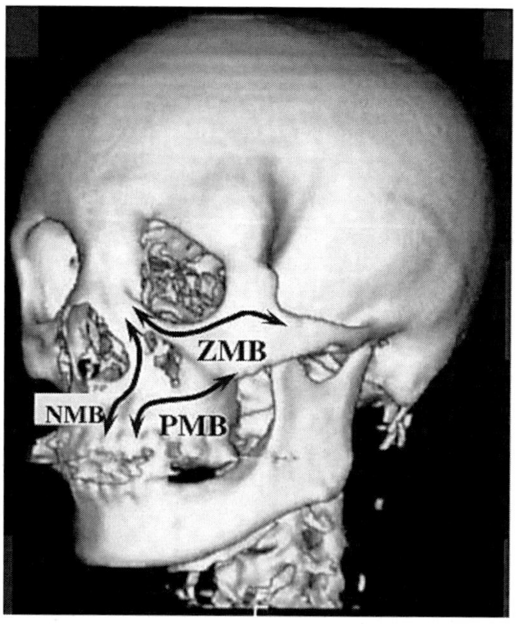

Figure 2. Vertical support wall. Nasomaxillary border (NMB), zygomaticomaxillary border (ZMB), and pterigomaxillary border (PMB) [2].

The muscles that control facial expressions are located in the midline and are covered by facial skin. The outer surface of the face is divided into the cheeks, nose, and lips. All of these units have different characteristics and require special attention during reconstruction. The parotid glands are another important structure on the medial surface and are located in the most lateral region. These glands do not only function as salivary glands but also provide soft tissue for facial contours [10].

The mid-facial blood supply primarily originates from the branch of the external carotid artery. The anastomosis of this artery, such as branching of the infraorbital artery and internal maxillary artery, provides good vascularization to the skin. This pattern of anastomosis branching is very important in the management of mid-facial reconstruction. Mid-facial innervation is provided by cranial nerves, namely, the facial and trigeminal nerves. The facial nerve is responsible for facial movements, and the trigeminal nerve is responsible for the mastication muscle. Sensory innervation of the facial muscles is supplied by the branches of the trigeminal nerve [10].

Facial skin and soft tissue receive arterial supplies from branches of the facial temporal artery, maxilla, and all branches of the external carotid artery. Blood supply to the forehead, eyelids, and upper part of the nose is supplied through the internal carotid system by the ophthalmic artery. Blood supply to the lip region is supplied by inferior and superior labial arteries. The facial artery near the medial canthus next to the nose is the angular artery. The maxillary artery is the terminal branch of the external carotid artery with three main branches: the mental, buccal, and infraorbital arteries. The mental artery is the terminal branch of the inferior alveolar artery that passes through the mental foramen to supply the chin and lower lip. The buccal artery crosses the buccinator muscle to supply the cheek tissue [12].

The infraorbital arteries reach the face through the infraorbital foramen and supply the eyelids, cheeks, and lower nose. The deep temporal artery is the terminal branch of the external carotid artery and crosses the superficial zygomatic arch in the superficial temporal fascia. The deep temporal artery is divided into anterior and posterior branches at 2 cm above the zygomatic arch. The anterior branch supplies the forehead and forms anastomosis with supraorbital and supratrochlear vessels, whereas the posterior branch supplies the parietal scalp and periosteum. The ophthalmic artery is a branch of the internal carotid system; its branches include the lacrimal, supraorbital, supratrochlear, infratrochlear, and external nasal arteries (Figure 3) [12].

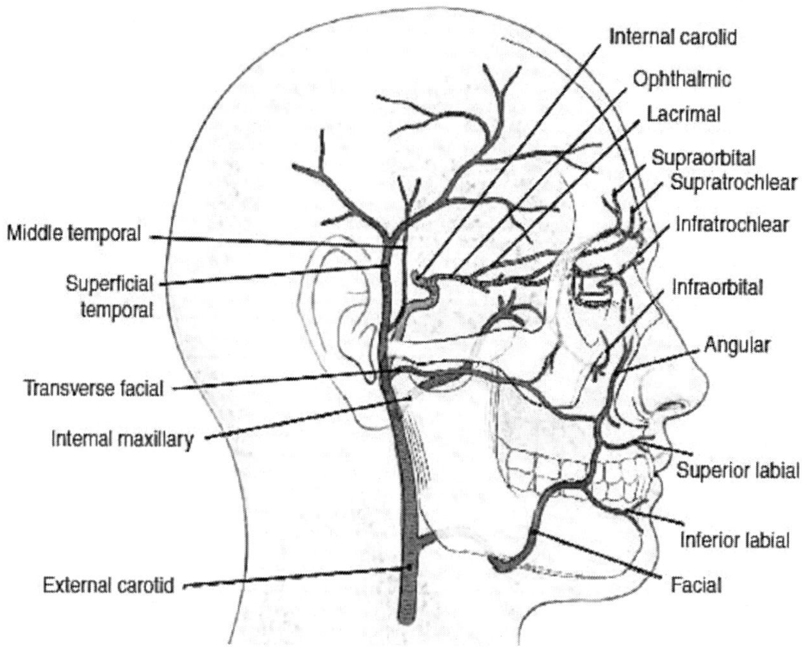

Figure 3. Scheme of facial arteries [12].

Facial Fat Compartments

Superficial Fat Tissue

The face has several compartments. Each compartment is separated by a network of fine fascia that forms a retaining ligament. The superficial facial fat layer consists of (1) the labial nasal fat compartment; (2) medial, middle, and lateral temporozygomatic fat pads; (3) medial, middle, and lateral temporozygomatic fat pads on the forehead; and (4) superior, inferior, and lateral orbital fat pads [12].

Nasolabial fat is located in the medial cheek adipose compartment and contributes to the nasolabial fold. The orbicularis retaining ligament below the inferior orbital plate borders the superior border of the nasolabial fat compartment and the medial cheek compartment. The middle fat compartment is limited by a group of fascia called the superior zygomatic septum on the superior side. The anterior border of the lateral temporal fat pads is the lateral zygomatic septum, which can be found during a facelift procedure with a dissection medial to the preauricular incision. The superior and inferior orbital fat compartments are located within the boundary of the orbicularis retaining ligaments located above and below the eye. These periorbital fat pads are separated from each other by the medial and lateral canthus. The lateral orbital fat compartment has two borders: the superior border, which is the inferior temporal septum, and the inferior border, which is the superior zygomatic septum. The main zygomatic muscle is attached to the superficial fat compartment [12].

The anatomy of the superficial subcutaneous fat compartment has an impact on the facial contour. Differences in the volume at each level will cause deviations in the facial contour and loss of facial concavity [12].

Deep Fat Compartment

The suborbicularis oculi fat has two parts: the medial and lateral parts. The medial component is located along the margins of the inferior orbit, from the medial limbus towards the lateral canthus. The lateral component runs from the lateral canthus to the temporal fat pad. The prezygomal space lies between the suborbicularis oculi fat and the zygomatic periosteum. This space has superior borders, which are the orbicularis retaining ligament and the zygomatic retaining ligament. The sublevator fat pad is located medially from the medial suborbicularis fat compartment and is the deepest infraorbital pad. This fat pad is a continuation of the buccal fat pad. The buccal fat pad is an important structure located in the posterolateral part of the superficial maxilla towards the buccinator muscle and extends deep into the anterior part of the masseter muscle. Functionally, the buccal fat pad facilitates the movement of masticatory muscles (Figures 4-7) [12].

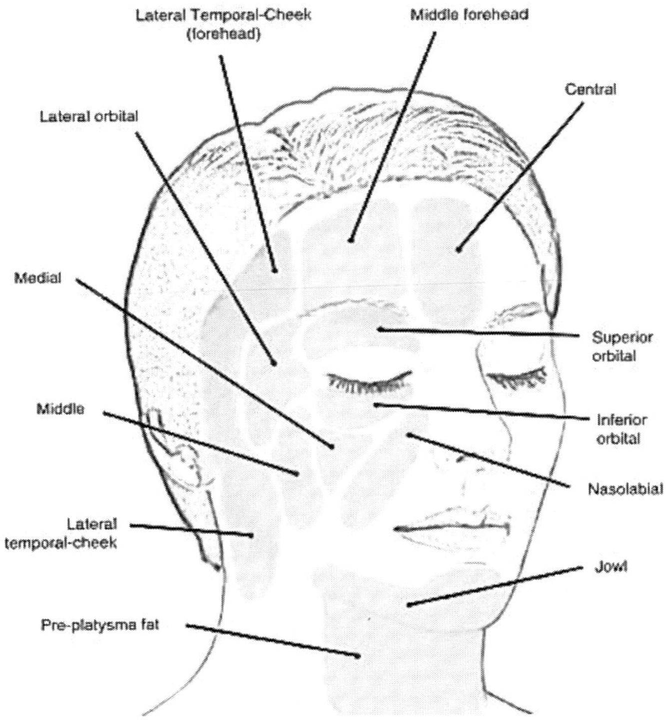

Figure 4. Superficial fat compartment [12].

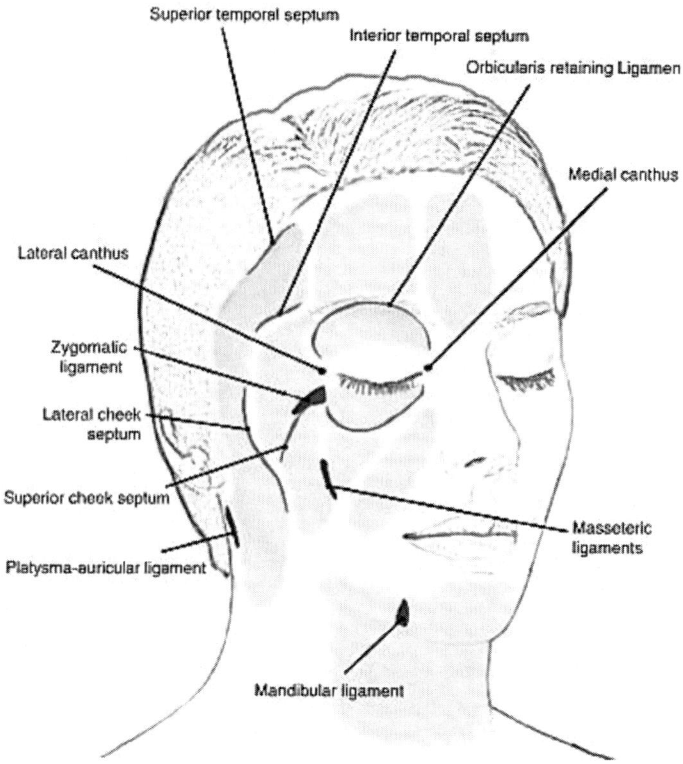

Figure 5. Ligaments between superficial fat compartments [12].

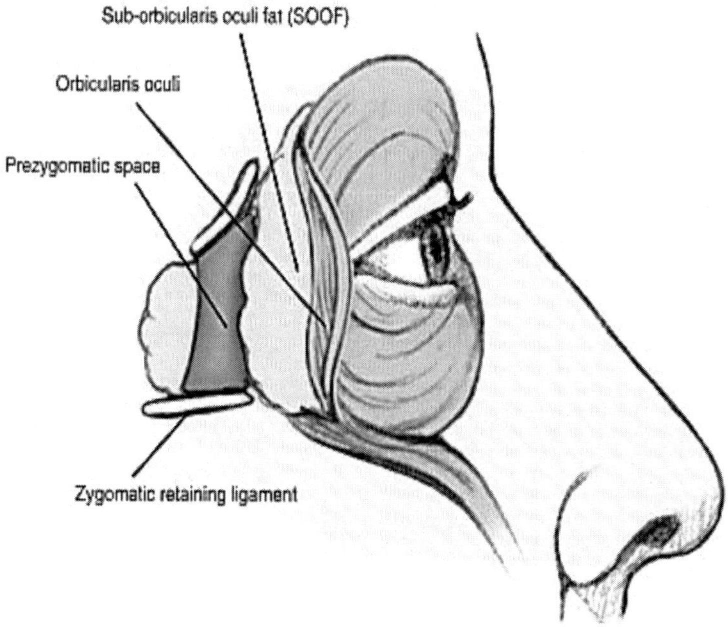

Figure 6. Suborbicularis oculi fat [12].

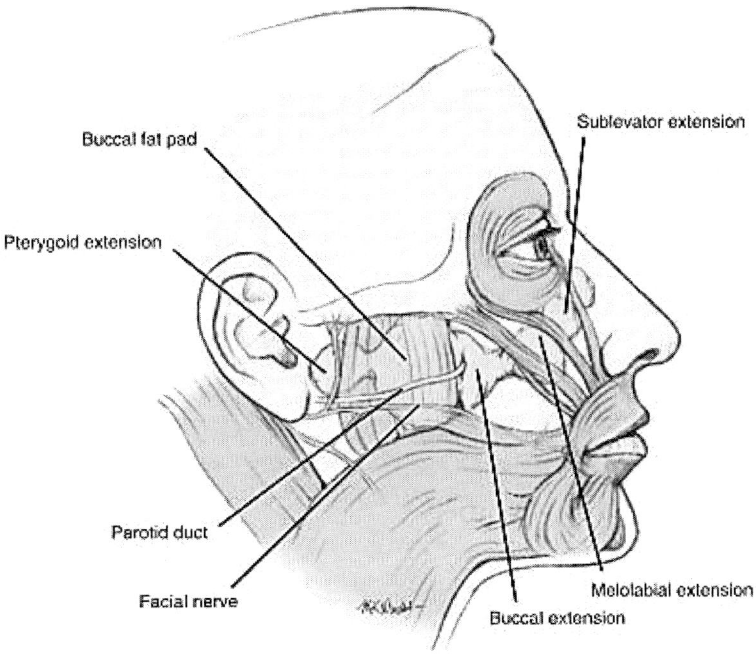

Figure 7. Buccal fat pad [12].

Fibrous Dysplasia

Fibrous dysplasia is an asymptomatic disease. The disease occurs in the maxilla more often than in the mandible. In the maxilla, fibrous dysplasia manifests with edema, no pain, and is sometimes followed by café-au-lait spots. The mass may be large enough to interfere with the chewing function. In the mandible, swelling can involve the labial, buccal, and lingual areas [6, 13].

Extensive maxillary lesions can involve the maxillary sinus, zygomatic bone, sphenoid bone, and orbital base. Unstable swelling that continues to increase for a long time can result in an asymmetrical face shape. Nasal obstruction can occur when the paranasal sinuses are involved. In some cases, exophthalmus and tooth dislocation can occur because of malocclusion. Lesions that extend to the temporal bone can cause hearing loss [13–15].

Fibrous dysplasia lesion is a fibro-osseous lesion. These types of lesions have three variants: monostotic, polystotic, and McCune–Albright syndromes, which are associated with endocrinopathy and hyperpigmentation. Fibrous dysplasia occurs from the mutation of the guanine nucleotide-binding protein alpha-stimulating activity polypeptide 1 (GNAS-1) gene. Proteoblasts are formed because of proliferation and differentiation triggered by c-AMP. The GNAS-1 mutation results in encoding of the α-subunit during transduction of the G-protein signal, which results in the increase of c-AMP production [16, 17].

The severity of the disease depends on when the gene mutation occurred during pregnancy or after birth. If the mutation occurred during the embryonic phase, the osteoblasts, melanocytes, and endocrine cells will carry the gene mutations and express the genes in the form of multiple bone lesions and pigmentation accompanied by endocrine disorders, leading to the McCune–Albright syndrome. Cells that mutate at the end of the embryonic phase will spread and fuse with bone to form multiple bone lesions, resulting in polystotic type fibrous dysplasia. Gene mutations that occur after birth will result in progenitor cell mutations that attach to one bone, resulting in monostotic type fibrous dysplasia [17,18].

FACIAL INCISION APPROACH

Surgical treatment for maxillectomy requires facial incisions to expose the maxillary bone. The type of incision depends on the tumor location, histology, and the surgeon's experience. Open surgery achieves good exposure of the tumor location, particularly for extensive resection [19].

Open surgery can be performed with various approaches. Five types of incisions can be employed to expose the maxilla: lateral rhinotomy incision, Weber–Ferguson incision, Weber–Ferguson incision with Lynch expansion, Weber–Ferguson incision with lateral expansion, and Weber–Ferguson incision with subciliary expansion [19].

Lateral rhinotomy is a basic incision that can be performed on the lesion without the involvement of the orbit or palate. The incision starts from the middle of the dorsum nasi to the medial canthus. The incision is performed following the shape of the face along the lateral edge of the nose to the ala nasi. The Weber–Ferguson incision is performed by continuing the incision in the ala nasi, curving through the nasal vestibule and then continuing with the upper lip edge incision on the philtrum from the nasolabial gap to the vermilion border followed by an incision in the gingivobuccal. After the incision is made and the facial bones are exposed, osteotomy is performed according to the location and size of the tumor. The approach requires calculation of the position of the nasal pyramid as an aesthetic consideration. A tumor that involves the entire nasal cavity and maxillary sinus with posterior sinus wall erosion can be treated using Weber–Ferguson's incision, which enables maximal exposure of the tumor [19, 20].

The Weber–Ferguson incision with Lynch expansion is performed by extending the incision in the middle of the medial canthus towards the lower border of the eyebrows. The aim is to expand the exposure to the ethmoid cells, frontal sinuses, nasolacrimal ducts, and medial canthus ligaments. The Weber–Ferguson incision with lateral expansion is performed by pulling an incision from the middle of the medial canthus to the lateral canthus through the skin folds of the inferior eyelid. The Weber–Ferguson incision with subciliary extension requires an incision just below the inferior eyelid cilia. The Weber–

Ferguson incision with lateral and subciliary expansion have a same goals to expanding the exposure of the infraorbital rim and the zygoma (Figure 8) [19].

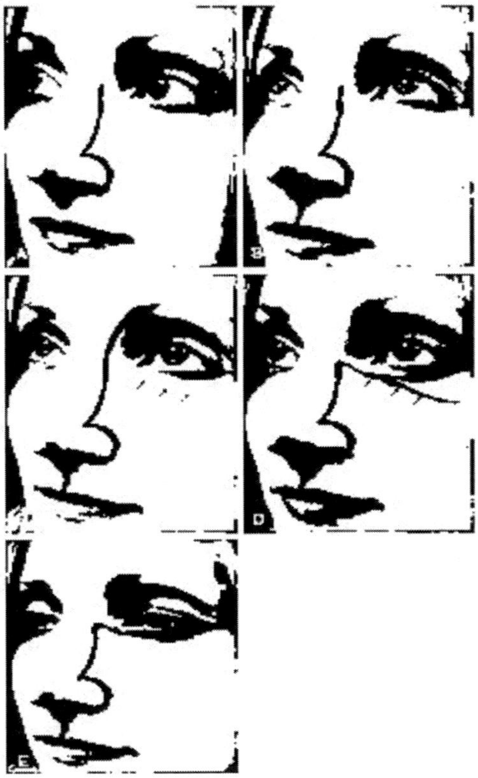

Figure 8. Facial incision scheme. (A) Lateral rhinotomy incision, (B) Weber–Ferguson incision, (C) Weber–Ferguson incision with Lynch expansion, (D) Weber–Ferguson incision with lateral expansion, and (E) Weber–Ferguson incision with subciliary expansion [19].

MAXILLECTOMY

The maxillectomy procedure was first performed in 1820 and was first documented by Liston in 1841 in patients with nasopharyngeal angiofibroma. The aim of this surgical technique is to manage tumors in the nasal cavity, the lateral wall of the nose, and the maxillary sinus by removing the maxillary sinus bone [21, 22].

Several types of maxillectomy have been identified. Based on the writing by Hanna [22], the long-known types of maxillectomy are medial maxillectomy, inferior maxillectomy, superior maxillectomy, subtotal maxillectomy, and total maxillectomy.

Medial maxillectomy involves removing the lateral nasal wall and the medial segment of the maxillary bone, which is bordered by the infraorbital nerve on the lateral side accompanied by a sphenoetmoidectomy. Intracellular maxillectomy is a procedure that involves inferior resection of the maxilla under the infraorbital nerve plane. This technique is most commonly used for tumors in the maxillary alveolar process with minimal extension to the maxillary antrum and hard palate lesions. The combination of sublabial and palatal incisions is used to expose the maxilla followed by osteotomy. Mid-facial degloving can be used for lesions that cross in the midline and bilaterally involve the inferior maxilla [22].

Suprastructure maxillectomy is a procedure performed by maintaining the structure of the hard palate while resecting the floor of the orbit and the upper part of the maxilla. This procedure requires reconstruction of the orbital floor so that the eyeball does not fall towards the maxilla. Subtotal maxillectomy is a variation of maxillary resection in which the resection is carried out depending on the location of the tumor. Total maxillectomy involves resection of the entire maxilla, orbital floor, and palate (Figures 9-11) [22].

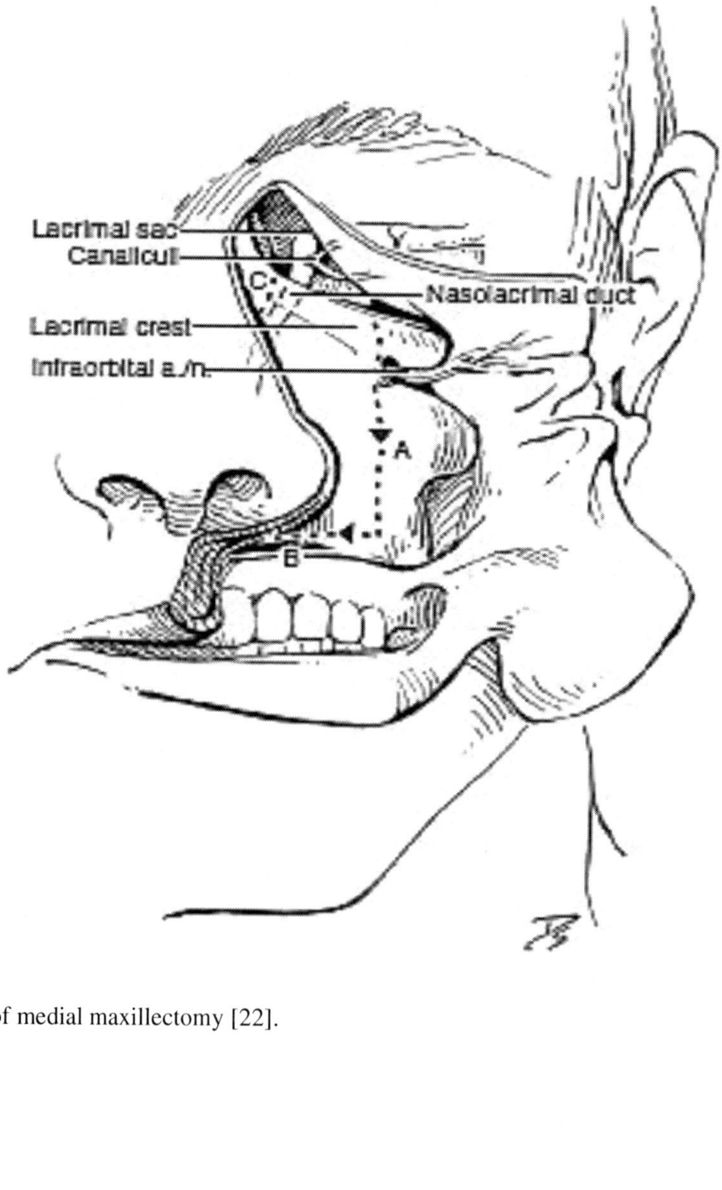

Figure 9. Scheme of medial maxillectomy [22].

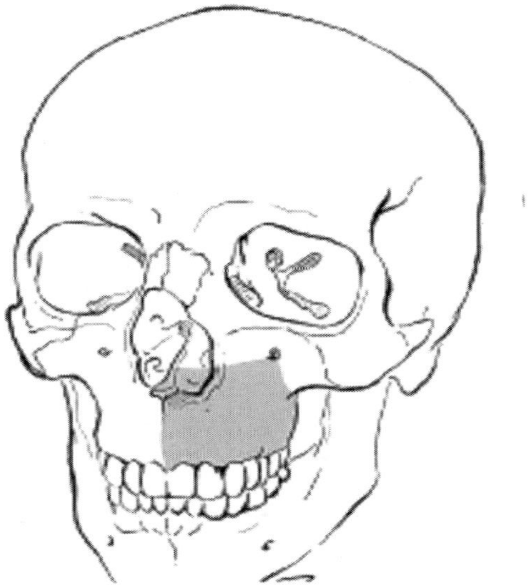

Figure 10. Scheme of inferior maxillectomy [22].

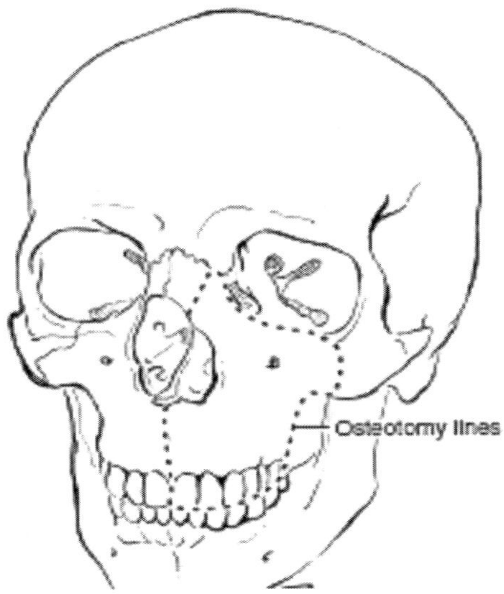

Figure 11. Scheme osteotomy lines of total maxillectomy [22].

Spiro et al. [23] reported another maxillectomy classification based on a study of 403 patients who fulfilled one of the three criteria for maxillectomy. These criteria were related to the number of maxillary walls resected and can be defined as limited, subtotal, and total maxillectomy.

Limited maxillectomy refers to all types of maxillectomy involving resection of only a maxillary wall in the antrum, usually the medial wall or maxillary base. Subtotal maxillectomy is a procedure in which at least two maxillary walls are resected, including the maxillary antrum floor, but resection does not reach the posterior maxillary wall.

This procedure includes resection of the pterygoid plate, soft palate, contralateral maxilla, zygoma, and nasal complex. Total maxillectomy is the removal of the maxilla accompanied by an orbital exenteration [23].

Post-Maxillectomy Defect

There are various classifications of post-maxillectomy defects proposed to describe the resulting damage. These classifications were developed to guide reconstruction and rehabilitation [21].

Bidra et al. [24] concluded that the classification of defects must meet surgical and prosthodontic needs, be simple, comprehensive, easy to use, and be able to guide clinicians regarding reconstruction and rehabilitation options. Post-maxillectomy defects are classified into six criteria: dental defects, oronasal or orantral defects, defects of the soft palate and surrounding tissue, defect expansion to the superoinferior area, defect expansion to the anteroposterior area, and defect expansion to the mediolateral area.

Expansion of the superoinferior defect may originate from the oroantral fistule, giving rise to a defect that borders the skull base superiorly and the tongue inferiorly. Therefore, superior and inferior expansion of the defect will extend into the alveolar level, palatal level, paranasal sinuses, orbit, and the anterior base of the skull bone. The size of the defect determines the technique used for reconstruction. The expansion of the anteroposterior defect occurs in the horizontal and sagittal fields with the involvement of the right-left posterior region, and the right-left anterior maxilla. An anterior defect can cause reduced lip movement, scar tissue on the lips, and the collapse of the nose when the nasal bone is removed.

Expansion of the mediolateral defect can cause a unilateral defect involving only one maxillary bone, whereas the bilateral defect involves both maxilla. Unilateral defect reconstruction requires less tissue than the reconstruction of bilateral defects. However, this depends on the tissue conditions, and the reconstruction can be followed by implant placement [24].

Brown et al. [25] classified post-maxillectomy defect into two categories, namely, vertical and horizontal defects. This classification is also reported in the literature review conducted by Bidra et al. [24] Vertical defects are divided into six types: maxillectomy without oronasal fistula, maxillectomy without orbital involvement, maxillectomy with orbital tissue involvement, maxillectomy with orbital enucleation, orbitomaxillary defect, and nasomaxillary defect. Horizontal defects are divided into four types: palate defect without alveolar involvement, unilateral defects less than or equal to half the palate, bilateral defects less than or equal to half the palate, and bilateral defects greater than half the palate (Figures 12, 13).

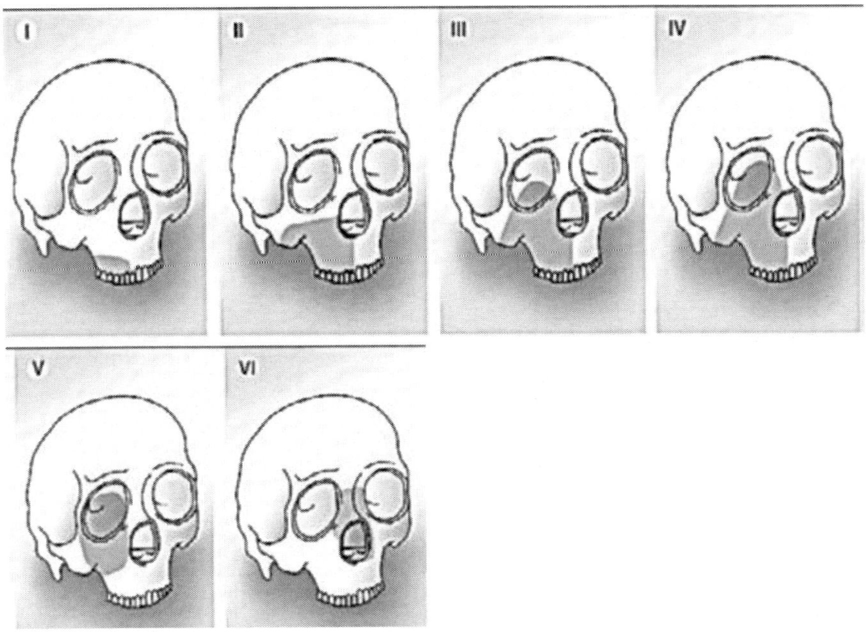

Figure 12. Vertical defect. (I) Maxillectomy without oronasal fistule, (II) maxillectomy without orbital involvement, (III) maxillectomy without orbital tissue involvement, (IV) maxillectomy with orbital enucleation, (V) orbitomaxillary defect, and (VI) nasomaxillary defect [25].

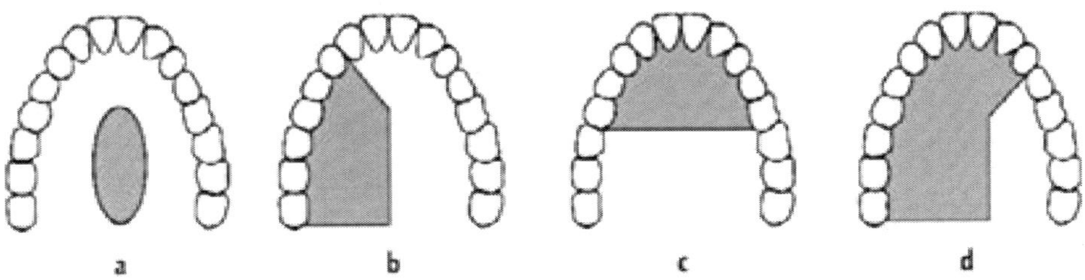

Figure 13. Horizontal defect. (a) Palate defect without alveolar defect, (b) unilateral defects less than or equal to half the palate, (c) bilateral defects less than or equal to half the palate, and (d) bilateral defects greater than half the palate [25].

SUPRASTUCTURE MAXILLECTOMY RECONSTRUCTION

Maxillofacial reconstruction can be performed with various materials, such as titanium mesh, hydroxyapatite gel, silica gel, bone, and ribs. Use of autologous material for maxillofacial reconstruction will aggravate the condition after maxillectomy due to injuries to the corresponding donor site [26].

The main goal of mid-facial reconstruction is to improve facial contours, eye volume, and position. The irregularity and thinness of the facial and eye anatomy as well as the contours of the face present obstacles to maxillofacial reconstruction. Titanium mesh is the most commonly used material for maxillofacial and orbital reconstruction. The advantages of using titanium mesh for reconstruction include good fabrication quality, stability, tool flexibility, the absence of tissue damage due to donor requirements, and the short duration of surgery. Post maxillectomy and resection, the defect is always extensive from the maxilla towards the zygoma and orbital floor, thus requiring diverse mesh and plates as well as tissue to protect the mesh [26].

The successful reconstruction of orbital floors with titanium mesh depends on two factors. First is the formation recovery of the individual orbital floor, and the second is the precise position of the titanium mesh installation. Important parameters for mid-facial reconstruction with good aesthetic results are contour recovery, maxillary volume, and eyeball position, as well as rehabilitation of the infraorbital area contour. The eyeball position is maintained by a balance between the orbit volume and intraorbital soft tissue. Balance disorders will cause a decrease in orbital content and can cause enophthalmus, which is a post-maxillectomy problem [26].

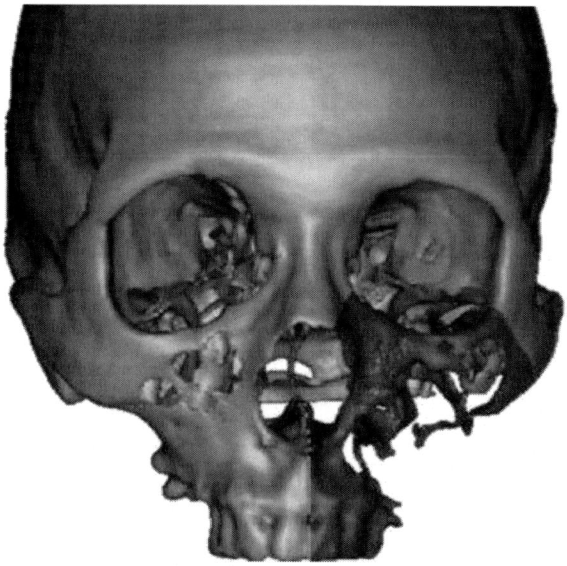

Figure 14. Virtual image of post-maxillectomy defect [26].

Alloplastic materials used for reconstruction must be able to integrate with the body. Titanium is a metal material first discovered by William Gregor in 1791 and used commercially in 1950. It was first used for a medical purpose in 1980. This material is anti-corrosive, elastic, unaffected by temperature changes, and has good bio-compatibility. The chemical composition of this material is capable of producing good integration between titanium and bone without causing fibrosis. Titanium will not inhibit tissue growth even with extensive defects in the maxillofacial region because the material interacts well with the soft tissues of the body [27, 28].

Although titanium mesh is an ideal choice for the reconstruction of orbit floors, some risks remain. The main risks are infection and exposure to titanium mesh, especially for tumor patients undergoing radiotherapy. Hypovascular tissue and extensive fibrosis after radiotherapy increase the risk of infection and exposure to titanium mesh (Figures 14, 15) [27].

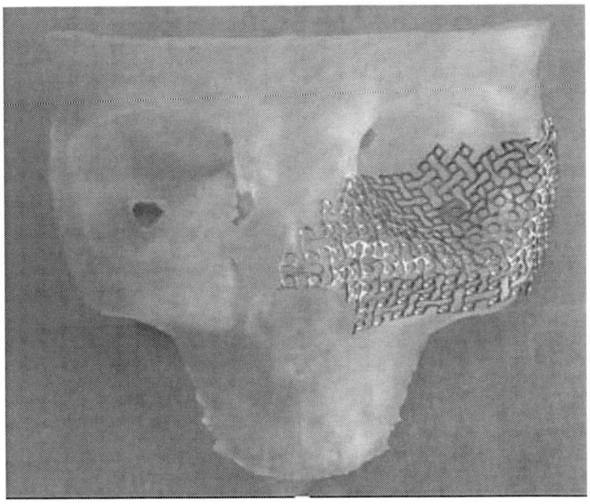

Figure 15. Titanium mesh used in the reconstruction of post-maxillectomy defect [26].

CASE REPORT

This paper presents the case of a patient with fibrous dysplasia treated with suprastructure maxillectomy. Reconstruction was later performed using titanium mesh and muscular buccal muscle slings.

An 11-year-olds girl was referred to the Oncology ENT division for reconstruction after the removal of a left maxillary tumor through suprastructure maxillectomy. The patient had a complaint of swelling in the left cheek accompanied by left eye exophthalmus and decreased vision starting 6 months earlier. She also complained of nasal congestion without nosebleeds and pain starting 4 months before hospital admission.

The patient was examined with computer tomography, which showed the compacting of the maxillary sinus, ethmoid and left sphenoid, with multiple calcification complexes in the ethmoid sinus accompanied by ethmoid, maxillary, and left sphenoid bone destruction extending to the left retrobulbar region, suspected as a sinonasal mass. Examination of magnetic resonance imaging shows a suspected benign solid tumor of the left ethmoid sinus with left orbital thrusting and a left osteomeatal complex that causes left proptosis, left sphenoid, and maxillary sinusitis (Figures 16).

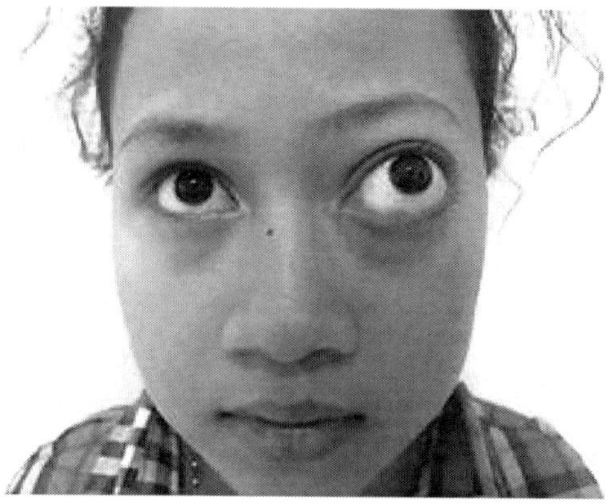

Figure 16. Asymetrical and protrution eye.

The patient was diagnosed with suspected maxillary fibroma, and suprastructure maxillectomy was planned by Oncology division Department of Otorhino-laryngology Head and Neck Surgery. The tumor tissue was sent to the Anatomy Pathology Department for histopathological examination. Post-maxillectomy, enophthalmus was found in the left eye with a posterior movement when the eyes were tightly closed. The patient was referred to the Plastic Recontruction division Department of Otorhinolaryngology Head and Neck Surgery for post-maxillectomy defect reconstruction.

After tumor removal surgery, defects occurred in several locations, including the anterior maxillary wall, medial maxillary wall, inferior wall of the left orbital rhyme, and enophthalmus, with a posterior movement when the eyes were closed firmly. At the beginning of the reconstruction, a sharp dissection was performed to expose the left buccal mucosa and muscle. Afterwards, a sling was created by sewing the end of the muscle to the medial canthus to form eye pads, followed by suturing the left septal mucosa to the medial canthus of the left eye. A titanium plate was sewn onto the buccal muscle sling to match the projection of the nasal lateral wall and form the medial wall of the left maxilla. The titanium mesh was shaped in accordance with the shape of the anterior maxillary wall and then sewn and fixed using screws. The reconstructed defect was closed using subcutaneous sutures following the directions for the Weber–Ferguson incision with Lynch extension to the gingivobuccal.

After the surgery, the patient was given ceftriaxone 2 gr once a day, ranitidine 50 mg twice a day, ketorolac 30 mg three times a day, and tranexamic acid 500 mg three times a day. The patient was fed a liquid diet through the nasogastric tube. An edema of the left orbit appeared and decreased on the second day after surgery, and the left eye appeared parallel to the right. The patient was treated for 5 days in the hospital after the procedure, and the sutures were removed 1 week later. The histological result showed that the fibro-osseous lesion was in accordance with fibrous dysplasia (Figures 17-23).

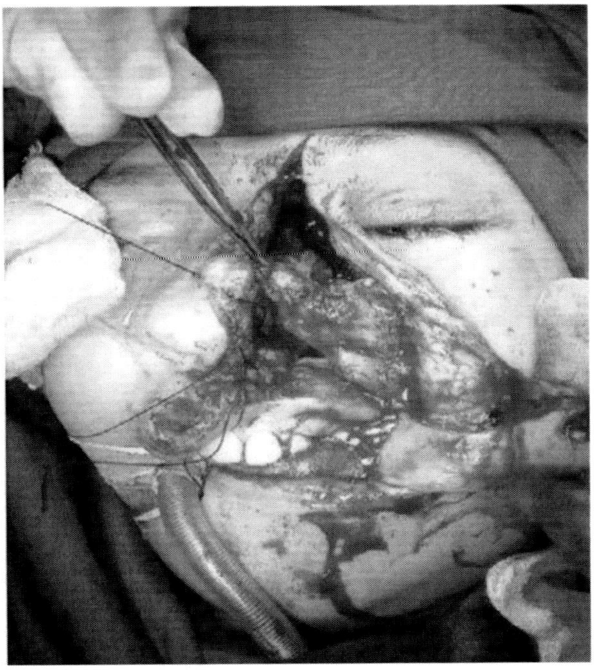

Figure 17. Buccal muscle sling.

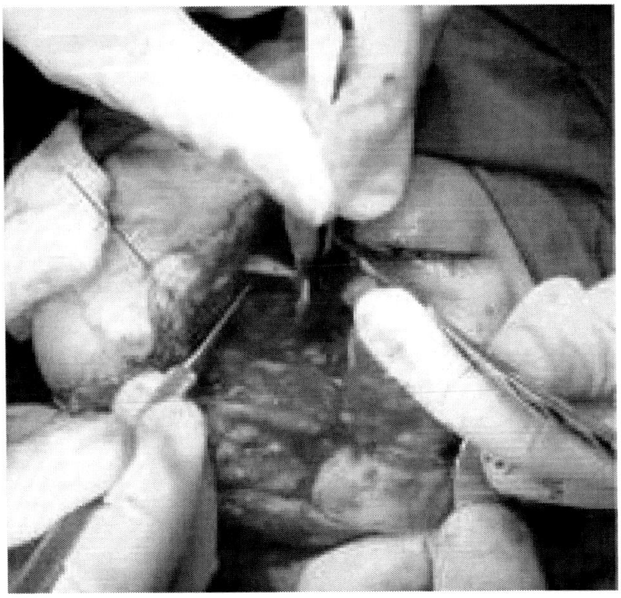

Figure 18. Elevation of the mucosa of the left nasal septum.

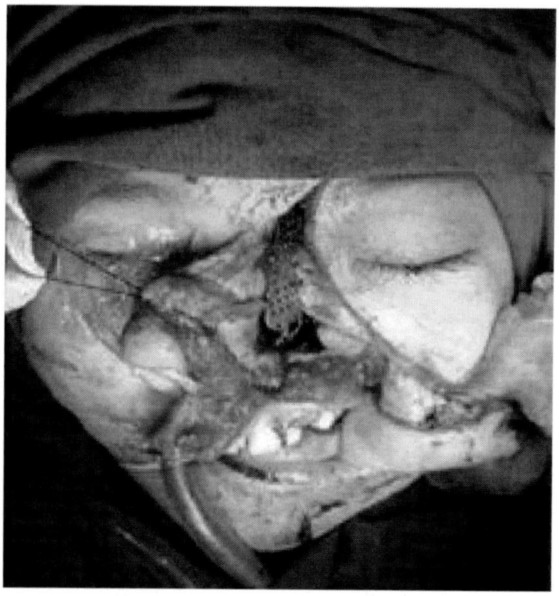

Figure 19. The plate was used to reconstruct the medial wall of the left maxilla.

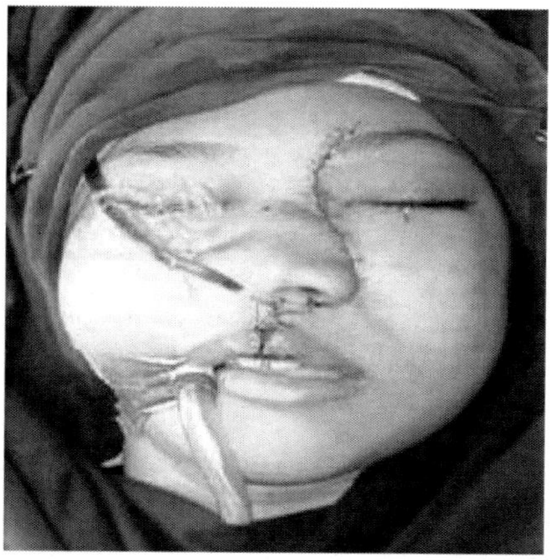

Figure 20. Suturing of Weber–Ferguson incision with Lynch expansion after suprastructure maxillectomy and reconstruction.

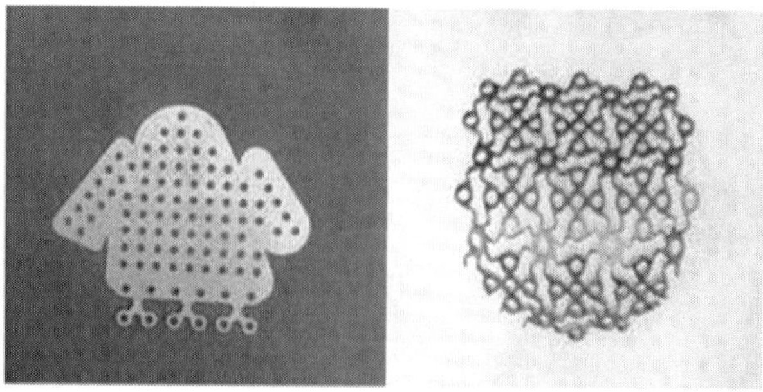

Figure 21. Orbital plate and titanium mesh.

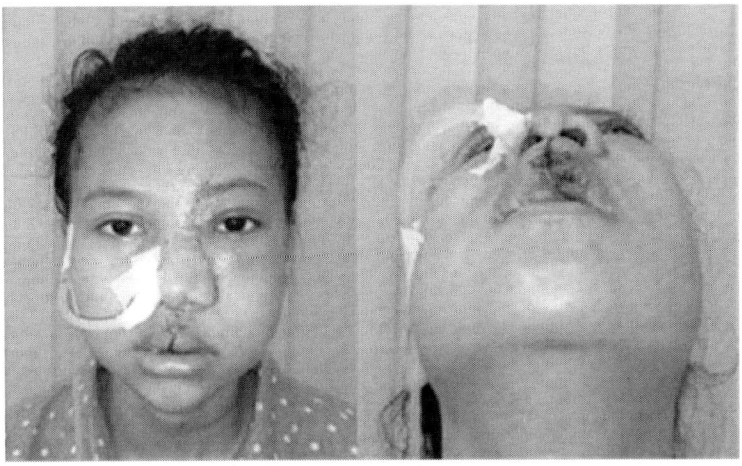

Figure 22. Five days after reconstruction.

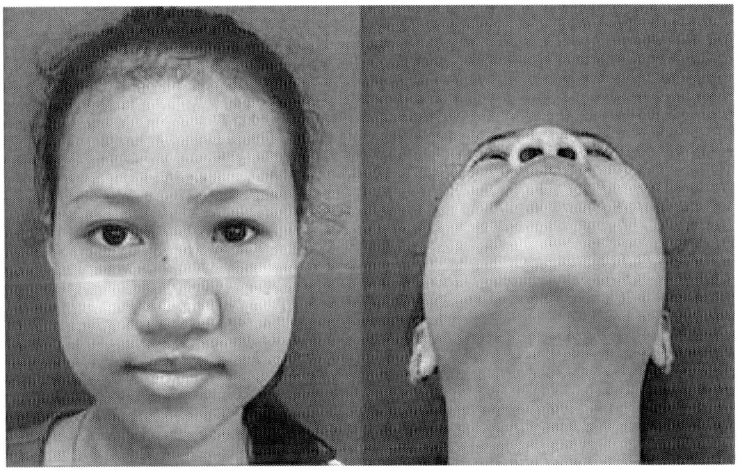

Figure 23. Three months after reconstruction.

LITERATURE SEARCHING METHOD

A literature search of PubMed, ScienceDirect, and ClinicalKey was performed. The keywords used were "maxillary and orbital floor defect reconstruction" and "titanium mesh," with clinical questions regarding the effect of titanium mesh use in the surgical management of suprastructure maxillectomy. The search yielded 310 articles. After screening the results for the latest articles, multiple publications, and compatibility to clinical questions, three relevant articles were obtained (Figure 24).

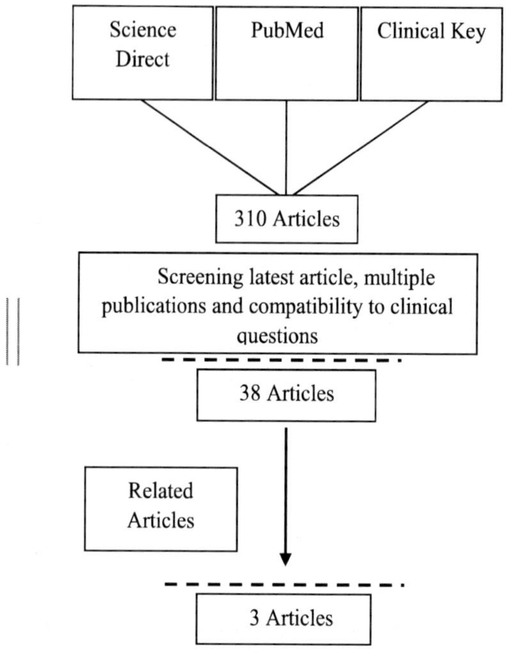

Figure 24. A literature search of PubMed, ScienceDirect, and ClinicalKey with clinical questions regarding the effect of titanium mesh use in the surgical management of suprastructure maxillectomy.

On the basis of the research by Zhang et al. [26], the use of titanium mesh material is more advantageous than the use of autograph materials. The material provides good results for maxillary and orbital reconstruction due to the complex characteristics of the cheeks and orbit contours. Titanium mesh can follow the contour and is therefore very good at closing defects. Expertise and caution during reconstruction are essential when performing facial reconstruction.

The use of titanium mesh for defect reconstruction after removal of the maxillary tumor leads to good results in repairing the anterior maxillary wall and the orbit base according to the report by Lv et al. [29].

A report by Motiee-Langroudi et al. [28] described the use of titanium mesh for maxillary and orbital base defect reconstruction. The combination of the use of fascia with titanium mesh prevents the fall of orbital fat through the titanium mesh hole.

Discussion

Defect reconstruction post-suprastructure maxillectomy for patients with maxillary fibrous dysplasia is a difficult and complicated procedure. According to the report by Duan et al. [5], the incidence of fibrous dysplasia is equal to 1:30,000 individuals, comprising 7.5% of all benign bone tumors. The percentage of benign tumors managed using the open maxillectomy technique was 26.4% among the 65 cases recorded from 2000 to 2009 in Malaysia.

The mid-facial area is an important structure on the face due to its anatomical and structural characteristics and functions related to breathing, phonation, chewing, swallowing, vision, and smelling.

The maxillary supporting wall, which is divided into vertical and horizontal supporting walls, is an important component of the facial structure. Vertical walls play a role in maintaining the mid-facial area in an upright position.

The main symptom of fibrous dysplasia is painless swelling of the facial bones, especially the maxilla and mandible. Symptoms of the eyes and nose can occur along with the growth of the lesion. Pushing towards the eyes will result in visual disturbances, whereas pushing towards the nose will result in nasal congestion. These symptoms are in accordance with fibrous dysplasia. Open surgery with maxillectomy is the treatment of choice, and maxillectomy has a variety of classifications. According to the classification proposed by Hanna et al. [22], the appropriate technique for fibrous dysplasia treatment is suprastructure maxillectomy. However, according to the criteria proposed by Spiro et al. [23], the appropriate technique is subtotal maxillectomy. The purpose of open surgery for maxillectomy is to remove the tumor by resecting the maxillary wall involved.

Brown et al. [25] suggested the classification of post-maxillectomy defects with the aim of facilitating reconstruction and guiding the clinician through the process. Bidra et al. [24] conducted a literature review of the classification proposed by Brown et al. The review yielded positive results because the classification divides the types of defects into vertical and horizontal types. The patient in this case report was classified as having a type V vertical defect because she suffered from left-sided facial defects covering the anterior maxillary wall, medial maxillary wall, and inferior orbital rhyme. She also suffered from left eye enophthalmus, which led to the occurrence of orbitomaxillary defects after suprastructure maxillectomy.

The orbitomaxillary defect is caused by attachment of the tumor to the maxilla and tissue around the orbit. The tissues surrounding the nose, maxilla, and orbit are elevated when suprastructure maxillectomy is performed. Suborbicularis fat, orbital retaining ligaments, and part of the orbital base are lifted after maxillectomy, which leads to enophthalmus. Reconstruction is aimed at not only closing the defect but also restoring the function and aesthetics of the face. Therefore, expertise and caution are necessary for good results. The use of mesh plates in post-maxillectomy reconstruction is in accordance with the study by Zhang et al. [26], in which a titanium mesh was used during reconstruction on post-maxillectomy patients with orbital floor defects.

Titanium materials are widely used in reconstruction, not only in the maxillofacial region but also through the body. Titanium is an alloplastic substance that is biocompatible and causes minimal allergic reactions due to the calcium-like chemical composition. The material achieves good integration with bone without causing fibrosis as described by Schubert et al. [27].

The patient described here was treated using a modified titanium mesh plate and muscle sling. Modification of management techniques following reconstruction is sometimes necessary to close the occurring defect. A muscle sling was employed to provide resistance and replace the orbital hanging ligaments, preventing enophthalmus. Reconstruction continued with the installation of titanium mesh as the orbital base while simultaneously reconstructing the anterior maxillary wall defect to obtain a shape that resembles the wall. The medial maxillary wall defect was reconstructed using a plate to keep the eyeball stable and to form the construction of the lateral nasal wall. The management process for this reconstruction is consistent with the reports by Zhang et al. [26], Lv et al. [29], and Motiee-Langroudi et al. [28] with a little modification to use muscle slings as orbital anchors. The final step involved suturing by observing the aesthetic contours of the face according to the facial fat compartment as described by Prendergast et al. [12].

REFERENCES

[1] Hanasono MM, Skoracki RJ. Mid-facial reconstruction. In: Hanasono MM, Robb GL, Skoracki RJ, Yu, P, editors. *Reconstructive Plastic Surgery of the Head and Neck*. 1st ed. New York: Thieme Medical Publishers Inc; 2016. p. 100–16.

[2] Yamamoto, Y. Mid-facial reconstruction after maxillectomy. *Int J Clin Oncol* 2005, 10, 218–22.

[3] Eachempati, P, Aggarwal, H, Shenoy, V, Baliga, M. Multidisciplinary approach for management of a patient with fibrous dysplasia of maxilla. *Br Med J*. 2015, (6), 1–4.

[4] Tinoco P, Pereira JCO, Filho RCL, Silva FB, Ruela KP. Fibrous Dysplasia of Maxillary Sinus. *Int Arch Otorhinolaryngol*. 2009, 13(4), 214–7.

[5] Duan C, Dai Q, Liu Q, Yu H. Characteristics of sinonasal fibrous dysplasia: experience from a single department. *Acta Otolaryngol*. 2017, (8), 1–6.

[6] MacDonald DS. Maxillofacial fibro-osseous lesions. *Clin Radiol* [Internet]. 2015; 70(1):25–36.

[7] Formete B, Agbara R, Osunde OD, Ogbeifun JO. Maxillectomy and its surgical indications in a tertiary health care centre in north-western Nigeria: Analysis of 66 cases. *J Oral Maxillofac Surgery*; Med Pathol. 2017, 29(3), 198–202.

[8] Mazlina S, Putra SHAP, Shiraz MARM, Hazim MYS, Roszalina R, Abdul ARR. Maxillary sinus tumours - A review of twenty-nine patients treated by maxillectomy approach. *Med J Malaysia*. 2006, 61(8), 284–7.

[9] Peled M, Leiser Y, Wolff A, Abu-El Naaj I. Our experience with maxillectomies - A 10-year retrospective study. *Oral Oncol*. 2011, 47:S146.

[10] Ozkan O, Coskunfirat OK, Ozkan O. Midface Reconstruction. *Semin Plast Surg*. 2010, 1(212), 181–7.

[11] Hopper RA, Salemy S, Sze RW. Diagnosis of Midface Fractures with CT: What the Surgeon Needs to Know. *Radiographics*. 2006, 26(5), 783–94.

[12] Prendergast PM. Cosmetic surgery: Art and techniques. In: Shiffman MA, Di Giuseppe A, editors. *Cosmetic Surgery: Art and Techniques*. 1st ed. Berlin: Springer-Verlag Berlin Heidelberg; 2013. p. 29–45.

[13] El-Mofty SK. Fibro-Osseous Lesions of the Craniofacial Skeleton: An Update. *Head Neck Pathol*. 2014, 8(4), 432–44.

[14] McCarthy EF. Fibro-Osseous Lesions of the Maxillofacial Bones. *Head Neck Pathol*. 2013, 7(1), 5–10.

[15] Suarez-Soto A, de la Hermosa M-CB-R, Minguez-Martínez I, Floría-García LM, Barea-Gámiz J, Delhom-Valero J, et al. Management of fibro-osseous lesions of the craniofacial area. Presentation of 19 cases and review of the literature. *Med Oral Patol Oral Cir Bucal*. 2013, 18(3), 479–85.

[16] Lee J, FitzGibbon E, Chen Y, Kim H, Lustig L, Akintoye S, et al. Clinical guidelines for the management of craniofacial fibrous dysplasia. *Orphanet J Rare Dis*. 2012, 7(1): S2.

[17] Srichinthu KK, Yoithapprabhunath TR, Chitturi RT, Yamunadevi A, Potsangbam AD, Singh DN. Fibro Osseous Lesions – Classifications; Pathophysiology and Importance of Radiology: A Short Review. *Int Biol Biomed J*. 2016, 2(1), 11–20.

[18] DiCaprio MR, Enneking WF. Fibrous Dysplasia. Pathophysiology; Evaluation; and Treatment. *J Bone Jt Surg*. 2005, 87(8), 1848.

[19] Ho AS, Zanation AM, Ganly I. Malignancies of the Paranasal Sinus. In: Flint PW, Haughey BH, Lund V, Niparko JK, Robbins T, Thomas R, et al., editors. *Cummings Otolaryngology Head and Neck Surgery*. 6th ed. Philadelpia: Elsevier Saunders; 2015. p. 1176–201.

[20] Tang IP, Shashinder S, Gopala Krishnan G, Narayanan P. Juvenile nasopharyngeal angiofibroma in a tertiary centre: ten-year experience. *Singapore Med J*. 2009, 50(3), 261–4.

[21] Durrani Z, Hassan SG, Alam SA. A study of classification systems for maxillectomy defects. *J Pak Prosthodont Assoc*. 2013, 1(2), 117–24.

[22] Hanna E. Maxillectomy. In: I Cohen J, L Clayman G, editors. *Atlas of Head and Neck Surgery*. VII. Philadelpia: Elsevier Saunders; 2016. p. 419–26.

[23] Spiro RH, Strong EW, Shah JP. Maxillectomy and its classification. *Head Neck*. 1997, 19(4), 309–14.

[24] Bidra AS, Jacob RF, Taylor TD. Classification of maxillectomy defects: A systematic review and criteria necessary for a universal description. *J Prosthet Dent.* 2012, 107(4), 261–70.

[25] Brown JS, Shaw RJ. Reconstruction of the maxilla and midface: Introducing a new classification. *Lancet Oncol.* 2010, 11(10), 1001–8.

[26] Zhang W, Mao C, Liu X, Guo C, Yu G-Y, Peng X. Outcomes of orbital floor reconstruction after extensive maxillectomy using the computer-assisted fabricated individual titanium mesh technique. J *Oral Maxillofac Surg*. 2015, 73(10), 1–15.

[27] Schubert W, Gear AJL, Lee C, Hilger P a, Haus E, Migliori MR, et al. Incorporation of titanium mesh in orbital and midface reconstruction. *Plast Reconstr Surg*. 2002, 110(4), 1022–30.

[28] Motiee-Langroudi M, Harirchi I, Amali A, Jafari M. Reconstruction of midface and orbital wall defects after maxillectomy and orbital content preservation with titanium mesh and fascia lata: 3- year follow-up. *J Oral Maxillofac Surg*. 2015, 73(12), 2447.

[29] Lv M, Li J, Shen Y, Wang L, Sun J. The "Drawer-Like" Resection and Reconstruction with Titanium Mesh: A Novel Surgical Technique for Treatment of Giant Ossifying Fibroma in the Maxilla. *J Oral Maxillofac Surg*. 2017, 75(8), 1752–61.

In: Case Reports in Surgery
Editors: Ahmad Jabir Rahyussalim et al.
ISBN: 978-1-53616-582-1

Chapter 14

CLEFT PALATE WITH VELOPHARYNGEAL INSUFFICIENCY: A CASE REPORT

Mirta H. Reksodiputro**, *Shally Adhina Putri*, *Dini W. Widodo and Trimartani Koento
Department of Otorhinolaryngology Head and Neck Surgery,
Faculty of Medicine Universitas Indonesia –Cipto Mangunkusumo General Hospital,
Central Jakarta, Indonesia

ABSTRACT

Cleft palate is a congenital abnormality of the face, in which the palate does not develop normally during pregnancy. It is caused by failure of the fusion of the lateral palatine procesuss, resulting in the persistence of a slit-like opening between the oral and nasal cavities. Velopharyngeal insufficiency is the inability of the velopharyngeal valve to close owing to a deficit in the velopharyngeal structure, and one of the causes is cleft palate. The activities of swallowing and speaking depend on the ability to achieve adequate closure of the velopharyngeal valve. Here we present a 21-year-old man with cleft palate since birth. He had complaints of nasal sounds (rhinolalia) and water/food coming out from the nose every time he swallowed. He underwent surgery to correct this abnormality. Cleft palate closure was performed using the V-Y pushback technique and a posterior pharyngeal flap as this approach can extend the palate and effectively improve speech function. After the surgery, there were no disruptions in eating and drinking, and the patient spoke more clearly and was satisfied. A good understanding of the anatomy, physiology, and pathophysiology of cleft palate is very important for the appropriate management in order to achieve optimal and comprehensive treatment with regard to all aspects of aesthetics, speech, and swallowing ability.

* Corresponding Author's E-mail: citamirta@yahoo.com.

Keywords: Congenital abnormalities, cleft palate, velopharyngeal insufficiency

INTRODUCTION

Cleft palate is a congenital abnormality of the face, in which the palate does not develop normally during pregnancy. It is caused by failure of the fusion of the lateral palatine processes, resulting in the persistence of a slit-like opening between the oral and nasal cavities [1]. Cleft palate is more common in males than females. Additionally, it is more common in Asians (1–2.1/1000 births) than Africans (0.41/1000 births). The etiology of cleft palate is multifactorial. Genetic factors are involved in about 25% of patients with a family history of cleft palate; therefore, the chance is even greater for a future child to be born with a cleft. Environmental factors, such as drug consumption during pregnancy, infection during the first trimester of pregnancy, alcohol consumption, and vitamin deficiency, also contribute to cleft palate [1, 2, 3].

Velopharyngeal insufficiency is the inability of the velopharyngeal valve to close owing to a deficit in the velopharyngeal structure, and one of the causes is cleft palate. The activities of swallowing and speaking depend on the ability to achieve adequate closure of the velopharyngeal valve [4]. Treatment for these abnormalities includes surgery and a complete team approach to help with the multiple complications that can occur in such a case. Here, we present a man with cleft palate who had speech issues. Cleft palate closure was performed using the V-Y pushback technique and a posterior pharyngeal flap. This technique was selected because it can extend the palate and improve speech function [5-6].

CASE REPORT

A 21-year-old man with cleft palate since birth presented with a complaint of nasal sounds (Figure 1A). He also mentioned that water/food came out from the nose every time he swallowed. He had never been treated, as he was not disturbed by the abnormality. However, when he started working, he experienced problems communicating with his coworkers and supervisor. In July 2018, he underwent cleft palate surgery using the V-Y pushback technique. After surgery, he could speak more clearly, although there were still nasal sounds (Figure 1B). After 2 months postoperatively, a small fistula (around 3 mm in diameter) was noted in the surgical area (Figure 1C). Thus, in October 2018, he underwent revision surgery using the V-Y pushback technique and a posterior pharyngeal flap (Figure 2A, B).

After the surgery, there were no disruptions in eating and drinking, and he could speak more clearly and was satisfied. In January 2019 (3 months after the revision surgery), he underwent speech assessment, including the mirror test (Figure 3) and kutugajah test to evaluate nasal air emission. He could not correctly pronounce the nasal consonants. There was dew on the mirror; however, he could not correctly pronounce the letters k, i, q, c, j, z, r, d, a, and s. Speech therapy was planned. He was trained several times to pronounce the nasal consonants, and a palatometer was used. Further evaluation is planned 1 month later.

DISCUSSION

In patients with cleft palate, one of the problems is speech function/communication [5]. Our patient with cleft palate underwent surgery using the V-Y pushback technique and a posterior pharyngeal flap, as this approach can extend the palate and improve speech function well [6-9]. In this case, the patient underwent alatoplasty in adulthood, which is usually performed at the age of 10–18 months. Subsequently, the patient received speech therapy to improve nasal air emission and training to pronounce the nasal consonants [10]. In our center, most patients with cleft palate undergo an audiological examination, and if the results are within normal limits, a nasometric examination is performed. Then, palatoplastyis performed, and after 1 month postoperatively, nasometry/ nasopharyngoscopy is performed to evaluate the velopharyngeal valve and assess the presence of speech disorder.

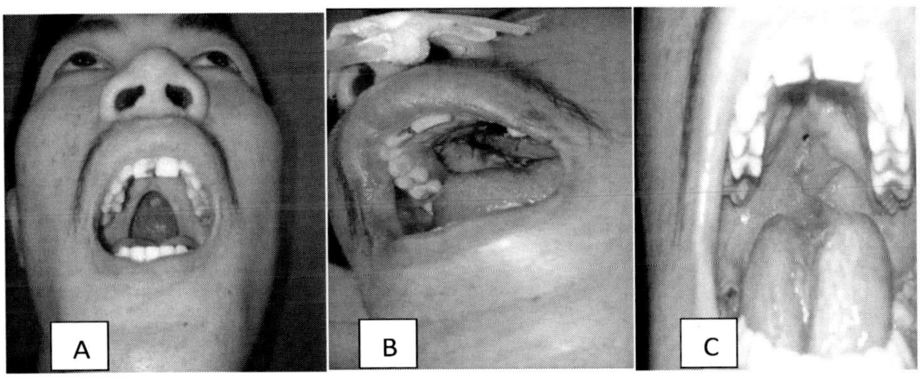

Figure 1. Cleft palate appearance. (A) Before surgery; (B) 3 days after surgery; and (C) 2 months after surgery.

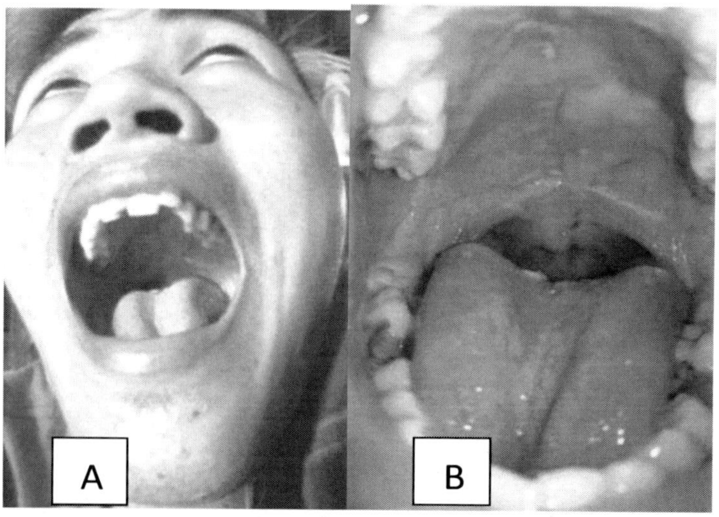

Figure 2. Cleft palate appearance after revision surgery. (A) Fourteen days after revision and (B) 2 months after revision.

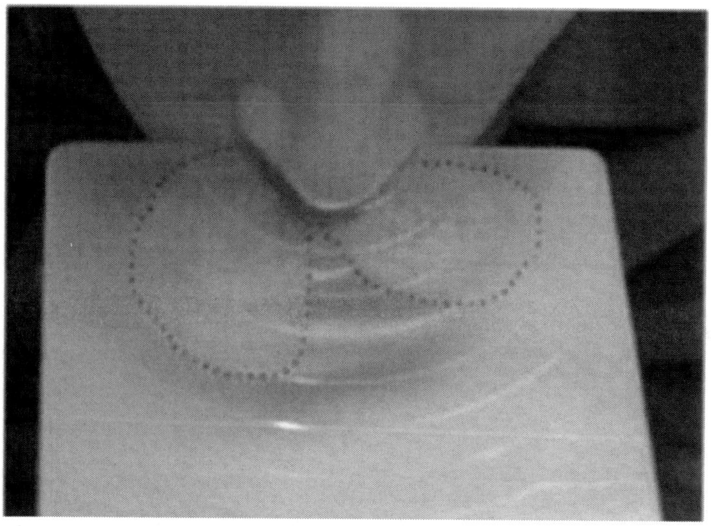

Figure 3. Mirror test.

CONCLUSION

In patients with cleft palate, speech function should be examined before and after palatoplasty. Cleft palate is a congenital disorder often found in the social community. A good understanding of the anatomy, physiology, and pathophysiology of cleft palate is very important for appropriate management in order to achieve optimal and comprehensive treatment with regard to all aspects of aesthetics, speech, and swallowing ability.

REFERENCES

[1] Dixon, M. J. & Marazita, M. L. (2011). Cleft lip and palate: synthesizing genetic and environmental influences. *Nature Reviews Genetics*, 12 (3): 168-178.

[2] Khan, M., Ullah, H., Naz, S., Iqbal, T., Ullah, T., Tahir, M. and Ullah, O. (2013). A revised classification of the cleft lip and palate. *The Canadian journal of plastic surgery*, 21 (1): 48-50.

[3] Hagberg, C., Larson, O., Millerad, J. (2008). Incidence of cleft lip, palate and risks of additional malformations. *Cleft Palate Craniofacial Journal*, 35(1): 40–45.

[4] Kummer, A. W. (2014). Resonance and Velopharyngeal dysfunction (VPD). In A. W. Kummer (Ed.), Cleft palate and craniofacial anomalies: *Effects on speech and resonance.* Clifton Park, NY: Cengage Learning. 188-224.

[5] Isik, D., Bora, A., Yuce, S., Davran, R., Kocak, O., Canbaz, Y., Avcu, S. and Atik, B. (2015). Comparison of the effect of the rotation palatoplasty and V-Y pushback palatoplasty techniques on palate elongation with magnetic resonance imaging. *International Journal of Oral and Maxillofacial Surgery*, 44 (6): 738-744.

[6] Sato, F.R, Silva, M. L., Moreira, M. W. (2016). Evaluation of two palatoplasty techniques in patients with cleft palate. *Journal of Otorhinolaryngology Head Neck Surgery*, 1(5): 119-121

[7] Andersson, E. M., Sandvik, L., Semb, G., Abyholm, F. (2018). Palatal fistulas after primary repair of clefts of the secondary palate. *Scandinavian Journal of Plastic and Reconstructive Surgery and Hand Surgery*, 42 (6): 296.

[8] Lu, Y., Shi, B., Zheng, Q., Hu, Q., Wang, Z. (2010). Incidence of palatal fistula after palatoplasty with levatorvelipalatiniretro positioning according to Sommerlad. *British Journal of Oral Maxillofac Surgery*, 48(8):637–40.

[9] Cervenka, B. & Rubistein, B. (2015). Surgical repair of the cleft palate. *Journal of Otolaryngology - Head & Neck Surgery*, 26 (3): 121-126.

[10] Watterson, T., Lewis, K., Brancamp, T. (2015). Comparison of Nasalance scores obtained with the Nasometer 6200 and the Nasometer II 6400. *The Cleft Palate-Craniofacial Journal*, 42 (5): 574-579.

In: Case Reports in Surgery
Editors: Ahmad Jabir Rahyussalim et al.
ISBN: 978-1-53616-582-1

Chapter 15

TONGUE EDEMA AFTER PALATOPLASTY: A CASE REPORT

Rahendra*[*] *and Pradini
Department of Anesthesiology and Intensive Care, Faculty of Medicine Universitas Indonesia and Cipto Mangunkusumo National Central Hospital, Jakarta, Indonesia

ABSTRACT

Palatoplasty is a commonly performed procedure in children. A complication of palatoplasty is tongue edema owing to the use of a mouth gag. Tongue edema can compromise the airway and be dangerous for the patient. The objective of this case report was to increase awareness that tongue edema may arise after palatoplasty and to explain how to manage it. We present the case of a 17-month-old female who presented with tongue edema after palatoplasty. Massive tongue swelling developed 2 hours post-surgery. The patient showed signs of upper airway obstruction and was reintubated. The patient was under observation in the intensive care unit for three days until the tongue size returned to the original. A longer observation period in the recovery room after surgery may be required to prevent occurrence of hazardous events after palatoplasty.
Keywords: tongue edema, palatoplasty, airway obstruction

INTRODUCTION

Palatoschisis is a frequently occurring congenital craniofacial disorder. The Centers for Disease Control and Prevention (CDC) has estimated that 2.650 babies are born every

[*] Corresponding Author's E-mail: rahend2k@yahoo.com.

year with palatoschisis in the United States [1, 2]. Palatoschisis can cause swallowing, talking, and breathing disorders in sufferers. Palatoplasty needs to be performed to correct this disorder and is typically performed at the age of 9-18 months. Corrections performed in palatoplasty include repair procedures in the hard palate and mole palate. Almost all palatoplasty procedures involve the use of a mouth gag to separate the tongue and cheeks from the surgery area, making it easier for the surgeon to access the operating area [1, 3, 4].

Although the use of a mouth gag in this procedure has been shown to ease surgery, there are many reports of complications arising from suppressing mouth gags to surrounding structures [2, 5, 6]. A complication that arises owing to the suppression of mouth gag is edema of the tongue. Although rare, edema of the tongue can cause upper airway obstruction, which, if not treated properly, has the potential to be life threatening [7-9]. This case report aimed to discuss the management of patients who develop post-palatoplasty tongue edema.

CASE REPORT

A healthy 17-month-old, 10-kg female was scheduled for palatoplasty. The patient had labiopalatoschisis since birth and had undergone surgery for labioschisis at the age of 6 months. Based on the patient's history and examination, there were no complaints or abnormalities other than palatoschisis. She was assessed as ASA 2 with congenital anomaly (palatoschisis). In the operating room, anesthesia was induced by using sevoflurane 8%, which was titrated down to 2.5%. A 24-G infusion line was secured in the patient's left hand. Fentanyl 2.5 mcg/kg (25 mcg) and atracurium 0.5 mg/kg (5 mg) were administered to facilitate intubation. Intubation was performed using direct laryngoscopy, with endotracheal tube size 4 (non-kinking type), fixed at 12 cm. The cuff was not inflated owing to pediatric airway consideration. A throat pack was inserted by the anesthesiologist. The ventilator setting was VC (Volume Control) 80/4/20/40%. No difficulties were faced while performing intubation.

After intubation, the patient's head was placed in a hyperextended position. A mouth gag was inserted by the surgeon. During the surgery, the surgeon changed the mouth gag position several times and increased the pressure because the visualization of the operating field was difficult. However, hemodynamically, the patient was stable with an estimated total blood loss of 50 mL. The surgery lasted for 3.5 hours. Anesthesia was maintained with administration of 2%-2.5% sevoflurane in air with 45% oxygen. At the end of surgery, the throat pack was removed, and the surgeon stitched a palatum pack to block unanticipated bleeding from the surgical site.

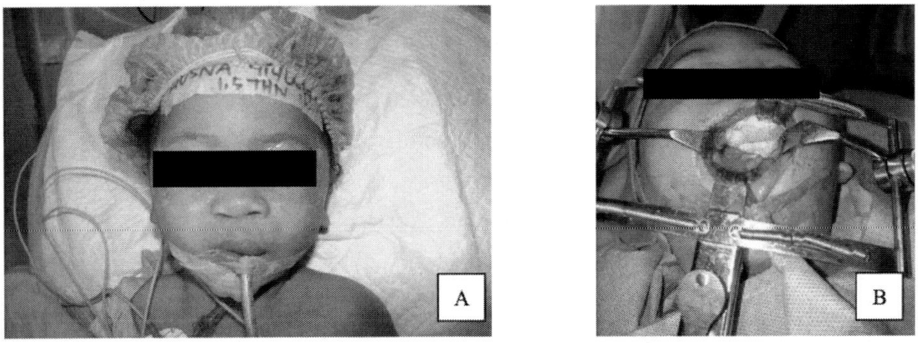

Figure 1. Intraoperative Position. (A) After intubation. (B) After mouth gag insertion.

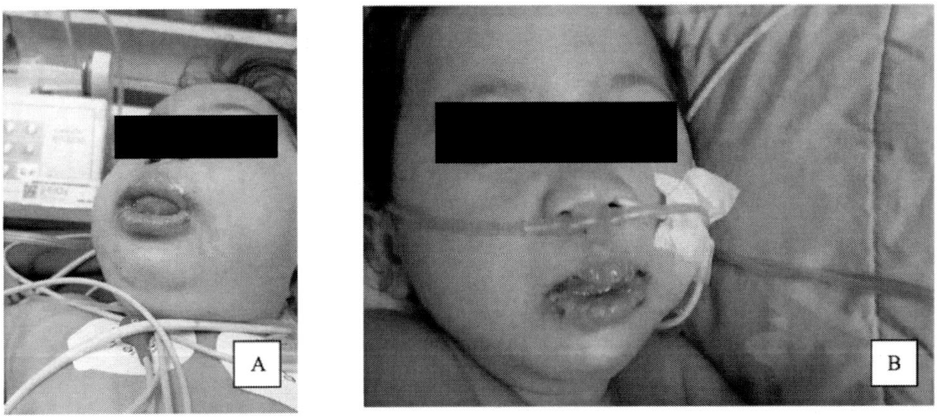

Figure 2. Tongue swelling. (A) More massive tongue swelling 2 hours post-surgery. (B) Decreased tongue swelling 3 days post-surgery.

At the end of the procedure, the residual neuromuscular block was antagonized, spontaneous ventilation was assessed to be adequate, and extubation was performed. Soon after extubation, the patient showed labored breathing with intercostal retraction. Oxygen saturation decreased to 88%; 100% oxygen was administered via the face mask, but the saturation continued to decrease until 76%. Propofol (25 mg) was injected to sedate the patient, and an LMA was inserted to provide adequate ventilation.

Soon after insertion of LMA, oxygen saturation increased to 100%. The anesthesiologist decided to wait until the effect of propofol subsided. Naloxone 0.01 mg/kg (0.1 mg) was added to reverse any residual opioid. The decision to exert the LMA was made after the patient gained consciousness and spontaneous ventilation was adequate. However, soon after LMA exertion, the patient showed labored breathing with intercostal retraction again, and oxygen saturation decreased to 90%. An oropharyngeal airway sized 0 was inserted, which solved the issue. Oxygen saturation quickly increased to 100%. A quick re-evaluation of the patient's airway was done, and a mild lingual edema was found. The anesthesiologist asked the surgeon to remove the palatum pack, so that air could flow through the oral cavity despite the presence of mild lingual edema. The child could then breathe normally without a period of desaturation. It was decided that the patient would be observed for longer period of time in the recovery room.

Two hours post-surgery, the patient developed a more massive lingual edema and produced a stridor sound, indicative of an impending airway obstruction. The decision to re-intubate the patient was made; reintubation was extremely difficult and was performed within two attempts using C-MAC and bougie. Soon after the intubation, an emergency lingual exploration was performed by the surgeon, which found no bleeding, hematoma, or laceration on the tongue. The patient was transferred to the intensive care unit (ICU) for observation. Dexamethasone was injected daily to reduce tongue swelling. After a 72-h in ICU, the tongue size slowly returned to normal. The patient was then extubated.

Discussion

Airway compromise following palatoplasty may be owing to tongue swelling, laryngeal edema, pharyngeal secretions, blood clots, a retained throat pack, prolonged action of anesthetic agents, or a combination of factors [1, 2, 5, 9]. Tongue swelling is an unusual sequel to cleft palate repair. Ischemia induced by the pressure arising from prolonged use of a mouth gag results in necrosis of the tongue muscle, venous stasis, and lymphedema, resulting in lingual swelling, which indicates tongue ischemia with reperfusion hyperemia and capillary leakage as important mechanisms [3, 4]. Hyperextension of the head may also contribute to an impaired blood flow to the tongue, producing more lingual venous stasis and swelling, necessitating immediate reintubation, which may be extremely difficult [2, 5, 6].

The onset of tongue edema can be insidious over a 2–2.5-h period [3, 8, 9]. This is potentially dangerous because by then, the patient is likely to have been discharged to the general ward. Tongue examination prior to extubation is needed after every palatoplasty surgery. It is important to maintain airway patency until the tongue size returns to normal.

Conclusion

Massive tongue swelling can compromise the airway. Periodic release of the mouth gag during palatoplasty prevents prolonged ischemia to the tongue. Once lingual edema develops, it is important to maintain airway patency until the tongue size returns to normal. It is important to keep in mind that reintubation is often difficult. A longer observation may be required especially in an ambulatory setting to prevent a hazardous event.

REFERENCES

[1] Rajesh, M. C., Kuriakose, S., Sukumar, J., Ramdas, E. K., (2013). Massive lingual swelling following cleft palate repair. *J. Anaesthesiol. Clin. Pharmacol.* 29, 262-263.

[2] Dell'oste, C., Savron, F., Pelizzo, G., Sarti, A. C., (2004). Acute airway obstruction in an infant with Pierre Robin syndrome after palatoplasty. *Acta Anaesthesiol. Scand.* 48, 787-789.

[3] Aziz, S. R., Ziccari, V. B., (2009). Severe glossal edema after primary palatoplasty. *J. Oral Maxillofac. Surg.* 67, 1326-1328.

[4] Sherif, R. D., Paymo, S. M., Taub, P. J., (2018) Lingual pressure during dingman-assisted cleft palate repair: an investigatory case series. *Cleft Palate Craniofac. J.* 55, 312-315.

[5] Lees, V. C., Pigott, R. W., (1992). Early postoperative complications in primary cleft lip and palate surgery - how soon may we discharge patients from hospital? *Br. J. Plast. Surg.* 45, 232-234.

[6] Gupta, R., Chhabra, B., Mahajan, R. K., (2001). Macroglossia following palatoplasty causing upper airway obstruction: Case report. *J. Oral Maxillofac. Surg.* 59, 940-941.

[7] Mukozawa, M., Kono, T., Fujiwara, S., Takakura, K., (2011). Late onset tongue edema after palatoplasty. *Acta Anaesthesiol. Taiwan.* 49, 29-31.

[8] Chan, M. T., Chan, M. S., Mu, K. S., Ho, B. P., (1995) Massive lingual swelling following palatoplasty. *Anaesthesia*, 50, 30-34.

[9] Prakash, S., Usha, G., Thakur, P., Mullick, P., (2016) Postoperative supraglottic edema following palatoplasty. *Anaesth. Pain & Intensive Care* 20, 89-91.

In: Case Reports in Surgery
Editors: Ahmad Jabir Rahyussalim et al.
ISBN: 978-1-53616-582-1

Chapter 16

NON-SYNDROMIC UNILATERAL TESSIER NO. 3 FACIAL CLEFT: A RARE CONGENITAL DISEASE

Mirta H. Reksodiputro**, *Tara C. Mariska*, *Dini W. Widodo and Trimartani Koento
Department of Otorhinolaryngology, Head and Neck Surgery,
Faculty of Medicine, Universitas Indonesia,
RSUPN Dr. Cipto Mangunkusumo, Jakarta, Indonesia

ABSTRACT

Facial clefts are extremely rare congenital anomalies. There are various types of clefts, and classifications are required for their description. Nasal anomalies are rare and, currently, there are no standard methods for the management of such defects. The number of operations and types of surgical intervention vary widely according to the pattern and complexity of the deformity. The aim of this case report is to formulate a standardized procedure for there pair of the nasal component of Tessier no. 3 clefts. A nasal dorsum advanced rotational flap was used to close the cleft of ala nasi during the first-stage surgery. Second-stage surgery involved an osteotomy and septoplasty to obtain a better shape for the nasal dorsum. During the third operation, we reconstructed the ala nasi to obtain improved symmetry. The nasal dorsum rotation flap showed good healing over the lateral surface of the nose and in the subciliary region. The closure of the nasal defect was accomplished using a composite downward rotation flap of the ala based on the lateral cleft wall. An advanced rotation-transposition flap was used in the management of a Tessier no 3cleft. We also recommend the use of a superiorly based transposition for extensive lateral nasal wall involvement. In the present case, we performed osteotomy and septoplasty to obtain an improved shape for the nasal dorsum. Although the symmetry between the two nostrils was not ideal, it was acceptable.

* Corresponding Author's E-mail: citamirta@yahoo.com.

Keywords: Tessier no. 3 cleft, advanced rotation-transposition flap

INTRODUCTION

Facial clefts are extremely rare congenital anomalies. There are numerous variations and classifications of clefting. The cleft nasal deformity is mostly associated with cleft lip and palate [1]. The goals of cleft nasal surgery are to re-establish normal nasal tip projection and align the nares and the position of the nasal base. Various techniques have been considered to repair these defects [1, 2].

A facial cleft is an opening or gap in the face, or a malformation of a part of the face. Nasal deformity involves the skin, cartilage, mucosa, and skeletal platform [1, 2]. Fortunately, congenital clefts of the nose, whether isolated or associated with other craniofacial clefts, are rare.

The exact incidence remains unknown. The incidence of craniofacial clefts, other than cleft lip and palate, is reported to be 1.4–4.9 cases per 100,000 live births. Even among these cases, a cleft of the nose is rare [3]. Several studies reported that congenital nasal anomalies are rare, with an incidence of one case per 20,000–40,000 livebirths [4]. Nasal anomalies are rarely observed, which may account form is diagnosis and treatment plans that result in a less than satisfactory outcome. Nasal defects are also part of craniofacial clefts and other various well-documented syndromes.

Several theories have been proposed to explain the etiology official clefts. At present, an established theory is the mesodermal penetration theory, which states that clefts occur along potential lines of fusion due to the lack of mesodermal penetration. Without this reinforcement, epithelial breakdown and separation may occur [4].

Facial clefts have been classified according to their pathology, etiology, pathomorphology, topographic anatomy, and time of development. The most commonly used classification for craniofacial clefts is the Tessier classification, proposed by Paul Tessier in 1976 [1]. This classification is based on specific axes (0–14) along the face and the cranium.

The orbit divides the cranial clefts (9–14) from facial clefts (0–7), and facial clefts have cranial extensions. Tessier clefts involving the nose are types 0, 1, 2, and 3 with their cranial counterparts. The patterns of nasal clefts are variable, ranging from simple notch or asymmetry of the alar margin to complex complete craniofacial cleft involving the lip, nose, eyelid, brow, forehead, and underlying bones [1, 5, 6].

Case Presentation

We present an 18-year-old female with a Tessier no. 3 facial cleft. She did not have a history of nasal obstruction or cyanosis at birth. The patient had an isolated unilateral cleft of the left ala nasi, without other congenital abnormalities (Figure 1).

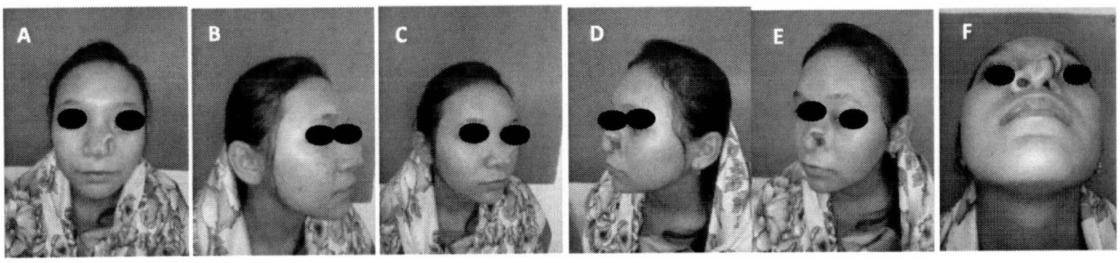

Figure 1. A female patient with a left Tessier no. 3 cleft. (A. Anterior view, B. Right lateral view, C. Right oblique view, D. Left lateral view, E. Left oblique view, F. Basal view).

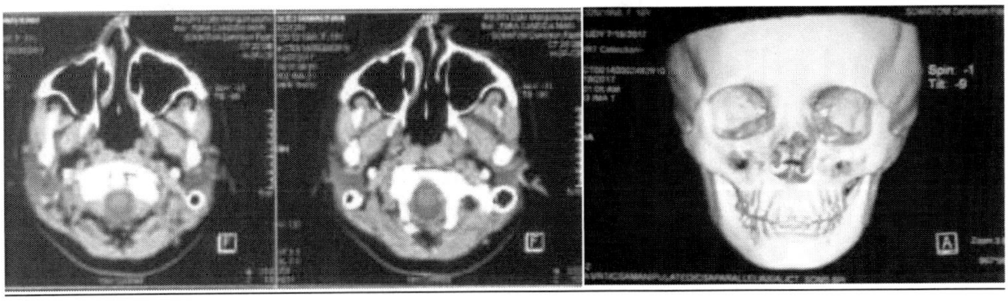

Figure 2. Computed tomography findings showed no abnormality in bone structure.

Computed tomography showed only deformities on the mucosa of the ala nasi, without cartilage deformities. Deviation of the nasal septum was observed. However, there were no structural defects of the hard tissue (Figure 2).

In this study, we used an advanced rotational local flap for the management of the patient. The incision design was made to obtain an improved symmetry and remove unnecessary structures. We set three reconstructive goals (i.e., reconstruction of the alar rim without a discernible notch, achieving symmetry with the normal side, and closing the secondary defect using local tissues).

The open rhinoplasty approach was performed to locate congenitally deformed anatomical landmarks, especially the cartilaginous framework of the nose. Nasal dorsum advanced rotational flaps were literally based from advanced rotation flaps. This flap design was in the shape of a pattern using ala from the other side. The medial incision was superficial, and a dissection was performed subcutaneously toward the nasomaxillary suture area. A deep dissection was continued lateral to the nasomaxillary suture area to mobilize the flap.

Open rhinoplasty was performed to open the anterior nasal area. This process exposed the alarcartilages. The lateral crura of the affected alarcartilage were dissected away from the nasal mucosa. The lining of the nasal mucosal was stretched and attached anteriorly to close the cleft. The lateral crus of the affected alarcartilage was repositioned laterally to be contiguous with the lateral crus of the lower lateral cartilage. The pedicled skin flap was rotated downward to recreate the alar rim. However, the limitation of this approach was that the flap was unable to rotate too far away to prevent the flap to stretch away and also to make sure the flap got good vascular feeding. (Figure 3). We inserted a nasal tampon to fixate the flap for 3 days.

A follow-up examination performed 1 month after surgery indicated that the flap was in good condition. However, it required additional intervention to obtain an improved ala symmetry. Second-stage surgery (refinement) was performed7 months after the first-stage surgery.

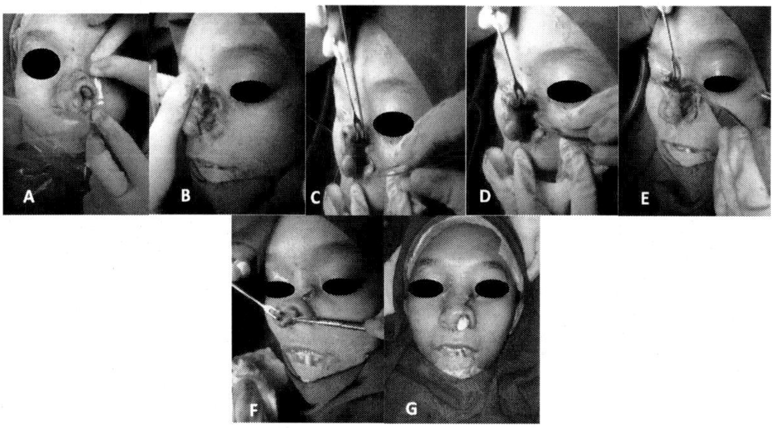

Figure 3. First-stage surgery. (A. Design of incision was to obtain symmetry). (B-E. Superficial and deep dissection and open rhinoplastyof the Nasal dorsum rotational flaps for correction of Tessier no. 3 facial cleft) (F. Removal of unneeded cartilage and mucosa). (G. Closure of the nasal dorsum rotational flaps for correction of Tessier no. 3 facial cleft).

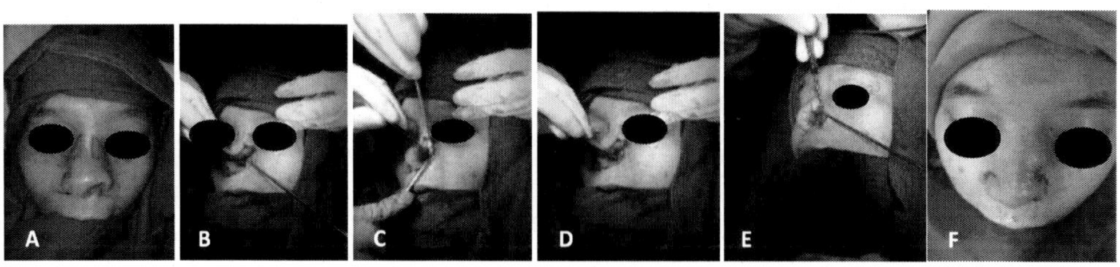

Figure 4. Second-stage surgery. (A. Marking of dorsum and ala nasi incision). (B-E. Undermined ala nasi and removed unneeded structure) (F. Superior view of second stage surgery shows a good shape of dome and ala nasi).

During second-stage surgery, osteotomy was performed to undermine the mucosal segment of the nasal dorsum. We used septoplasty to recreate the ala. In addition, we undermined the ala nasi to reconstruct the dome of ala nasi and obtain an improved shape and good symmetry. Although the symmetry between the two nostrils was not ideal, it was acceptable. Multiple procedures were performed to ensure a good healing process of the graft and closure of the secondary defect (Figure 4).

The results of the nasal dorsum rotation flap showed good healing over the lateral surface of the nose and in the subciliary region. However, scarring over the alarcartilage was suboptimal. The closure of the nasal defect was accomplished using a composite downward rotation flap of the ala based on the lateral cleft wall (Figure 5). The main defects were closures using advanced nasal dorsum rotational flap, while the secondary defect is closed after assessment of tissue availability and the remaining scars. Multiple approaches were performed to obtain an improved shape and symmetry of both nostrils.

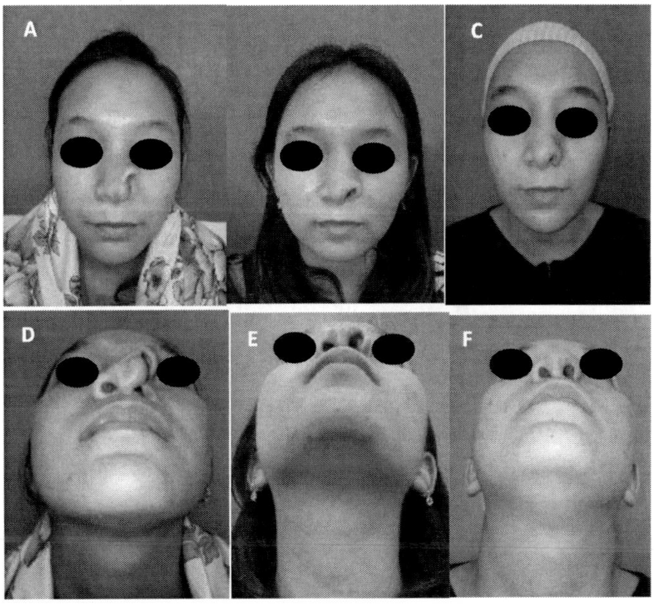

Figure 5. Anterior and lateral views prior to surgery (A and D), and 1 month after surgery (B and E) and 2 months (C and F) after second-stage surgery.

DISCUSSION

Paul Tessier studied facial clefts, and his clinical classification has become the current international standard. The cleft crosses the nasal ala between the tail of the alarcartilage and the alarbase, and the tip [1]. The most distinguishing characteristics of the Tessier no. 3 facial clefts are: medial orbital maxillary clefts, characterized by displacement of the medial canthus, superior displacement of the ala nasi cleft lip, alveolus and palate, coloboma of the lower eyelid, nasolacrimal abnormalities, disruption of the medial wall of the antrum, a cleft in the medial wall of the orbit, and teleorbitism.

Considering the rarity and lack of standard guidelines, the management of patients with such facial clefts is challenging. Depending on the degree of malformation, a staged procedure is currently considered the treatment of choice. However, various surgical protocols have been described in the literature, and the selection of approach has not been standardized [3]. The Australian Craniofacial Unit Treatment Protocol, which is one of the most widely accepted protocols for the management official clefts, has suggested early repair of the soft tissue defects and prevention of exposure keratitis. In addition, the protocol states that bone grafting if needed, orthognathic surgery, and rhinoplasty maybe performed after the patient reaches adulthood. Moreover, this protocol propounded the role of tissue expansion in the cheek to accommodate bone grafts. Numerous different types of flaps may be used to repair such lateral defects of the nose, depending on the size, shape, and site of the defects [3].

The main surgical goal in the treatment of patients with Tessier no. 3 clefts is nasal symmetry, which is rarely achieved. Surgeons have proposed different techniques for the repair of Tessier no. 3 facial clefts. Madaree et al. [7] used five local flaps, with two pairs utilizing the "z" plasty principle to achieve lengthening and the fifth being a turnover flap for additional nasal lining. A full thickness flap of the alar rim was rotated downward, thereby equalizing the external nares. The medially based turnover flap was used to close the gap. Monasterio et al. [8] used a local transposition flap to correct skin shortening between the medial canthus and the eye. A medial flap was rotated to elevate the dystopic canthus, and cheek flaps were advanced to close the gap and lengthen the nose [9, 10].

In the present case, we found that this flap improved alarsymmetry; however, it decreased the nostril area. The main limitation of this technique is the notch in the affected ala that required multiple corrective procedures. Similar results were obtained by Monasterio et al. [8]. These investigators suggested the need for multiple refining procedures and claimed that severe clefts extending along the whole length may be corrected by rotation of longer nasal flaps alone or in combination with forehead flaps.

Conclusion

We recommend the use of the advanced rotation-transposition flap for the management of nasal defects associated with Tessier no 3 clefts. We also recommend the use of a superiorly based transposition for cases with extensive lateral nasal wall involvement. In our case, we performed osteotomy and septoplasty to obtain an improved shape for the nasal dorsum. Surgeons may infrequently observe such cases. Consequently, they may not possess the necessary expertise to individualize the corrective procedure. The present technique is simple and can be easily incorporated in the armamentarium of surgeons. A number of studies reported that several surgical procedures are required to obtain an improved shape and nasal symmetry. In the present case, three procedures were performed to achieve acceptable symmetry between the two nostrils.

REFERENCES

[1] Tessier, P. (1976). Anatomical classification facial, cranio-facial and latero-facial clefts. *Journal of Maxillofacial Surgery*, *4*, 69-92.

[2] Zhou, Y. Q., Ji, J., Mu, X. Z., Zhang, R. H., Wei, M. & Yu, Z. Y. (2006). Diagnosis and classification of congenital craniofacial cleft deformities. *Journal of Craniofacial Surgery*, *17*, 198-201.

[3] Kawamoto, H. K. Jr. (1990). Rare craniofacial clefts, plastic surgery. Philadelphia, PA: Saunders.

[4] Losee, J. E., Kirschner, R. E., Whitaker, L. A. & Bartlett, S. P. (2004). Congenital Nasal Anomalies: A Classification Scheme. *Plastic and Reconstructive Surgery*, *113*(2), 676-689.

[5] Nishimura, Y. (1993). Embryological study of nasal cavity development in human embryos with reference to congenital nasal atresia. *Acta Anatomica (Basel)*, *147*, 140.

[6] Arey, L. Developmental Anatomy: A Textbook and Laboratory Manual of Embryology. 7th Edition. Philadelphia: Saunders, 1965.

[7] Madaree, A., Morris, W. M. & McGibbon, I. C. (1992). A method of repairing the no 3 facial cleft. *British Journal of Plastic Surgery*, *45*, 44-46.

[8] Ortiz Monasterio, F., Fuente del Campo, A. & Dimopulos, A. (1987). Nasal clefts. *Annals of Plastic Surgery*, *8*, 377.

[9] Ortega, J. & Flor, E. (1969). Incomplete naso-ocular cleft. Case report. *Plastic and Reconstructive Surgery*, *43*, 630-636.

[10] Jinka, J. R., Chekuri, H. & Annavarapu, G. (2012). Isolated cleft of the ala nasi: A report of seven cases. *Indian Journal of Plastic Surgery*, *45*, 512-515.

SECTION 3. ORTHOPEDICS AND TRAUMATOLOGY

In: Case Reports in Surgery
Editors: Ahmad Jabir Rahyussalim et al.
ISBN: 978-1-53616-582-1

Chapter 17

OUTCOMES OF RESECTION ARTHRODESIS FOR KNEE MALIGNANCIES

***Yogi Prabowo*[1]*, Afif Alhadi*[2] *and Adisa Yusuf Reksoprodjo*[2,*]**
[1] Department of Orthopedic and Traumatologic, Faculty of Medicine, RSUPN Dr. Cipto Mangunkusumo, Universitas Indonesia, Jakarta, Indonesia
[2] Orthopaedic and Traumatology Residency Program, Faculty of Medicine, Universitas Indonesia, Jakarta, Indonesia

ABSTRACT

Limb salvage surgery with tumor resection and endoprosthesis insertion is currently the preferred treatment for malignancies of the extremity. However, this procedure is not feasible in many cases and requires expensive implants that may not be available or affordable for many patients, such as in developing countries. We present three cases with distinct malignancies of the knee, osteosarcoma, metastatic bone disease due to lung cancer, and spindle cell carcinoma, treated by resection arthrodesis. After wide excision of the tumor, the combination of plates crews and K-nails with bone cement was used for arthrodesis. Functional outcomes were evaluated using the Lower Extremity Functional Scale (LEFS) score. LEFS scores were 24, 30, and 2 6 out of 80, respectively. These low scores reflected substantial loss of limb immobility. Resection arthrodesis is a viable treatment option for limb salvage in cases of knee tumor for which resection and endoprosthesis insertion are not feasible, but functional outcome is limited.

Keywords: limb salvage, resection arthrodesis, functional outcome

---

* Corresponding Author's E-mail: adisayr@gmail.com.

Introduction

Musculoskeletal tumors are relatively rare, accounting for less than 1% of all malignancies [1]. However, the majority of lower extremity tumors affect the knee, a critical joint for full limb function. Wide resection is reserved for a small subset of patients with biologically more aggressive, recurrent, and extensive tumors. Wide resection and mobile joint reconstruction are preferable for treating tumors around the knee. In certain situations, resection arthrodesis or amputation is suggested. Limb salvage surgery with tumor resection and endoprosthesis insertion is the preferred treatment, but the expensive implants may be unattainable, especially in developing countries. Resection arthrodesis is currently considered a less attractive option due to loss of joint mobility. However, resection arthrodesis does provide a stable limb, and the patient is unlikely to require revision surgery [2, 3]. In this case series, we examined the outcomes of resection arthrodesis for three distinct knee malignancies.

Case Series

The first case (Table 1) was a 15-year-old male who reported pain in his left leg for 18 months before presentation (Figure 1). The patient was diagnosed with osteosarcoma and referred to CiptoMangunkusumo Hospital, where he received four cycles of neoadjuvant chemotherapy before limb salvage surgery with wide excision and ELIAS cancer immune therapy in January 2016 (Figure 2). The wound became infected, however, requiring two corrective surgeries, but neither was successful. In May 2016, the cement was exposed. The patient then underwent knee arthrodesis in December 2016. The postoperative outcome as measured by LEFS score was 24 out of 80, indicating substantial disability (Figure 3).

The second case was a 60-year-old male who reported left leg pain for the past year before presentation. There was no history of trauma or prolonged fever, although he reported a history of weight loss. There was progressive swelling of his left knee (Figure 1). The patient was diagnosed with lung cancer in 2014 and had received curettage and bone cement surgery in December 2015. Pathological examination revealed micro-metastases of adenocarcinoma. Three months later, pain re-emerged in the same region, and X-ray examination confirmed metastatic bone disease of the left distal femur (Figure 2). In October 2016, the patient underwent limb salvage surgery using resection arthrodesis. Postoperative LEFS score was 30 (Figure 3).

The third case was a 16-year-old male who reported pain in his right knee, starting six months before presentation. His knee was swollen and painful, although he could still stand and walk (Figure 1). The patient received three treatments from a bonesetter. Two months later, a nascent lump on the knee had enlarged to the size of a tennis ball. The growth was painful and firm. In April 2016, the patient received a core biopsy, and histopathological examination revealed conventional osteosarcoma (Figure 2). At that time, the lump had grown to the size of a volleyball with no clear margin; was painful, firm, wih solid consistency; and felt warmer than the surrounding tissue. The patient then decided to receive neoadjuvant chemotherapy for three cycles with a regimen of cisplatin, ifosfamide, and adriamycin. After finishing chemotherapy, the lump was still expanding, although no inflammation or ulceration was noted. The patient agreed to limb salvage surgery including wide excision and reconstruction using right knee arthrodesis. Postoperative LEFS score was 26 (Figure 3).

Table 1. Summary of patient information

Patient	Diagnosis	Location of lesion	Time from initial complaint to arthrodesis	Other treatments	Postoperative LEFS score
Male, 15 y	Osteosarcoma	Left leg	16 months (August 2015–December 2016)	4 cycles of neoadjuvant chemotherapy Wide excision and ECI[1] Debridement and implant removal	24
Male, 60 y	Metastatic bone disease from lung carcinoma	Left thigh	2 years (2014–2016)	Chemotherapy for lung carcinoma Curettage and bone cement application	30
Male, 16 y	Osteosarcoma	Right knee	Approximately 1 year (2015–2016)	Neoadjuvant chemotherapy by cisplatin, ifosfamide, and adriamycin	26

y: year, ECI: ELIAS cancer immunotherapy.

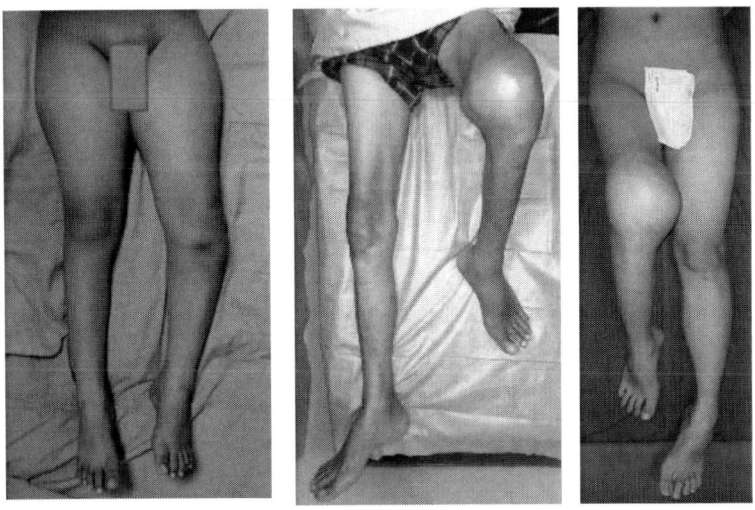

Figure 1. Clinical images of the first, second, and third patients (from left to right, respectively).

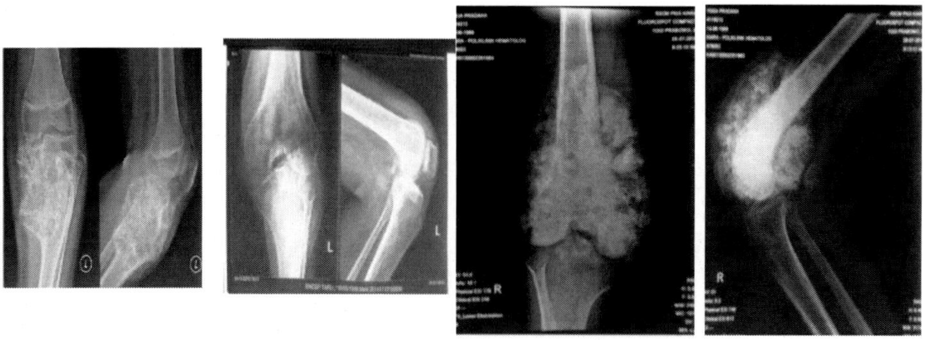

Figure 2. Preoperative X-ray images of the first, second, and third patients (from left to right).

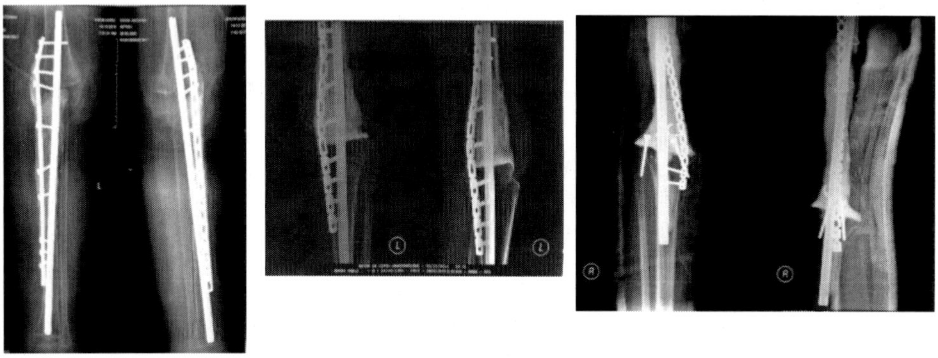

Figure 3. Postoperative X-ray images of the first, second, and third patients (from left to right).

DISCUSSION

The primary goals of knee tumor excision are to prevent recurrence and prolong life, which generally requires wide-margin resection, whereas functional preservation or restoration is secondary [4]. The choice of reconstruction strategy after resection of a tumor around the knee joint is based on many factors. Arthrodesis provides stable, durable, and predictable reconstruction that preserves some leg motion but at the expense of flexion and extension at the knee. Once the decision has been made to perform arthrodesis, the specific technique selected should have demonstrated success with few complications, as this group of patients will probably receive postoperative chemotherapy and some will have limited life expectancy [5].

Enneking and Shirley [6] proposed the following indications for resection arthrodesis: 1) a recurrent benign, potentially malignant, or malignant lesion that involves the distal end of the femur, the knee joint, or the proximal end of the tibia; 2) a tumor location with an adequate plane of uninvolved tissue between the lesion and posterior neurovascular structures for surgical resection according to the degree of aggressiveness of the tumor; and 3) a vigorous patient whose expectations and lifestyle require a stable, painless extremity capable of withstanding demanding function. All three of our cases were deemed suitable for resection arthrodesis based on these criteria [6].

Kwan [7] evaluated the outcomes and complications associated with resection arthrodesis for 22 primary bone tumors (13 giant cell tumors and nine osteosarcomas) around the knee and reported that of 14 patients who returned for final evaluation, 79.8% had satisfactory outcomes according to the Musculoskeletal Tumor Society grading system. A study by Alam [8] evaluating functional outcomes in children with a malignant tumor around the knee joint also supported the efficacy of resection arthrodesis, particularly for pediatric sarcomas around the knee and for cases in which endoprosthesis insertion is not feasible because of young age or lack of resources. In a study by Bassiony et al. [9], all patients receiving resection arthrodesis achieved functional results comparable with endoprosthetic patients. This result was confirmed by Harris et al. [10], who reported that patients functioned similarly and walked with comparable velocities, efficiencies, and oxygen consumption rates whether treated by arthrodesis or arthroplasty.

In our cases, the outcome was measured using the LEFS, which consists of 20 items evaluating the ability to perform everyday tasks, each with a maximum score of 4[11] The LEFS results in our cases indicated substantial functional limitations after arthrodesis. Nonetheless, resection arthrodesis appears preferable to amputation. Shih et al. [12] reported a 5-year survival rate of 39% following arthrodesis for knee osteosarcoma, which was lower than following endoprosthetic insertion (60%) but higher than after amputation (13%).

CONCLUSION

Resection arthrodesis is a viable treatment option for limb salvage in patients with tumors around the knee, although the functional outcome is limited. However, for cases in which prosthesis replacement is unobtainable, arthrodesis with wide excision still salvages a tumorless limb with some functional capacity.

REFERENCES

[1] Siegel R, Miller KD, Jemal A. Cancer Statistic 2016. *CA Cancer J Clin.* 2016; 66(1): 7-30.

[2] Salai M, Neurabay J, Caspi I, Horoszowski H. Resection arthrodesis of the knee in the treatment of tumours – a long-term follow-up. *Int Orthop.* 1997; 21(2): 101-3.

[3] Bassiony AA, Abdelrahman M, Abdelhady A, Assal MK. Resection arthrodesis for the management of aggressive giant cell tumor of the distal femur. *Indian J Orthop.* 2009; 43(1): 67-71.

[4] Chao EY, Sim FH. Functional results following resection arthrodesis about the knee. In *New Developments for Limb Salvage in Musculoskeletal Tumors.* Tokyo: Springer; 1989. p. 567-71.

[5] Kapoor SK, Tiwari A. Resection arthrodesis for giant cell tumors around the knee. *Indian J Orthop.* 2007; 41(2): 124-8.

[6] Enneking WF, Shirley PD. Resection-arthrodesis for malignant and potentially malignant lesions about the knee using an intramedullary rod and local bone grafts. *J Bone Joint Surg Am.* 1977;59(2):223-36.

[7] Kwan MK, Ng ES, Penafort R, Saw A, Sengupta S. Resection arthrodesis for primary bone tumor about the knee. *Med J Malaysia.* 2005;60(C): 66-71.

[8] Alam S. *Functional outcome in children undergoing resection-arthrodesis for malignant tumors around the knee joint.*

[9] Shalaby S, Shalaby H, Bassiony A. Limb salvage for osteosarcoma of the distal tibia with resection arthrodesis, autogenous fibular graft and Ilizarov external fixator. *J Bone Joint Surg.* 2006;88(12):1642-6.

[10] Harris IE, Leff AR, Gitelis S, Simon MA. Function after amputation, arthrodesis or arthroplasty for tumors about the knee. *J Bone Joint Surg Am.* 1990;72(10):1477-85.

[11] Binkley JM, Stratford PW, Lott SA, Riddle DL. The Lower Extremity Functional Scale (LEFS): scale development, measurement properties, and clinical application. *Phys Ther.* 1999;79(4):371-83.

[12] Shih HN, Shih LY. Resection arthrodesis of the knee for osteosarcoma: An alternative when mobile joint reconstruction is not feasible. *Chang Gung Med J.* 2005; 28(6): 411.

In: Case Reports in Surgery
Editors: Ahmad Jabir Rahyussalim et al.
ISBN: 978-1-53616-582-1

Chapter 18

Total Sacrectomy and Spinopelvic Reconstruction of Sacrococcygeal Chordoma

***Yogi Prabowo*[1]*, Afif Alhadi*[2]*, and Rizky Priambodo Wisnubaroto*[2,*]**

[1]Department of Orthopedic and Traumatologic, Faculty of Medicine, RSUPN Dr. Cipto Mangunkusumo, Universitas Indonesia, Jakarta, Indonesia

[2]Orthopaedic and Traumatologic, Faculty of Medicine, Universitas Indonesia, Jakarta, Indonesia

Abstract

Chordoma is a low-to-intermediate-grade malignant tumor encapsulating the notochord. It is rare, insidious in onset, and frequently diagnosed late. Due to its size, location, and nature, surgical treatment becomes challenging. Here we report a case of sacral chordoma in a 33-year-old woman treated with a combined anterior and posterior approach to remove the tumor enbloc, followed by posterior stabilization using rod–screw system. Total sacrectomy and spinopelvic reconstruction is the treatment of choice for sacral chordoma. We were able to achieve complete resection of the tumor mass with no recurrence after six months of follow-up.

Keywords: sacrum, chordoma, combined posterior and anterior approach, sacrectomy

[*] Corresponding Author's E-mail: risky.wisnubaroto@gmail.com.

Introduction

Chordoma is a low-to-intermediate-grade malignant tumor encapsulating the notochord. It accounts for 1%–4% of all primary malignant bone tumors, is insidious in onset, and frequently has a late presentation. Most chordomas present after the age of 30, with one-third occurring in the sixth decade [1]. This is a slow-growing but locally aggressive tumor and originates from primitive notochordal elements. This tumor is mainly found along the midline from the base of the skull to the sacrococcygeal region of the pelvis [2].

The treatment goal for sacral chordoma is to achieve en bloc excision with tumor-free margins to maximize local tumor control and survival. However,this is challenging in some cases, as sacral chordomas are difficult to excise entirely because preservation of sacral stability and sacral nerve pathways to the rectum and bladder limits the extent of the surgery [2, 3]. The prognosis for these patients correlated with negative surgical margins, which almost always results in a poor prognosis in patients with intralesional resection [2, 4].

We report a case of sacral chordoma in a 33-year-old woman presenting with radiating pain and bladder obstruction as the primary symptoms. Due to the nature of the tumor involvement, we performed an en bloc sacral resection with the Galveston technique using a combined anterior and posterior approach, achieving stability with pedicle screw and rod fixation.

Case Report

A 33-year-old female patient presented to our office with a chief complaint of ongoing pain in her left hip for four years. The symptoms started with periodic cramps in the hip that radiated to her feet. Though the pain was initially abated with the use of over-the-counter pain killers, some degree of pain remained. Approximately two years ago, the patient started experiencing lower urinary tract symptoms along with worsening hip pain, which had now extended to her left knee. She consulted with an internist and was diagnosed with a urinary tract infection and treated accordingly. However, shortly after that, she was unable to pass urine and was eventually hospitalized. A complete workup was performed, including a CT scan, which revealed an abdominal mass. She was referred to an obstetrician-gynecologist, and a working diagnosis of uterine myoma was made. A follow-up MRI was performed, which showed the bony origin of the tumor. Next, the patient was referred to our outpatient clinic for treatment at CiptoMangunkusumo Hospital.

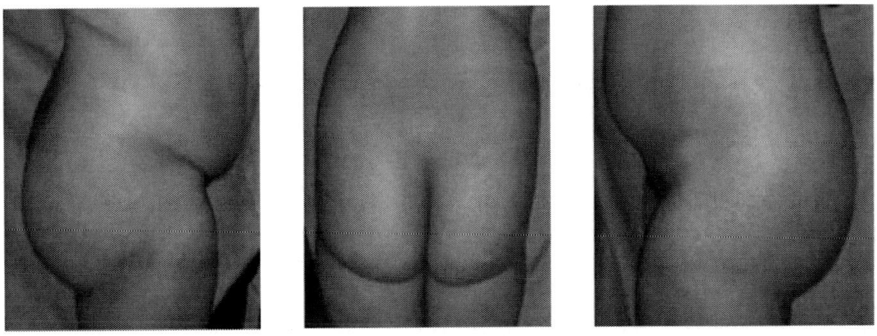

Figure 1. Lateral and anteroposterior view of the sacrum. No remarkable features were noted during the physical examination.

No remarkable features were noted during the physical examination. Examination of the lower back revealed no palpable mass, minimal tenderness of the lower back with palpation, and a visual analog scale score of 2–3. Also, she had a normal range of motion of the hip, knee, and ankle joints. Neurological examination revealed a sensory deficit in the left lower extremity, particularly the lateral aspect of the foot, along with hypoesthesia in the perianal region. Motor examination of the lower extremity identified slight weakness of the gastrocnemius and peroneus muscles of the left foot (motor score 4/5). In addition, the patient exhibited catheter dependency of the bladder with normal bowel function.

We conducted a pelvic X-ray and an MRI of the whole abdomen and the lumbosacral area. From the plain radiograph of the pelvis, we identified a mass extending to the right sacroiliac joint (S1–S5) that was suggestive of a chordoma.

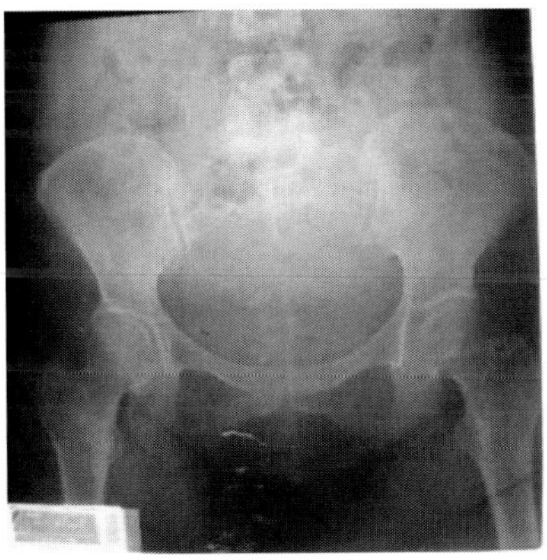

Figure 2. Anteroposterior and lateral view of the pelvis. The mass extends from S1 to S5, with possible involvement at the right sacroiliac joint.

Next, we obtained an MRI of the lower abdominal and pelvic region, which revealed a dense, lobulated mass with active hemorrhage from S1 to S5, extending to the anterior and posterior, obliterating the anterior visceral organs and spinal cord, respectively, suggestive of chordoma. The mass also appeared to involve the sacrum, the Coccygeus, and part of the left iliac ostium.

A follow-up was done with a CT-guided biopsy of the lesion. The pathology results matched the initial suspicion of the diagnosis, with features characteristic of a chordoma.

From the medical history, physical examination, imaging, pathologic examination, and conferences with a range of specialists, we diagnosed the tumor as sacral chordoma. Surgery is the treatment of choice; thus, the orthopedic and spinal oncology teams performed total sacrectomy and spinopelvic reconstruction, respectively.

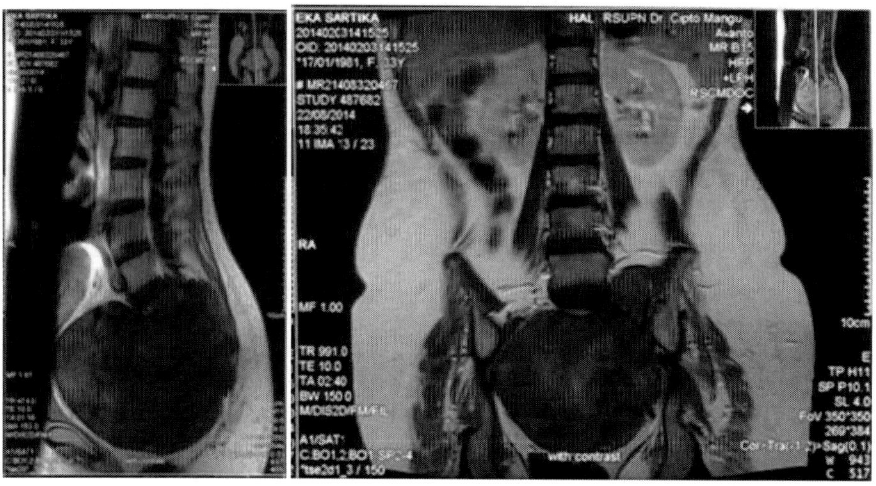

(A) (B)

Figure 3. MRI of the lumbar spine and pelvic region demonstrating the extent of the lesion. (a) Sagittal view showing involvement at L5–S5 and obliteration of the spinal canal. (b) AP view showing the lesion extending to both sacroiliac joints and involving the gluteus minimus and medius muscles.

We elected to divide the operation into two stages. For the first stage, the tumor was resected, and posterior instrumentation of the cervical spine was performed. For the second stage, pelvic reconstruction with fibular graft was performed in hopes that the patient can sit independently.

In the first stage of the operation using an anterior approach, we made a midline incision along the abdomen to remove the anterior part of the tumor, incising the rectus abdominis and the internal and external oblique muscles. There, we obtained a view of the tumor, which was putting pressure anteriorly on the intraperitoneal organs. Next, we released the anterior mass of the tumor, whereas the vascular team performed ligation of the internal iliac and median sacral arteries. The gastroenterology team preserved the sigmoid colon, created the stoma, and closed the wound. We prepared the patient in pronation to remove as much of the tumor as possible to ensure a clear margin.

For the second stage of the operation, we continued the posterior approach to release the posterior portion of the tumor and remove the sacrum and the tumor mass. A longitudinal incision was made through the midline of the sacrum from L2 to the coccyx. The tumor mass extended to the bilateral S1 joints. We removed the tumor and a small amount of the surrounding tissue. The L2–L5 nerve roots were compressed within the tumor mass.

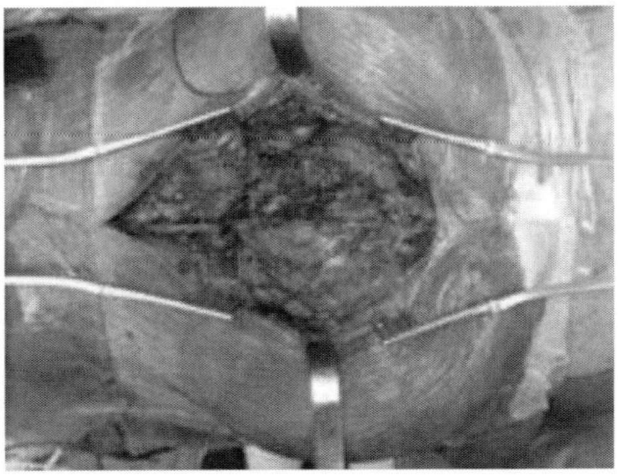

Figure 4. Posterior view of the chordoma extending from S1 to S5. Note the presence of nerve roots within the mass.

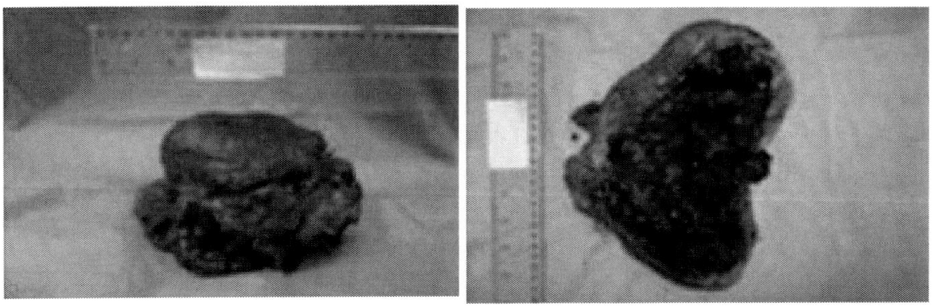

(A) (B)

Figure 5. (a) gross view of the chordoma. (b) The cross-sectional view of the tumor. Note the lobulated mass with fat lobules separated by fibrous bands.

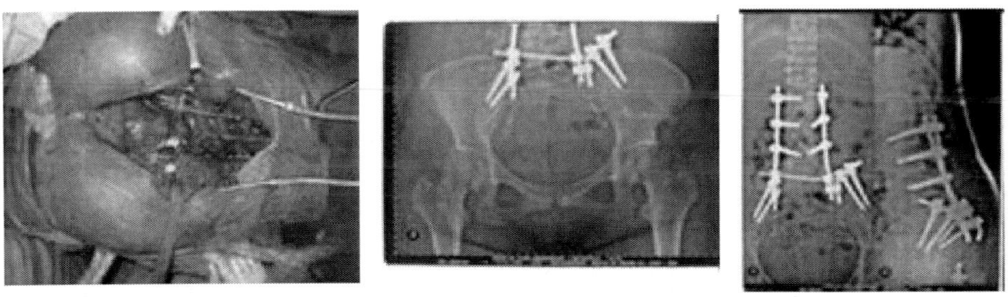

(A) (B) (C)

Figure 6. (a) Direct view of the screws. The allograft used to promote bone healing is not shown. (b) Anteroposterior view of the hip post-operation. (c) Anteroposterior and lateral view of the hip post-operation.

To stabilize the site, we installed pedicle screws at the L2–L4 level, and at the bilateral sacroiliac joint (Galveston technique). We performed laminectomy between L5 and S1 and ligation of the thecal sac, followed by an osteotomy at L5–S1. We removed the tumor and placed the fibular bone allografts. Finally, we closed the wound and installed a closed-suction drain.

The tumor mass was sent for pathological evaluation. The results were consistent with chordoma, macroscopically, and also microscopically, with the appearance of lobulated cell mass separated by fibrous bands. Besides, the presence of "physaliphorous cells" (pale vacuolated cytoplasm) suggested a chordoma.

DISCUSSION

The clinical features of a chordoma correlate with the location and spread of the neoplasm. As this is a slow-growing tumor, it usually produces-characteristic signs and symptoms, making diagnosis difficult. Pain in the sacrococcygeal region is the most common presenting symptom. The pain is dull and may be felt on the lower back or the tip of the spinal column. Constipation or anuria may be experienced due to the obstruction [1]. The degree of obstruction in the patient made her dependent on the catheter until the time of surgery.

Currently, surgery is still the mainstay of treatment for sacral chordomas. Enbloc excision remains the central tenet in the surgical management of chordoma [5]. Kaiser et al. reported that local recurrence was almost twice as high in patients who underwent en bloc resection with dissection of the tumor capsule at the time of surgery compared with those who had complete en bloc excision without violating the tumor capsule [6]. Today, more aggressive surgery and wider surgical margins have improved the local control of sacral chordomas [7].

Before the operation, we talked to the patient about all of the possible consequences of the operation, including recurrence, reoperations, and diminished functional outcomes [8]. We also acted quickly before the tumor occupied more space in the pelvic area, and before more symptoms occurred and became a further risk to the patient.

For this patient, we used a combined anterior and posterior approach due to the extensive nature of the tumor. This approach is used only for tumors with radiological suspicion of anterior involvement. In most cases, chordomas are extremely difficult to excise completely [9]. A combined anterior and posterior procedure allows for an intralesional/marginal resection of the tumor and the involved vertebra. En bloc resection of primary malignant bone tumors, including chordoma, is shown to increase the survival rate of patients and is a crucial part of the treatment regimen [3].

The extent of sacral resection determines pelvic stability and the need to undergo reconstruction. We performed an osteotomy at L5–S1 and removed the tumor involving the S1 joints. Such a procedure may cause spinopelvic dissociation, resulting in gross instability in the rotational and vertical planes. Therefore, reconstruction and reinforcement are needed to ensure stability [10]. We placed iliac screws and screws at L2–L3–L4 to maintain stability.

Even though our patient received meticulous care, there were some complications. The patient developed a fever with pain at the surgical site. The allografts were identified as the primary cause of infection; thus, we debrided the wound and removed the graft. Also, despite our best efforts at prevention, early signs of decubitus ulcer (bed sore) were noted on the left buttock.

The complication rate after total sacrectomy is quite high, mainly related to wound healing. A second or even third surgery may be required to remove deep wound infection or flap necrosis [11]. Postoperatively, the patient retained her neurological status and experienced less pain. There was no recurrence of the tumor after six months of follow-up.

CONCLUSION

Chordoma is a rare primary bone tumor. Clinicians of different specialties need to recognize these conditions early, as the symptoms are not characteristic and are site-dependent — adequate surgical treatment results in substantial improvement in neurological function and symptoms. Extensive tumor removal using a combined anterior and posterior approach followed by a stable reconstruction may achieve a favorable clinical outcome [3]. Even with strict adherence to protocol, the risk of infection is high,and a second operation may be required [4, 9, 10].

REFERENCES

[1] Mirra, J. M. N. S., Rocca Della, C., Mertens, F. *Pathology and Genetics of Tumours of Soft Tissue and Bone.* (Fletcher CDM, U. K., Mertens F (ed.)). Lyon: IARC Press, 2002.

[2] Rao, B. S. S., Menezes, L. T., Rao, A. D. & John, S. K. (2005). Sacral chordoma–a report of two cases. *Indian journal ofsurgery, 67.*

[3] Jung, Y. Y., &S hin, H. (2009). Combined anterior and posterior en bloc vertebrectomy for lumbar chordoma, *Journal ofkorean neurosurgical society, 45,* 243-245.

[4] Hulen, C. A., Temple, H. T., Fox, W. P., Sama, A. A., Green, B. A., Eismont, F. J. (2006) Oncologic and functional outcome following sacrectomy for sacral chordoma. *JBJS, 88,* 1532-1539.

[5] Walcott, B. P., Nahed, B. V., Mohyeldin, A., Coumans, J.-V., Kahle, K. T., Ferreira, Chordoma., M. J. (2012). Current concepts, management, and future directions. *The Lancet oncology. 13,* e69-e76.

[6] Kaiser, T. E., Pritchard, D. J. & Unni, K. K. (1984). Clinicopathologic study of sacrococcygeal chordoma. *Cancer, 53,* 2574-2578.

[7] Hsieh, P. C., Xu, R., Sciubba, D. M., McGirt, M. J., Nelson, C., Witham, T. F., Wolinksy, J. P. & Gokaslan, Z. L. (2009). Long-term clinical outcomes following en bloc resections for sacral chordomas and chondrosarcomas: a series of twenty consecutive patients. *Spine, 34,* 2233-223.

[8] Gallia, G. L., Haque, R., Garonzik, I., Witham, T. F., Khavkin, Y. A., Wolinsky, J. P., Suk, I. & Gokaslan, Z. L. (2005). Spinal pelvic reconstruction after total sacrectomy for en bloc resection of a giant sacral chordoma. *Journal of neurosurgery: Spine, 3,* 501-506.

[9] Cheng, E. Y., Özerdemoglu, R. A., Transfeldt, E. E. & Thompson Jr, R. C. (1999). Lumbosacral chordoma: prognostic factors and treatment. *Spine, 24,* 1639.

[10] Okaji, R. Y., Silveira Jr, J. M. D., Nakano, M. K., Kiuti, L. T. & Maiorano, M. C. N. T. (2008). Sacral chordoma en-bloc resection and lumbar-iliac stabilization. *Arquivos de neuro-psiquiatria, 66,* 400-401.

[11] Varga, P. P. & Lazary, A. (2010). Chordoma of the sacrum: "en bloc" total sacrectomy and lumbopelvic reconstruction. *European Spine Journal, 19,* 1039-1040.

In: Case Reports in Surgery
Editors: Ahmad Jabir Rahyussalim et al.
ISBN: 978-1-53616-582-1

Chapter 19

LOW BACK AND LEG PAIN INDUCED BY DURAL SCAR FORMATION AFTER LAMINECTOMY FOR LUMBAR CANAL STENOSIS: CASE REPORT AND LITERATURE REVIEW

Ahmad Jabir Rahyussalim[1,2,3,*], Aria Adhitya[1], Tri Kurniawati[2,3] and Khairul Hukmi[1]

[1]Department of Orthopaedic and Traumatology, Faculty of Medicine, Universitas Indonesia-Cipto Mangunkusumo General Hospital, Jakarta, Indonesia
[2]Stem Cell and Tissue Engineering Cluster, IMERI Faculty of Medicine, Universitas Indonesia, Jakarta, Indonesia
[3]Stem Cell Medical Technology Integrated Service Unit, Cipto Mangunkusumo General Hospital, Jakarta, Indonesia

ABSTRACT

Introduction: Dural scarring may develop after laminectomy, resulting in persistent back and leg pain. Laminectomy for decompression exposes the dura mater, stimulating the growth of scar tissue on the dural surface. Such scarring can impair nerve conduction and induce chronic pain, localized according to the affected spinal levels. *Case Presentation:* A single case of back pain and pain radiating to the lower limbs is reported 12 months following laminectomy at L4–L5. Magnetic resonance images revealed new soft tissue in the posterior region pressing on the dura. *Discussion:* Re-operation was performed for decompression. Intraoperative examination revealed scar tissue around the dural surface at the previous laminectomy site. Decompression and scarectomy were conducted, but the outcome was unsatisfactory because it proved impossible to remove all

* Corresponding Author's E-mail: rahyussalim71@ui.ac.id.

the scar tissue from the dura without increasing the risk of nerve root damage. As a result, low back pain was mitigated, but the leg pain persisted. *Conclusion:* Laminectomy can result in dural scar formation and chronic pain that is intractable to reparative surgery. Thus, it is critical to institute perioperative procedures that reduce the risk of subsequent dural scar formation.

Keywords: Dura scar, laminectomy, leg pain, fibrosis

INTRODUCTION

Postoperative dural scar formation, involving the paravertebral musculature, thecal sac, and nerve roots, is a frequent cause of recurrent symptoms and pain after lumbar disk surgery [1, 2]. Such dural lesions result from the destruction of epidural fat, intra-spinal hematoma, and advancement of the spinal erector muscles into the spinal canal, [3] and are a major cause of lumbar pain and sciatic irritation after lumbar surgery. The mechanical tethering of nerve roots to the dura by epidural adhesions may contribute to persistent back and leg pain after lumbar laminectomy, termed failed back syndrome [4, 5].

Non-invasive treatments are being developed to reduce neural adhesion to scar tissue. Absorbable, oxidized, regenerated cellulose (Inter-ceed) reduced neural adhesion in a rabbit model following experimental laminectomy [6]. In addition, intraoperative neuromonitoring (IONM) can predict the risks of adverse outcomes, such as paraparesis, paraplegia, and quadriplegia, following spinal surgery [7]. Nonetheless, prevention and treatment of dural scar formation remain substantial challenges for spinal surgeons.

We report a case of dural scar following laminectomy that resulted in progressively worsening low back and radiating leg pain. This case highlights potential complications that should be anticipated before primary surgery and re-operation for scar excision, including preventing a dural tear, as well as the importance of IONM.

CASE ILLUSTRATION

A 36-year-old male with no history of spinal trauma presented with complaints of worsening back pain, radiating to the right and left legs, for the previous two months. It was described as continuous sharp pain with intermittent tingling that was influenced by activity and disappeared in the resting position. He had reported back pain four years earlier, described as dull intermittent pain without spread or tingling, which was treated using pain relievers and physiotherapy. Two years before the current presentation, he reported back pain and was examined by a neurosurgeon, who diagnosed lumbar disc herniation at L4–L5 and performed fenestration and laminectomy. The patient reported being pain free until the previous two months, when he began to experience back pain in the same place.

He also suffered weakness during dorsiflexion. An orthopedic spine surgeon recommended reparative surgery after conducting a full examination. The patient provided informed consent to publish anonymized clinical results.

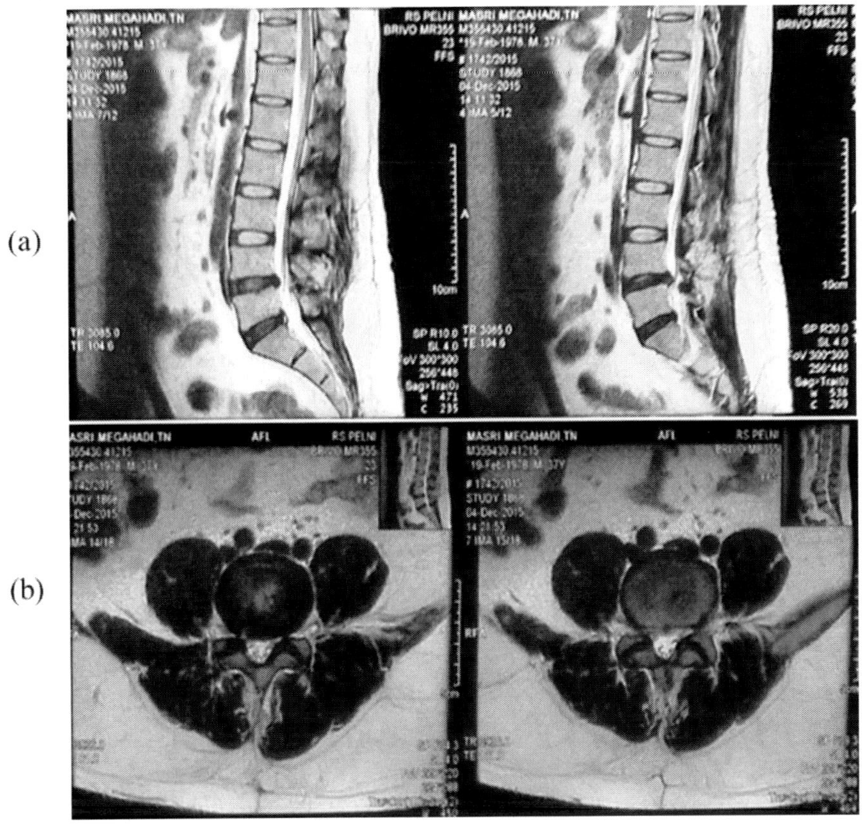

Figure 1. Preoperative MRI. (a) Sagittal projection showing disk protrusion at the L4–L5 level and a hyperintense defect posterior to L3–L5. (b) Axial projection showing canal stenosis and inflammation of facet joints and flavum ligaments.

At presentation, lumbosacral MRI showed compression of the right thecal sac and nerve roots caused by right posteroparacentral protrusion of L4 and L5 intervertebral discs (Figure 1). There was also a hyperintensity region on the posterior side of the L3–L5 intervertebral discs from suspected scar tissue. A myelograph revealed mild spinal canal indentation at the same level as intervertebral discs L4 and L5, which was diagnosed as lumbar canal stenosis due to disk herniation and scar formation (Figure 2).

Surgery was performed, using the posterior approach, at L4–L5. Scar tissue was attached to the entire dural surface field, measuring about 1.5 cm2 and extending to the edge of the lamina. After pedicle screw fixation (Figure 3), we attempted to free the dural surface of scar tissue. Unfortunately, this proved impossible, so we performed a partial scarectomy and carefully created a floating dura (Figure 4). After surgery, pain symptoms were reduced, sensorimotor functions were normal, and the patient was able to return to his normal activities. However, leg pain persisted during follow-up.

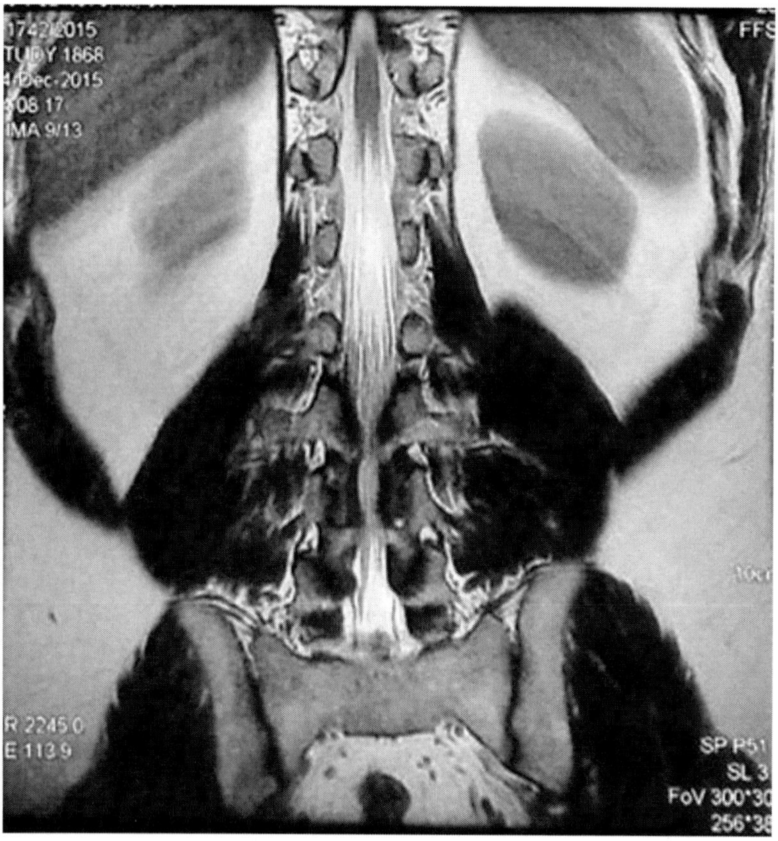

Figure 2. Myelograph showing mild indentation of the spinal canal at the level of intervertebral discs L4 and L5.

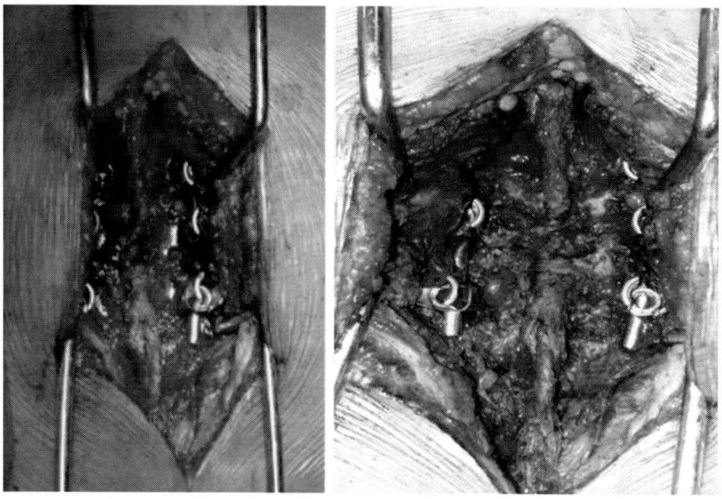

Figure 3. Intraoperative findings. (a) Posterior stabilization with pedicle screw fixation. (b) Exposed dural scar at spinal level L4–L5.

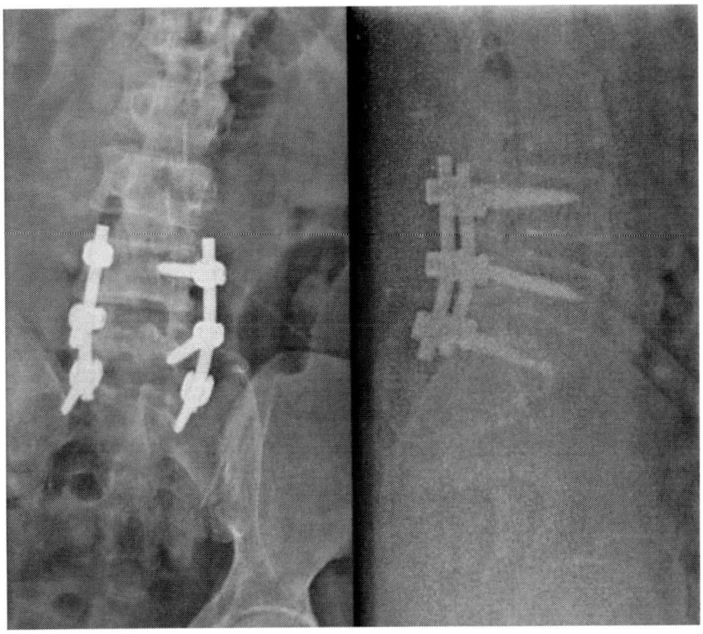

Figure 4. Postoperative X-ray (anteroposterolateral projection). Pedicle screw stabilization at spinal levels L4, L5, and S1.

DISCUSSION

Scar formation around the dura and the nerve root may cause clinically intractable complications following laminectomy. Post-laminectomy scar tissue is formed mainly by invasive fibrous connective tissue from the posterior paraspinal muscles into the postoperative hematoma [6]. Connective tissue from the bony edges of the laminectomy margins may also contribute to a limited extent. Scar tissue invasion into the vertebral canal is suppressed when epidural fatty tissue is present. Even if absent, invasion of scar tissue into the vertebral canal is not very marked. However, the scar tissue may adhere strongly to the dura. Therefore, separating the postoperative hematoma from vertebral canal tissues, including the dura, may inhibit scar tissue from invading the vertebral canal and adhering to the dura [2]. The current case underscores the importance of preventing scar formation in the perioperative period. Intraoperative neuromonitoring is critical for this purpose.

Monitoring during structural spine and spinal cord surgeries may include somatosensory evoked potentials (SSEP), motor evoked potentials (MEP), and electromyography (EMG, free running and stimulated) [8]. MEP directly monitors the motor pathway itself. The persistence of full muscle MEP amplitude usually indicates good central motor function preservation, while substantially reduced MEPs or elevated thresholds can indicate partial, transient, or even permanent central motor deficits. It is currently difficult to explain these different outcomes following MEP reduction. Partial weakness can be difficult to assess in the acute postoperative patient and so may be overlooked, while documented weakness may recover slowly. Thus, long-term evaluation is critical for identifying intraoperative MEP signs of more severe and lasting damage. Note, however, that a partial central motor deficit is possible even without any appreciable intraoperative muscle MEP alteration [8]. Somatosensory evoked potentials (SSEP) are generated by stimulation of afferent peripheral nerve fibers by electrical, vibrational, or tactile stimuli. Following either mixed nerve or sensory nerve stimulation, SSEPs can be recorded over more proximal portions of the peripheral and central nervous system, including the peripheral nerves, spinal cord, and/or brain [7].

CONCLUSION

A dural scar is a fibrotic lesion that can form after laminectomy and cause recurrence of back pain and (or) radiating leg pain. Scarring is favored by factors such as the fibrous organization of hematomas, keloid reaction, and technical faults in the operation, and may develop into a hypertrophic, enveloping membrane. Pain severity and distribution depends on the dural scar's size and location. Attempts to limit tissue formation involve surgical technique variations, microdiscectomy, anti-inflammatory medications, and several biologic and synthetic materials. However, preventing epidural fibrosis after laminectomy remains a major challenge in spinal surgery.

REFERENCES

[1] Benoist, M; Ficat, C; Baraf P; Cauchoix J. Postoperative lumbar epiduroarachnoiditis. Diagnostic and therapeutic aspects. *Spine*, 1980 5, 432-436.

[2] Lee, CK; Alexander, H. Prevention of post laminectomy scar formation. *Spine*, 1984 9, 545-550.

[3] LaRocca, H; Macnab, I. The laminectomy membrane: Studies in its evolution, characteristics, effects and prophylaxis in dogs. *J. Bone Joint Surg. Br.* 1974 56, 545-50.

[4] Ross, JS; Robertson, JT; Frederickson, RCA. Association between peridural scar and recurrent radicular pain after lumbar discectomy: magnetic resonance evaluation. *Neurosurgery*, 1996 38, 855-861.

[5] Boot, DA; Hughes, SPF. The prevention of adhesions after laminectomy. Adverse results of Zenoderm implantations into laminectomy sites in rabbits. *Clin. Orthop.*, 1987 215, 296-302.

[6] Ikeda, K; Yamauchi, D; Tomita, K. Preliminary study for prevention of neural adhesion using an absorbable oxidized regenerated cellulose sheet. *Hand Surg.*, 2002 7, 11-14.

[7] Takata, Y; Sakai, T; Higashino, K; Matsuura, T; Suzue, N; Hamada, D; Goto, T; Nishisho, T; Tsutsui, T; Goda, Y; Morimoto, M; Abe, M; Mineta, K; Kimura, T; Nitta, A; Hama, S; Higuchi, TC; Jha, S; Takahashi, R; Fukuta, S; Sairyo, K. Review: State of the art: Intraoperative neuromonitoring in spinal deformity surgery. *J. Med. Invest.*, 2015 62, 103-108.

[8] Park, JH; Hyum, SJ. Intraoperative neurophysiological monitoring in spinal surgery. *World J. Clin. Cases*, 2015 3,765-773.

In: Case Reports in Surgery
Editors: Ahmad Jabir Rahyussalim et al.
ISBN: 978-1-53616-582-1

Chapter 20

FUNCTIONAL AND RADIOLOGICAL OUTCOMES IN PATIENTS WITH SPONDYLITIS TUBERCULOSIS AND KYPHOTIC DEFORMITY TREATED USING A TWO-STAGE CORRECTION PROCEDURE: A CASE SERIES

***Ifran Saleh*[1] *and Auliya Akbar*[2,*]**

[1]Spine consultant of Orthopedic and Traumatology
Department of Cipto Mangunkusumo General Hospital,
Faculty of Medicine, Universitas Indonesia
Jakarta, Indonesia

[2]Resident of Orthopedic and Traumatology
Department of Cipto Mangunkusumo General Hospital,
Faculty of Medicine, Universitas Indonesia
Jakarta, Indonesia

ABSTRACT

Kyphotic deformity is a devastating complication of spondylitis tuberculosis as it can progress to more severe complications, such as cardiopulmonary dysfunction and nerve compression symptoms. Surgical correction is as important as local infection control itself (through debridement and abscess drainage). There are several approaches for spondylitis tuberculosis with kyphotic deformity, and all are based on the patient's condition and other

*Corresponding Author's E-mail: abay.jabz@gmail.com.

local considerations, such as hospital and national health policies. This report aims to provide information on the clinical and radiological outcomes after two-stage treatment for kyphotic deformity in patients with spondylitis tuberculosis. We present four cases of kyphotic deformity in patients with spondylitis tuberculosis who underwent two-stage surgery at Cipto Mangunkusumo National Hospital, Jakarta, Indonesia. All patients were female, with a mean age of 37.5 years. The mean follow-up period was 45 months. One patient had a lumbar lesion with loss of lordosis (less than 20° lordosis), and the remaining three had thoracic lesions with a kyphotic angle more than 45°. All patients underwent a two-stage surgery involving initial debridement, kyphotic correction, posterior stabilization, and fusion, followed by anterior fusion with a titanium cage and bone graft. The surgical outcomes were evaluated by comparing the preoperative and postoperative Oswestry Disability Index (ODI) scores and kyphotic angles. After surgery, all patients had good outcomes with reductions in the ODI score and kyphotic angle. The mean ODI score reduced from 20 preoperatively to 5 postoperatively. Additionally, the kyphotic angle reduced from 90° preoperatively to 22° postoperatively (after the second stage). Our two-stage procedure for the treatment of spondylitis tuberculosis with kyphotic deformity was associated with good functional and radiological outcomes at long-term follow-up. Thus, we recommend this two-stage procedure as a standard for cases similar to our reported cases.

Keywords: anterior fusion, kyphotic deformity, posterior stabilization, spondylitis tuberculosis

INTRODUCTION

Indonesia has the third highest tuberculosis (TB) endemicity, and spinal TB is quite common, although the exact prevalence of spondylitis tuberculosis (STB) in Indonesia is unclear [1]. The major problems associated with this disease are pain and deformity. Kyphotic deformity has been reported as a disabling complication of spinal infection, as progression causes additional pain, cardiopulmonary symptoms, and possible neurological deficit, in addition to the cosmetic problem itself [2].

Surgical debridement and stabilization are considered in many patients with progressive deformity and abscess formation with or without neurological deficit. Stabilization for deformity correction and maintenance can be achieved either with bone grafts alone or with a combination of grafts and posterior or anterior instrumentation [3].

Implant placement in an infected area remains controversial, partly because it is unclear whether implants interfere with infection control. This has led many authors to treat STB in two stages with initial debridement and bone grafting followed by delayed instrumented fusion. Although approach selection for the surgical treatment of thoracolumbar TB is still being debated, a combined anterior plus posterior approach can help overcome the stability-related drawbacks of the anterior approach alone. However, this approach entails two surgeries (single or staged) with additional morbidity [3].

This report aims to provide information on the clinical and radiological outcomes after two-stage treatment for kyphotic deformity in thoracic and thoracolumbar TB at our center. We present four cases of kyphotic deformity in STB patients who underwent first-stage debridement and decompression followed by second-stage anterior fusion with a titanium mesh cage and graft.

Case Series

Between 2011 and 2016, 15 patients with confirmed STB infection (nine females and six males; mean age, 34.3 years; age range, 13–65 years) were treated surgically with a two-stage procedure involving debridement, kyphotic correction, and stabilization followed by anterior fusion at Cipto Mangunkusumo National Hospital, Jakarta, Indonesia. However, 11 patients were lost to follow-up, and thus, we were able to collect data from only four patients. All four patients were female, and the mean age was 37.5 years. Of these four patients, one had lumbar loss of lordosis and the other three had kyphotic deformity.

In the first stage, we performed debridement, kyphotic correction, and stabilization. All patients were operated under general anesthesia and were placed in the prone position. A posterior midline approach was used in all patients. Debridement was performed by removing necrotic material within the body and disk by using curettes, and any paraspinal abscess was drained. Kyphotic correction was achieved by inserting bilateral pedicle screws at 2–3 cranial and caudal vertebrae. Further correction was achieved after completion of rod insertion by gradual compression between the screws toward the apex of the deformity. Finally, posterolateral fusion was performed by trimming the facets and laminae of the diseased vertebral segments. The bone materials obtained in the trimming process were used as bone grafts.

In the second stage, we performed anterior fusion by the anterior approach. All patients were operated under general anesthesia and were placed in the supine position. Thoracotomy was performed, and then, anterior reconstruction of the vertebral body was performed using a titanium mesh or anterior cage filled with cancellous bone grafts from the iliac spine.

Before surgery and after the first and second stages, we evaluated the kyphotic angle using Subroto Angle Aid (Figure 1 and 2). Subjectively, we determined the disability level using the Oswestry Disability Index (ODI) questionnaire before surgery and at follow-up (more than 6 months) (Figure 3). The ODI questionnaire includes questions that assess a patient's ability to perform activities of daily living.

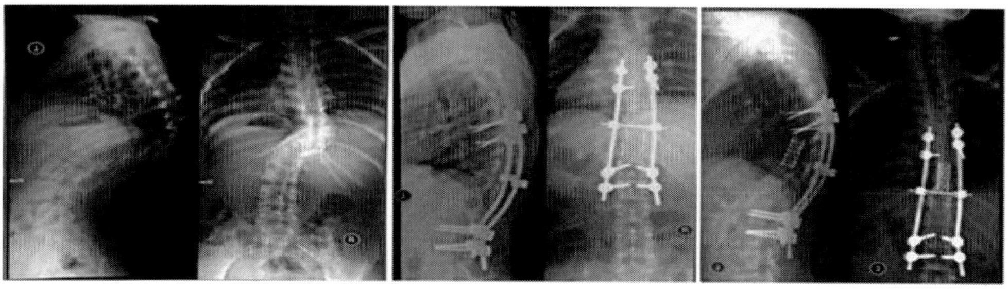

(a) (b) (c)

Figure 1. Radiography in patient 1. (a) Preoperative regional kyphotic angle, 96°; (b) Kyphotic angle after the second stage, 24°; (c) Kyphotic angle at a 4-year follow-up, 28°.

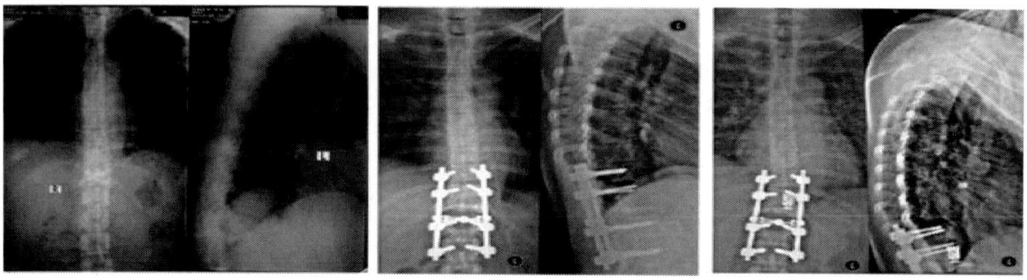

(a) (b) (c)

Figure 2. Radiography in patient 2. (a) Preoperative regional kyphotic angle, 66.74°; (b) Kyphotic angle after the first stage, 27.04°; (c) Kyphotic angle at a 2-year follow-up, 28.05°.

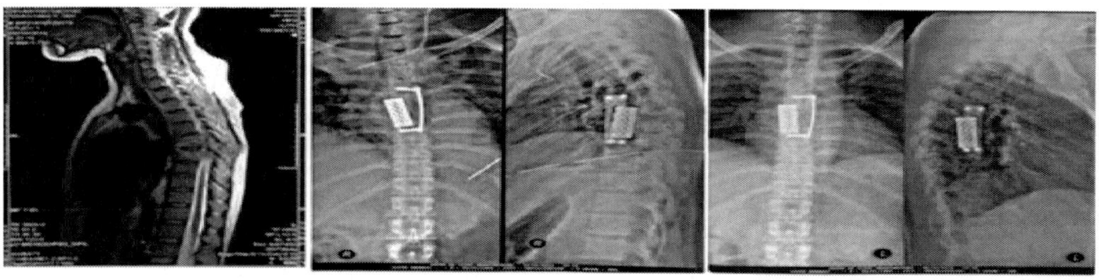

(a) (b) (c)

Figure 3. Radiography in patient 3. (a) Preoperative regional kyphotic angle, 53°; (b) Kyphotic angle after the second stage, 26.5°; (c) Kyphotic angle at a 2-year follow-up, 26.5°.

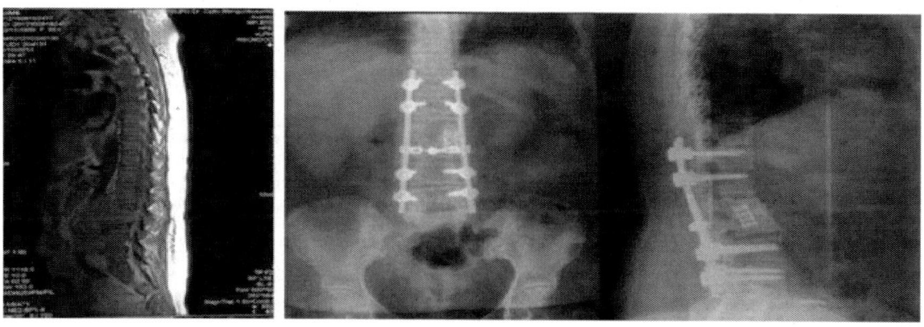

(a) (b) (c)

Figure 4. Radiography in patient 4. (a) Preoperative lumbar lordotic angle, 13°; (b) Lumbar lordotic angle at a 3-year follow-up, 23.5°; (c) MOHON DILENGKAPI.

SECTION 1 - PAIN INTENSITY

☐ I have no pain at the moment.
☐ The pain is very mild at the moment.
☐ The pain is moderate at the moment.
☐ The pain is fairly severe at the moment.
☐ The pain is very severe at the moment.
☐ The pain is the worst imaginable at the moment.

SECTION 2 - PERSONAL CARE (washing, dressing etc.)

☐ I can look after myself normally, without causing extra pain.
☐ I can look after myself normally, but it is very painful.
☐ It is painful to look after myself and I am slow and careful.
☐ I need some help, but manage most of my personal care.
☐ I need help every day in most aspects of self-care.
☐ I do not get dressed, wash with difficulty and stay in bed.

SECTION 3 - LIFTING

☐ I can lift heavy weights without extra pain.
☐ I can lift heavy weights, but it gives extra pain.
☐ Pain prevents me from lifting heavy weights off the floor, but I can manage if they are conveniently positioned (e.g., on a table).
☐ Pain prevents me from lifting heavy weights but I can manage light to medium weights if they are conveniently positioned.
☐ I can lift only very light weights.
☐ I cannot lift or carry anything at all.

SECTION 4 - WALKING

☐ Pain does not prevent me walking any distance.
☐ Pain prevents me walking more than 1 mile.
☐ Pain prevents me walking more than ½ of mile.
☐ Pain prevents me walking more than 100 yards.
☐ I can only walk using a stick or crutches.
☐ I am in bed most of the time and have to crawl to the toilet.

SECTION 5 - SITTING

☐ I can sit in any chair as long as I like.
☐ I can sit in my favourite chair as long as I like.
☐ Pain prevents me from sitting for more than 1 hour.
☐ Pain prevents me from sitting more than ½ an hour.
☐ Pain prevents me from sitting more than 10 minutes.
☐ Pain prevents me from sitting at all.

SECTION 6 - STANDING

☐ I can stand as long as I want without extra pain.
☐ I can stand as long as I want but it gives me extra pain.
☐ Pain prevents me from standing for more than 1 hour.
☐ Pain prevents me from standing for more than ½ an hour.
☐ Pain prevents me from standing for more than 10 minutes.
☐ Pain prevents me from standing at all.

SECTION 7 - SLEEPING

☐ My sleep is never disturbed by pain.
☐ My sleep is occasionally disturbed by pain.
☐ Because of pain, I have less than 6 hours of sleep.
☐ Because of pain, I have less than 4 hours of sleep.
☐ Because of pain, I have less than 2 hours of sleep.
☐ Pain prevents me from sleeping at all.

SECTION 8 - SEX LIFE (if applicable)

☐ My sex life is normal and causes no extra pain.
☐ My sex life is normal but causes some extra pain.
☐ My sex life is nearly normal but is very painful.
☐ My sex life is severely restricted by pain.
☐ My sex life is nearly absent because of pain.
☐ Pain prevents any sex life at all.

SECTION 9 - SOCIAL LIFE

☐ My social life is normal and causes me no extra pain.
☐ My social life is normal, but increases the degree of pain.
☐ Pain has no significant effect on my social life apart from limiting my more energetic interests, e.g., sports, etc.
☐ Pain has restricted my social life and I do not go out as often.
☐ Pain has restricted my social life to my home.
☐ I have no social life because of pain.

SECTION 10-TRAVELLING

☐ I can travel anywhere without pain.
☐ I can travel anywhere but it gives extra pain.
☐ Pain is bad but I manage journeys over 2 hours.
☐ Pain restricts me to journeys of less than 1 hour.
☐ Pain restricts me to short necessary journeys under 30 minutes.
☐ Pain prevents me from travelling except to receive treatment.

Figure 5. Oswestry Disability Index scale (in Bahasa).

The mean follow-up period was 45 months. All patients reported a better condition postoperatively. The mean preoperative ODI score was 20 (patients 1, 2, 3, and 4: 16, 22, 24, and 18, respectively), and the mean postoperative ODI score was 5 (patients 1, 2, 3, and 4: 2, 8, 4, and 6, respectively). The mean kyphotic angle reduced from 90° preoperatively to 30° after the first stage and 22° after the second stage.

DISCUSSION

Indonesia has the third highest TB incidence worldwide, with an incidence of approximately 1,020,000 (30 per 100,000 population). Although the exact incidence and prevalence of STB in most parts of the world are not known, in countries with a high burden of pulmonary TB, the incidence of STB is expected to be proportionately high [1].

STB is a disease of developing countries and is more likely related to the socio-economic status. Unfortunately, its morbidity involves nerve compromise that eventually results in tetraplegia or severe kyphosis, which can affect cardiopulmonary function.

Furthermore, this disease mostly affects young adults in their most productive years, and thus, it reduces productivity and triggers a vicious cycle of poverty. Because of these issues, effective and applicable treatments to prevent further morbidity are urgently required.

The main aims of STB treatment are as follows: (i) TB eradication using anti-TB drugs; (ii) general condition improvement; (iii) deformity prevention or correction using decompression and stabilization; and (iv) prevention or treatment of complications, such as neurological deficit.

Chemotherapy is highly effective for controlling tubercular infection. However, patients treated with chemotherapy alone have an average increase in kyphotic deformity of 15°, and 3%–5% of patients develop kyphosis greater than 60°. Severe kyphosis can lead to immense cosmetic and psychological disturbances in growing children and can cause costopelvic impingement, secondary cardiorespiratory problems, and late-onset paraplegia. Correction of established kyphosis is both difficult and hazardous, with a high rate of complications, even when performed by experienced surgeons. Deformity prevention should be an integral part of any treatment schedule for spinal TB [5].

The role of surgery in STB treatment is still controversial. Surgery is indicated when neurological and spinal deformities are progressive (more than ± 40° of segmental kyphosis, anteroposterior or lateral translation) or when conservative approaches fail to treat the neurological deficit and deformity, severe pain occurs owing to an abscess or spinal instability, and the diagnosis is uncertain (inability to diagnose microbiologically with microscopy, culture, or even polymerase chain reaction for the detection of mycobacterial DNA) [3, 5, 6].

Deformity prevention should be the primary aim in the treatment of spinal TB, as the availability of potent anti-tuberculous drugs has made uncomplicated TB a medical disease. The severity of deformity in spinal TB depends on the extent of vertebral destruction, level of the lesion, and age of the patient, with more severe deformities seen in children and in patients with lesions involving the thoracolumbar spine [7, 8].

Surgery for established deformity is difficult, and it might need to be staged. Additionally, it is hazardous with a significant complication rate. Even with a staged approach, Yau et al. reported a mortality rate of 10%, and the mean correction amount was only 28%. They advocated that corrective surgery should be performed only in patients with severe deformity, active disease, or imminent paraplegia or death from chest complications [5, 7, 8].

Refinement of surgical techniques, development of new approaches, and availability of rigid spinal instrumentation have made single-stage correction of established deformity relatively safe with good outcomes. Transpedicular decancellation osteotomy, pedicle subtraction osteotomy, and direct internal kyphectomy have been used to treat kyphosis in active as well as healed diseases. Jain et al. reported kyphosis correction through an extra-pleural, anterolateral (costotransversectomy) approach, with a mean kyphosis correction of

27.3° and no persistent neurological deficit. Bezer et al. used transpedicular decancellation osteotomy to correct post-tuberculous deformity, with no neural complications [7, 9, 10].

The two-stage surgery performed in our center was adjusted according to the National Health Insurance coverage policy. The outcomes regarding reductions in the ODI score and kyphotic angle were good and matched our aim for treating the patients. Thus, we recommend this two-stage procedure as a standard for cases similar to our reported cases.

CONCLUSION

Our two-stage procedure for the treatment of spondylitis tuberculosis with kyphotic deformity was associated with good functional and radiological outcomes at long-term follow-up. Thus, we recommend this two-stage procedure as a standard for cases similar to our reported cases.

REFERENCES

[1] Anandita, Y., Basri, C. & Besral, Budiono F. X. (2009). A brief history of TB control in Indonesia. *World Health Organization, 07.* (http://whqlibdoc.who.int/publications/2009/9789241598798_eng.pdf).

[2] Mbata, G. C., Ofondu, E., Ajuonuma, B., Asodike, V. C. & Chukwumam, D. (2012). Tuberculosis of the spine (Pott's disease) presenting as hemiparesis. *African Journal of Respiratory Medicine*, *8*(1), 18-20.

[3] Huang, Y., Lin, J., Chen, X., Lin, J., Lin, Y. & Zhang, H. (2017). A posterior versus anterior debridement in combination with bone graft and internal fixation for lumbar and thoracic tuberculosis. *Journal of Orthopaedic Surgery and Research*, *12*(150), 1-10.

[4] Issack, P. S. & Boachie-Adjei, O. (2012). Surgical correction of kyphotic deformity in spinal tuberculosis. *International Orthopaedics*, *36*, 353-357.

[5] Paudel, S. (2013). Kyphotic deformity in pott's spine. *Journal of Kathmandu Medical College*, *2*(4), 201-204.

[6] Jain, A. K. (2010). Tuberculosis of the spine: A fresh look at an old disease. *The Journal of bone and joint surgery*, *92*(B), 905-913.

[7] Rajasekaran, S. (2012). Kyphotic deformity in spinal tuberculosis and its management. *International Orthopaedics*, *36*(2), 359.

[8] Tuli, S. M. (1995). Severe kyphotie deformity in tuberculosis of the spine. *International Orthopaedics*, *19*, 327-331.

[9] Fukuta, H., Miyamoto, K., Masuda, T., Hosoe, H., Kodama, H., Nishimoto, H., et al. (2003). Two-stage (posterior and anterior) surgical treatment using posterior spinal instrumentation for pyogenic and tuberculotic spondylitis. *Spine*, *28*, 302-308.

[10] Zhang, H. Q., Li, J. S. & Guo, C. F. (2012). Two-stage surgical management using posterior instrumentation, anterior debridement and allografting for tuberculosis of the lower lumbar spine in children of elementary school age: minimum 3-year follow-up of 14 patients. *Archives of Orthopaedic and Trauma Surgery*, *132*, 1273-1279.

In: Case Reports in Surgery
Editors: Ahmad Jabir Rahyussalim et al.
ISBN: 978-1-53616-582-1

Chapter 21

MANAGEMENT OF NEGLECTED CONUS MEDULLARIS SYNDROME WITH LUMBAR CANAL STENOSIS

***Ahmad Jabir Rahyussalim*[1,2,3,*], *Sammy Saleh Alhuraiby*[1], *Tri Kurniawati*[2,3] *and Khairul Hukmi*[1]**
[1]Department of Orthopaedic and Traumatology, Faculty of Medicine, Universitas Indonesia-Cipto Mangunkusumo General Hospital, Jakarta, Indonesia
[2]Stem Cell and Tissue Engineering Cluster, IMERI Faculty of Medicine, Universitas Indonesia, Jakarta, Indonesia
[3]Stem Cell Medical Technology Integrated Service Unit, Cipto Mangunkusumo General Hospital, Jakarta, Indonesia

ABSTRACT

Conus medullaris syndrome is a complex disease entity that is difficult to define because of its location between the spinal cord and nerve roots. The presenting symptoms are not specific and are often missed by primary doctors, making diagnosis challenging. It is even more difficult because the time since onset plays a major role in the outcome. A 47-year-old female displayed neglected conus medullary syndrome due to a compression fracture of L1 that presented as bladder and defecating dysfunctions and leg pain due to lumbar canal stenosis of L4-L5. A decompression surgical procedure involving total laminectomy at the L1 level, posterior stabilization from T11 to L3, and laminotomy, flavectomy, and discectomy at L4 and L5 were performed in this patient. The patient experienced improved motor function after the operation. Her hypoesthesia also improved. However, her bladder and defecating problem were not resolved. Non-full function restoration likely occurred because of the patient's neglected conus medullaris. However, her function still improved; therefore, surgery was a better option.

* Corresponding Author's E-mail: rahyussalim71@ui.ac.id.

Keywords: conus medullaris syndrome, lumbar canal stenosis, spinal cord injury

INTRODUCTION

The conus medullaris is very susceptible to injury because of its proximity to the commonly injured thoracolumbar junction [1]. Conus medullaris syndrome results in a tremendous burden due to the resultant morbidity, expenses, and resources necessary to treat the disease. This disease affects an estimated 14,000 people in the United States annually [1].

Conus medullaris syndrome is a complex disease entity that is difficult to define because of its location between the spinal cord and nerve roots [2]. This disease manifests itself as back pain, unilateral or bilateral leg pain, weakness or paresthesia, and bladder or bowel incontinence [3]. In thoracolumbar or lumbosacral injuries, conus medullary syndrome should be distinguished from cauda equina syndrome: the latter presents as a spinal cord compression and dysfunction (upper motor neurons) whereas symptoms in the former present as lumbosacral radiculopathies (lower motor neurons) [3]. However, the lesions affecting the transition between the conus medullaris and cauda equina may present symptoms consistent with both upper and lower motor neurons [2, 3]. This research work has been reported in line with the Surgical Case Report criteria [4].

CASE ILLUSTRATION

A 47-year-old female came to the orthopedic clinic with a chief complaint of numbness on both legs and the perianal area that worsened during the month prior to her visit. Five years previously, the patient had fallen from a tree of 2–3 meters in height. She landed in a sitting position. The patient was unable to walk immediately after the fall, and she could not control her urge to urinate or defecate. The patient also felt numbness at the perianal area and the posterior part of both legs. At that time, the patient was still able to move her legs but was reluctant to walk because of back pain. The patient sought treatment at a nearby hospital, and a urinary catheter was inserted, but she was referred for further treatment. The patient continued treatment in the form of massages and was able to walk after 8 months of treatment. After those 8 months, the patient did not continue with the treatment and merely went to a nearby clinic for urinary catheter changes.

After 4 years, the patient went to a nearby hospital for defecation and micturition problems. She was then referred to a larger hospital and was treated by a rehabilitation specialist; however, she was only given analgesics. After 6 months, the patient discontinued treatment. Over the last month, numbness in both calves worsened, accompanied by a tingling sensation.

A physical examination of the spine revealed that there was no wound, deformity, or other evident issues (Figure 1). A neurological examination revealed impairment in sensory and motor function in the S1 region; her motor strength was a 4 (on a scale of 1 to 5), and her sensory function was a 1 (on a scale between 0 and 2). Her patellar (L4) and Achilles (S1) tendon reflexes were normal. Babinsky's reflex and clonus were not present in this patient (Figure 2). Her bulbocavernosus reflex was negative. Additionally, her autonomic nerve function (micturition and defecation control) was disturbed.

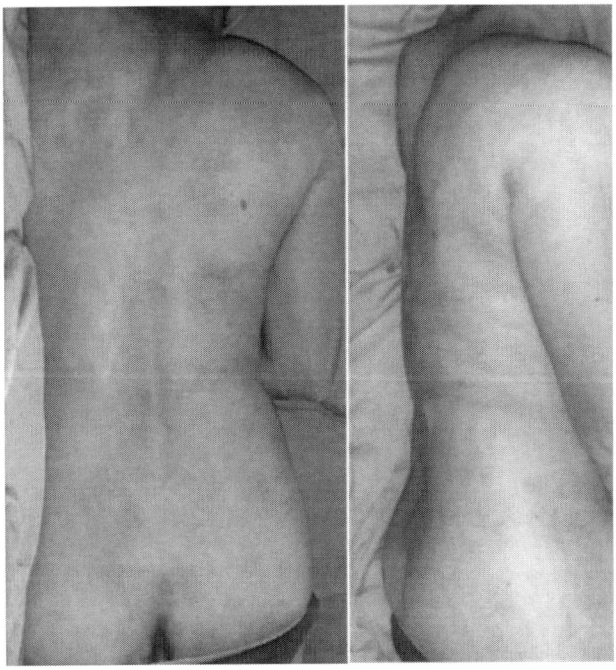

Figure 1. Clinical pictures of the patient before treatment.

The laboratory investigation results were unremarkable except for the increased erythrocyte sedimentation rate. A lumbosacral x-ray showed a thoracolumbar kyphotic deformity, osteophyte, loss of height, and sclerotic endplate at the first lumbar vertebrae, and good bone stock, accompanied by narrowed disc space in T12–L1 and L1–L2 (Figure 3). A magnetic resonance imaging (MRI) of the lumbosacral spine showed a compression fracture of the L1 vertebrae with suppression on the conus medullaris and myelopathy at the T12–L1 level. Spondyloarthrosis lumbar with a herniated nucleus pulposus at L2–L3 until L4–5 and nerve root compression at the L3–L4 and L4–L5 levels was also observed (Figure 4).

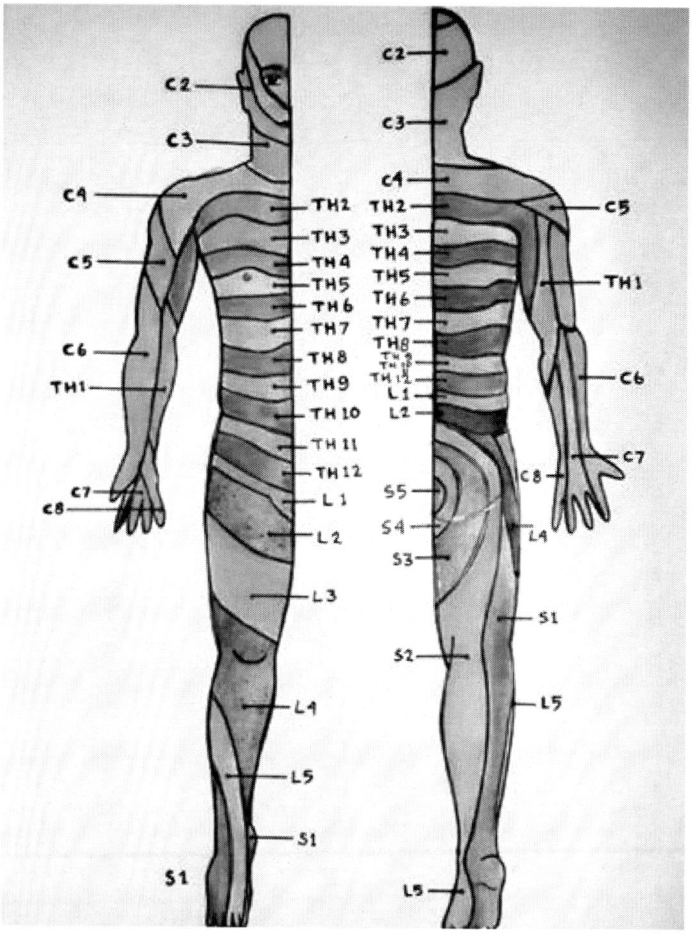

Figure 2. Neurologic examination showing sensory impairment at the S1 level.

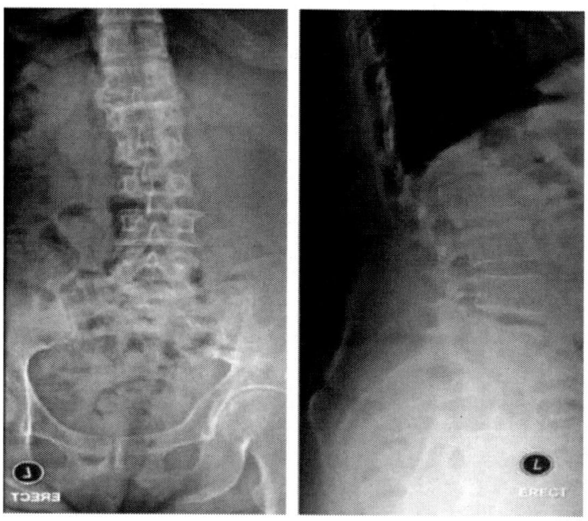

(a) (b)

Figure 3. X-ray of the lumbosacral spine: (a) posteroanterior projection and (b) lateral projection.

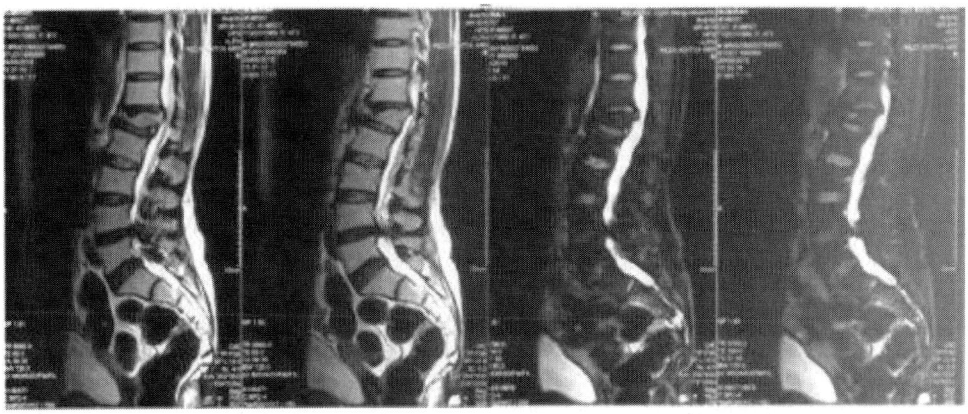

(a)

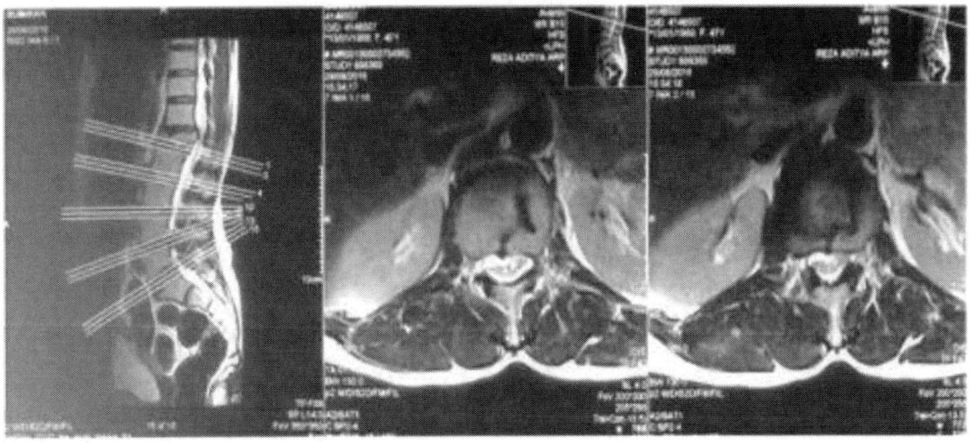

(b)

Figure 4. MRI of the lumbar spine. (a) T2-T1 sagittal projection shows a fracture at vertebrae L1. (b) Axial projection shows the fracture line and narrowing of the canal at that level.

Based on her history, physical examination, and laboratory and radiologic investigations, the patient was diagnosed with neglected conus medullary syndrome due to a compression fracture of L1 and leg pain due to lumbar canal stenosis of L4–L5. We had already performed a decompressive surgical procedure consisting of total laminectomy at the L1 vertebrae, posterior stabilization from T11 to L3, and laminotomy, flavectomy, and discectomy at L4 and L5. The surgery lasted three hours. The somatosensory evoked potential and motoric evoked potential were monitored throughout the surgery.

Her postoperative results showed improvement in both sensory and motor functions. In the lower extremities, both sensory function and motor strength at the S1 level increased to 2 and 5, respectively. Her neurological examination showed that the patella and Achilles tendon reflexes were unimpaired. Babinsky's reflex and clonus were still not present. However, the patient still complained of micturition and defecation, similar to the preoperative state.

DISCUSSION

Diagnostics

This patient presented to our clinic with symptoms and signs suggestive of conus medullaris syndrome. The findings from her history and physical examinations were supported by x-ray and MRI examinations that revealed compression at the level of the conus medullaris. However, the patient also presented with leg numbness, which is not consistent with conus medullaris syndrome. The MRI then showed lumbar canal stenosis at the L4 and L5 vertebrae, which is consistent with leg pain. These two clinical entities are seldom found in one patient, which makes this a unique case.

Because the two disorders appeared in one patient, we decided to perform decompression and stabilization for L1 (where the conus medullaris syndrome originated) and only decompression for L4–L5 (where the LCS appeared). Before the surgery, the patient was classified as Frankel D, which improved to Frankel E after the surgery. This is consistent with findings from Rahimi–Moghavar in which all patients classified as Frankel D improved to Frankel E after surgery [5].

Surgical Intervention

We elected to perform a laminectomy using a posterior approach to release the conus medullaris of the L1 from compression. The segment was stabilized using screws and rods (Figure 5). Despite being decompressed, the fourth and fifth lumbar vertebrae were not stabilized because intraoperatively, we determined that the segment was still stable. Neurological deficit and instability were the main indications for surgery, as stated in the literature. Posterior decompression, followed by an instrumentation two levels above and below the injury level are the most common surgical procedures performed [5]. The posterior approach provides excellent visualization and access to the dorsal sac, which is useful for the treatment of the concomitant fracture. The entrapped nerve root compression cannot be accessed through an anterior approach [2].

The results of a timely surgical procedure have not been established in patients with conus medullaris syndrome [6-9]. Immediate surgery has been associated with excessive bleeding, which has prompted surgeons to delay treatment for 2 to 3 days; however, this has not yielded significant differences in outcomes. Notably, in conus medullaris syndrome, the decision to perform immediate surgery does not correlate with better results compared with delayed surgery [8-10]. Therefore, the recommendation is to perform surgery within three days of injury to achieve a better prognosis with immediate decompression reserved for those with a progressive neurological deficit with significant thecal sac compression. However, currently, no studies have reported the outcome of surgery performed 5 years after the injury. This report indicates that even after 5 years, surgery for conus medullaris syndrome still results in improvement in sensory and motor functions [6-8].

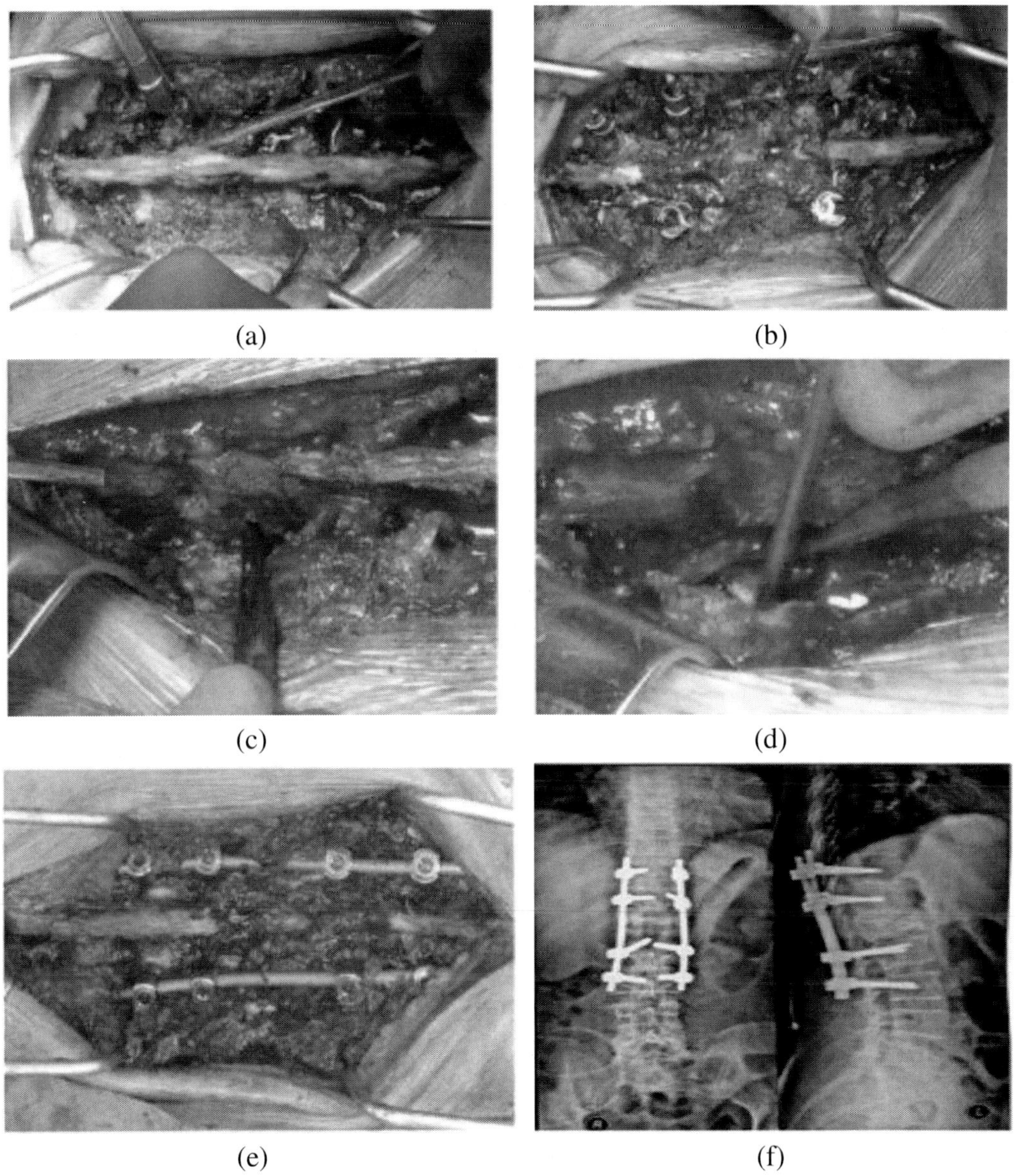

Figure 5. Intraoperative procedure. (a) Exposure; (b) pedicle screw placement and laminectomy of L1; (c) and (d) laminotomy, flavectomy, and discectomy of L4–L5; (e) final instrumentation; (f) X-ray of thoracolumbal post op Ap Lat.

Neurologic Impairment

Even after surgery, our patient still complained of poor bladder and bowel function. The results from another study also showed that bladder function displayed the least improvement compared with motor or sensory function. Transfeldt reported that although neurologic improvement occurred in 68% of patients who underwent surgery within 2 years, only 27% of patients reported improvement in bladder function. Although these lesions often have a devastating effect on the quality of life, they do not significantly shorten the lifespan [6-8, 11]. A good outcome was recorded if there was a recovery of one or more motor-root levels in the lower extremities or partial recovery of multiple levels. A fair result was recorded if there was a partial improvement of one or two motor-root levels, and a poor result was shown by no cord or root improvement; however, it would be adequately significant if the case was acute to compare the result, which was difficult to apply to our patient [11, 12]. Further workup and management is necessary to assess the bladder and defecating problems of patients. Several treatment options are available, but rehabilitation therapy is the mainstay of treatment. Currently, stem-cell based regenerative medicine is gaining popularity for spinal cord injuries because it may benefit patients; however, this option has several issues still at stake that must be resolved [13, 14].

Conclusion

The management of conus medullaris syndrome includes decompression of the spinal cord level that is injured and providing stability for the structure. Diagnosis is challenging, and management is even more difficult for patients because of its associated complications, particularly when neglected. We presented a case of conus medullaris syndrome due to a neglected compression fracture that coincidentally co-existed with lumbar canal stenosis. Surgery was the elected option, and it improved motoric functions, although the bladder and defecating function results were not satisfactory. Stem-cell-based therapy might benefit the latter problem.

Conflict of Interest

The authors declare that there are no conflicts of interest regarding publication of this paper.

Informed Consent

The authors have obtained consent from the patient.

References

[1] Bhandutia AK, Winek NC, Tomycz ND, Altman DT.. Traumatic conus medullaris syndrome: a case report and review of the literature. *JBJS Case Connect.* 2016;6(2):e38.

[2] Radcliff KE, Kepler CK, Delasotta LA, Rihn JA, Harrop JS, Hilibrand AS, Albert TJ, Vaccaro AR. Current management review of thoracolumbar cord syndromes. *Spine J.* 2011;11(9):884-92.

[3] Harrop JS, Hunt GE, Vaccaro AR. Conus medullaris and cauda equina syndrome as a result of traumatic injuries: management principles. *Neurosurg Focus* 2004;16(6):1-23.

[4] Agha RA, Fowler AJ, Saetta A, Barai I, Rajmohan S, Orgill DP and the SCARE Group. The SCARE Statement: Consensus-based surgical case report guidelines. *Int J Surg.* 2016;34:180-6.

[5] Rahimi-Movaghar V, Vaccaro AR, Mohammadi M. Efficacy of surgical decompression in regard to motor recovery in the setting of conus medullaris injury. *J Spinal Cord Med.* 2006;29(1):32-8.

[6] Podnar S. Epidemiology of cauda equina and conus medullaris lesions. *Muscle Nerve* 2007;35(4):529-31.

[7] Podnar S, Oblak C, Vodusek DB. Sexual function in men with cauda equina lesions: a clinical and electromyographic study. *J Neurol Neurosurg Psychiatry* 2002;73(6):715-20.

[8] Demetriades AK, Naik S, Gunasekera L. Conus medullaris syndrome from a transdural disc herniation at the thoracolumbar junction. *Acta neurochirur.* 2010;152(6):1081-2.

[9] Dawodu ST. Cauda equina and conus medullaris syndromes. *Medscape J Med.* 2013;1-14.

[10] Wostrack M, Shiban E, Obermuller T, Gempt J, Meyer B, Ringel F. Conus medullaris and cauda equina tumors: clinical presentation, prognosis, and outcome after surgical treatment. *J Neurosurg Spine.* 2014;20: 335-43.

[11] Fehlings MG, Arvin B. The timing of surgery in patients with central spinal cord injury. *J Neurosurg Spine* 2009;10(1):1-2.

[12] Chou D, Hartl R, Sonntag VK. Conus medullaris syndrome without lower-extremity involvement in L-1 burst fractures: report of four cases. *J Neurosurg Spine* 2006;4(3):265-9.

[13] Tewarie RSN, Hurtado A, Bartels RH, Grotenhuis A, Oudega M. Stem cell-based therapies for spinal cord injury. *J Spinal cord med.* 2009;32(2):105-14.

[14] Rahyussalim AJ, Saleh I, Armin MF, Kurniawati T, Safri AY. Pedicle screw position changing policy for nerve injury problems during screw insertion on thoracolumbar compression fractures. *Int J Surg Case Rep.* 2016;28:155-60.

In: Case Reports in Surgery
Editors: Ahmad Jabir Rahyussalim et al.
ISBN: 978-1-53616-582-1

Chapter 22

ANTERIOR INNOMINATE OSTEOTOMY FOR CLOSURE OF NEGLECTED BLADDER EXSTROPHY: A REPORT OF TWO CASES AND A BRIEF REVIEW OF THE LITERATURE

***Aryadi Kurniawan*[1,*] *and Andi Praja Wira Yudha Luthfi*[2]**
[1]Pediatric Orthopaedics Division,
Department of Orthopaedics and Traumatology, Faculty of Medicine,
RSUPN Dr. Cipto Mangunkusumo, Universitas Indonesia,
Jakarta, Indonesia
[2]Department of Orthopaedics and Traumatology, Faculty of Medicine,
University of Indonesia, RSUPN Dr. Cipto Mangunkusumo, Universitas Indonesia,
Jakarta, Indonesia

ABSTRACT

Congenital malformations in bladder and cloacal exstrophy involve the genitourinary tract, musculoskeletal tissue, and occasionally the gastrointestinal tract. Pediatric orthopedists and urological surgeons need to have substantial knowledge in order to properly manage such cases. The foremost goal of orthopedic reconstruction is to reduce pelvic diastasis, which enables closure of the bladder and abdominal wall, while reducing tension. Here, we report two cases of a seven-year-old boy and a 12-year old boy who were referred to our pediatric surgery service with the diagnosis of bladder exstrophy. Preoperatively, the pubic diastasis of the two patients was 6 and 9 cm, respectively. Bilateral anterior innominate osteotomy with external fixator placement was executed by the pediatric urological surgical team following bladder closure. Both patients remained

[*] Corresponding Author's E-mail: aryadi.paedortho@gmail.com.

hospitalized for two weeks on bed rest. Skin traction was not applied. External fixators were applied for eight weeks. Immediately after surgery, the diastases were reduced to 4 cm in the 7-year-old patient and 6 cm in the 12-year-old patient. No postoperative complications occurred in either patient and both were able to walk with normal gaits. Slight external leg rotation was noted. Urological abnormalities were improved. Despite the technique, it is difficult to achieve perfect closure of the pelvic diastasis in this age group. Pelvic osteotomy remains the most beneficial intervention for corrective exstrophy closure. The bilateral anterior technique is recommended for this procedure and is applicable in neglected cases. Further follow-up is needed to evaluate the effectiveness of this technique.

Keywords: pelvic osteotomy, bladder exstrophy

INTRODUCTION

Classic bladder exstrophy (CBE) is a congenital defect primarily involving the musculoskeletal system and genitourinary tract with an incidence of one case for every 10,000–50,000 live births. The intricacy of congenital malformations, which involves bladder and cloacal exstrophy, involves the genitourinary and musculoskeletal systems, and occasionally the gastrointestinal tract. Correct management of these conditions requires sufficient knowledge of pediatric orthopedists and pediatric urological surgeons. The most significant defect of this congenital malformation is cloacal exstrophy, or CBE with additional intestinal prolapse at the site of bladder exstrophy. In some cases, cloacal exstrophy is accompanied by lipomeningocele or myelomeningocele formation and other congenital malformations, such as anal atresia, colonic hypoplasia, genitalia anomalies, and omphalocele development [1–3].

The mechanism of CBE originates from a defect during embryologic development of the abdominal wall. The genetic and environmental origins of this defect remain unclear, although both are considered contributors. It is now hypothesized that throughout the initial embryonic period, the urogenital part of the cloacal membrane fails to regress caudally consequent to the abnormal caudad position of genital tubercles primordia. The urogenital part of the cloacal membrane fails to ventrally migrate and is displaced anteriorly against the abdominal wall. This position prevents migration of the mesenchyme to the midline of the lower abdominal wall, resulting in a shortage of mesenchyme-derived tissues in this area. Following cloacal membrane rupture to shape the urogenital and anal orifices according to the physiological sequence of embryologic events produces herniation of the viscera of the lower abdomen against the lower abdominal wall, which leads to numerous signs of the epispadias-exstrophy complex, as elaborated earlier [4, 5].

The usage of pelvic osteotomy for the reconstruction of bladder exstrophy deformities has been considerably debated over the past several years. Fundamental descriptive analysis of the bony pelvis and deficiencies and deformities of the muscular pelvic floor in patients with exstrophy have resulted in a better understanding of how reconfiguration of the pelvic ring could provide safe and dependable bladder posterior urethra placement within the pelvis. Over the past 20 years, surgery for bladder exstrophy management has progressed significantly, along with the development of different techniques to acquire good closure and optimal functional outcomes. The ultimate goal of orthopedic reconstruction is to reduce pelvic diastasis, thus allowing for closure of the bladder and abdominal walls, while lessening tension [3, 5, 6].

Here, we report two cases of neglected bladder exstrophy and the outcomes of pelvic osteotomy for exstrophy bladder repair with one-year follow-up. To the best of our knowledge, this is the first case series about the management of pubic diastasis in so-called neglected cases of bladder exstrophy.

CASE 1

Our first patient was a seven-year-old boy who was referred to our Orthopedic Pediatric Surgery Department for repair of anomphalocele and bladder exstrophy (Figure 1a) with a preoperative pubic diastasis size of 6cm (Figure 1b). Bilateral anterior pelvic osteotomy in the supine position was performed in August 2017. Salter osteotomy was performed, during which an oblique inguinal incision was made to the ilium and the innominate bone was bared by separation of the periosteum on each side. The posterior limit of the exposure was the sacroiliac joint and the inferior limit was the pectineal tubercle. The sciatic notch was distinctly recognized and an oblique osteotomy was executed with a saw from the iliac crest to the greater sciatic notch, while evading the sacroiliac joint. The oblique osteotomy resulted in adequate bone for placing external fixator pins into the distal and proximal pelvic segments without invasion of the sacroiliac joint. A number of four parallel 4-mm Shanz screws were subsequently inserted into the distal and proximal pelvic segments. The same procedure was completed on the contralateral side. Repair of the bladder and abdominal soft tissue was later accomplished by the urology team. Next, to complete the repair and reconstruction of the bladder, the fixator pins were connected and compressed using a triangular anterior fragment frame to reduce the diastasis (Figure 1c). An X-ray was obtained intraoperatively to confirm the reduction. No wires were used for fixation of the pubic symphysis.

Diastasis reduction to 4cm was accomplished immediately in the post-operative period (Figure1d). The patient was bed-rested in the hospital for one week without traction. An external fixator was applied for a total of eight weeks. There were no complications and the patient was able to walk with a normal gait and without any external leg rotation. The urological status of the patient was improved.

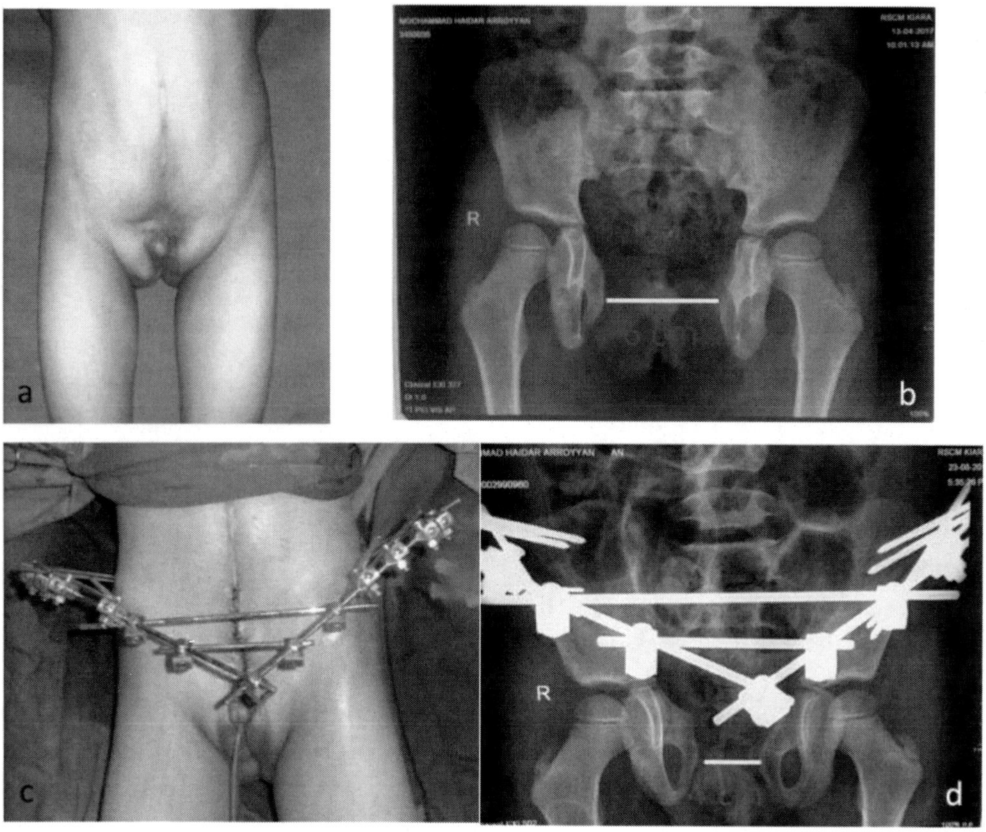

Figure 1. (a) Patient with bladder exstrophy and omphalocele; (b) initially with 6 cm of pubic diastasis; (c) bilateral anterior pelvic osteotomy was performed with external fixation; (d) after surgery, the diastasis was reduced to 4 cm.

CASE 2

Our second patient was a 12-year-old boy who was referred for epispadia correction and pelvic osteotomy. Cloacal exstrophy closure had been completed at another facility (Figure 2a). The patient had a preoperative pubic diastasis of 9cm (Figure 2b). Bilateral anterior pelvic placement with external fixators was performed in October 2017 using a previously described technique, following cloaca closure and repair procedure but parallel to epispadiarepair (Figure 2b). Diastasis reduction to 6 cm was accomplished immediately during the postoperative period (Figure 2d). The patient was hospitalized for two weeks with bed rest but no skin traction. An external fixator was applied for eight weeks. Urological status was improved and no postoperative complications were recorded. Preoperative external rotation of the patient's gait was marginally corrected at postoperative assessment.

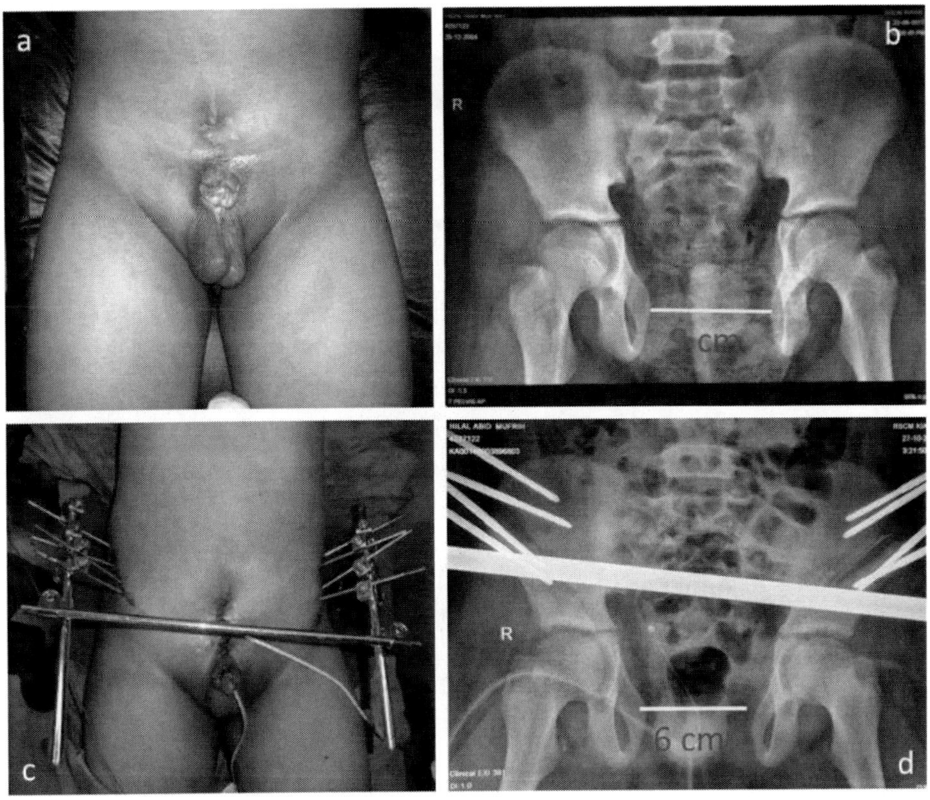

Figure 2. (a) Patient with bladder exstrophy that was performed at another hospital; (b) initial pubic diastasis was 9 cm; (c) bilateral anterior pelvic osteotomy with external fixation; (d) reduced the diastasis to 6 cm after surgery.

DISCUSSION

Despite its rarity, pediatric orthopedists should be familiar with bladder exstrophy so that proper treatment can be performed alongside urological or pediatric surgeons. Our institution has been conducting follow-up examinations of referred cases such as these. We concluded that pelvic osteotomy parallel to closure of a urological defect is significantly advantageous for gait development and prevention of arthrosis of the hip joints. This technique also supports the performance of urological procedures. In most cases, bladder exstrophy is diagnosed in patients younger than five years. These two cases are exceptional and advanced, due to the older ages of the patients upon presentation. These cases presented challenges to determine the best treatment option for diastasis reduction. Bilateral anterior pelvic osteotomy should be performed as soon as possible, but can be applied in older patients for better deformity correction [2–4, 7-11].

The primary objective of early exstrophy repair is closure of the pubic bones and anterior abdominal wall soft tissue while relieving any tension. Any type of osteotomy can avoid dehiscence of the repaired bladder and abdominal wall. There are numerous techniques for pelvic osteotomy available to fit the surgeon's personal experience and preferences. Anterior pelvic osteotomy for children with bladder exstrophy was first described by Frey and Cohen [12] who reported complications in two patients: partial bladder prolapses in one; and a deep wound infection with total breakdown of the reconstruction in a second. Anterior pelvic osteotomy has several benefits, including versatility for both primary and re-do cases without regard to the patient's age; reasonable surgical duration with no positional changes; and limited anesthetic exposure. Blood loss was also minimal, thus blood transfusion was seldom needed [6, 8–11].

The patient is conditioned in the supine position with elevation of the pelvis using a pad. The bladder is isolated with the use of a sterile drape. A 5cm incision is made 1–2cm distal to the anterior superior iliac spine, similar to the incision for Salter osteotomy. The lateral cutaneous nerve of the thigh was identified and protected. Both sides of the pelvis were subperiosteally exposed by the iliac wings to the extent of the sciatic incision, posteriorly to the extent that the medial ligaments of the sacroiliac joint end and caudally just over the triradiate cartilage (Figure 3) [9].

A small window is opened to the periosteum beside the iliac for control during osteotomy and pin insertion. Subsequent to insertion of a Hohmann spacer into the sciatic incision, oblique osteotomy is completed using an osteotome on the iliac. The lower segment of the pelvis afterward should move medially (Figure 4) [2, 3, 5, 12].

One, or occasionally two, fixator pins are inserted into the lower segment of the ilium and one to two pins into the upper segment of the ilium. The incisions are closed with absorbable intradermal sutures, thus making it possible for the pediatric urological surgeon to completely repair the genitourinary tract. Following the urological procedure, closure of the pubic diastasis can be performed in several ways, as determined by the urologist, using nylon 2-0 sutures, while turning the pelvis internally, thus supporting the sutures. In our cases of older patients or those cases of patients with more extreme diastasis, continuously adjusting the external fixator bar may be necessary for gradual closure of the pelvis. For abdominal wall closure, the bars of the external fixator are placed to retain the pelvis in the correct position [1, 7, 13].

We recommend the use of an external fixator for four to eight weeks. The original technique uses skin traction of both legs during fixation in order to avoid early release of the pins. Nevertheless, skin traction was not applied in the present cases because there is no significant benefit in this age group. Radiographic examination should be performed monthly. The pins are to be removed only upon radiographic evidence of consolidation.

The most common complications of this procedure include infection from the pins, transitory paralysis of the lateral cutaneous nerve of the thigh, and postponement of the consolidation process. Cutaneous traction may also cause complications. Less frequent complications include pseudarthrosis, arthrosis, lower-limb dysmetria, and lesions to the sciatic, femoral, and superior gluteal nerves, while deep infection is a relatively rare complication [10, 12–14].

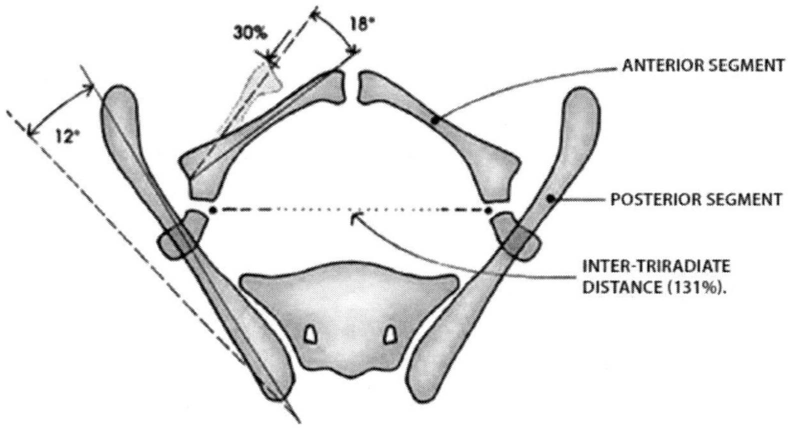

Figure 3. Pelvic anatomy in cases of bladder exstrophy.

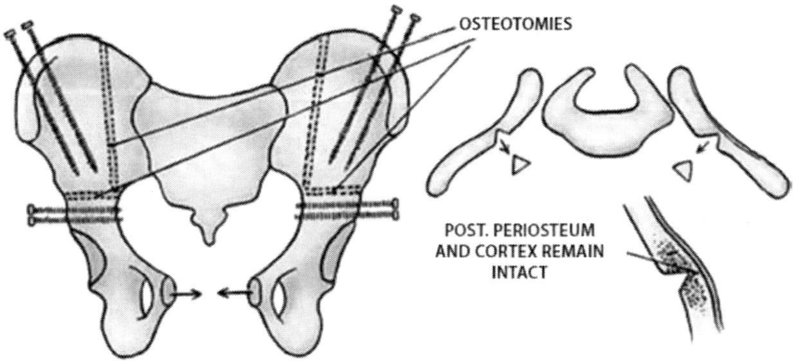

Figure 4. Pelvic anatomy in cases of bladder exstrophy.

Sponseller et al. [6] in their study described a new perspective on osteotomy for CBE treatment based on anterior innominate osteotomies performed from 1988 to 1996. The procedure was deemed effective with a postoperative continence rate of 76%. Nevertheless, the degree of pubic diastasis reduction was not significantly associated with continence. These findings suggest that while osteotomy could ensure continence by sling restoration of the pelvic floor muscles surrounding the urethra, the position of the pubic rami offers no significant benefit to achieve continence. It was also discovered that more diastasis correction would be retained during the procedure for older children. As the degree of pubic diastasis increases linearly to growth in patients with untreated CBE, younger patients are more likely to achieve lesser correction as a result of more considerable growth than older patients. When the main objective is to improve the widened perineum in CBE, delay of osteotomy until the age of eight years is recommended in order to achieve an optimal degree of correction [4–7].

CONCLUSION

Further techniques for the repair of bladder exstrophy in older children will be explained in the near future. Nonetheless, pelvic osteotomy is still the most beneficial intervention for the success of corrective exstrophy closure in older children. At present, the bilateral anterior technique is the most recommended for this procedure. However, further follow-up of this technique is needed.

REFERENCES

[1] Elsayed, ER, Alam, MN, Sarhan, OM, Elsayed, D, Eliwa, AM, Khalil, S. Closure of bladder exstrophy with a bilateral anterior pubic osteotomy: Revival of an old technique. *Arab J Urol*, 2011, 9, 203-206.

[2] Chiari, G, Avolio, L. Bilateral anterior pubic osteotomy in bladder exstrophy repair: report of increasing success. *Pediatr Surg Int*, 2001, 17, 160-163.

[3] Mattos, CB, Mendes, PH, Boechat, PR, Llerena Júnior, J, Guimarães, LD. Bilateral Anterior Pelvic Osteotomy for closure of bladder exstrophy : description of technique. *Rev Bras Ortop*, 2011, 46, 107-113.

[4] Wild, AT, Sponseller, PD, Stec, AA, Gearhart, JP. The role of osteotomy in surgical repair of bladder exstrophy. *Semin Pediatr Surg*, 2011, 20, 71-78.

[5] Baird, AD, Sponseller, PD, Gearhart, JP. The place of pelvic osteotomy in the modern era of bladder exstrophy reconstruction. *J Pediatr Urol*, 2005, 1, 31-36.

[6] Sponseller, PD, Gearhart, JP, Jeffs, RD. Anterior innominate osteotomies for failure or late closure bladder exstrophy. *J Urol,* 1991, 146, 137-140.

[7] Hassan, MA. Bladder exstrophy closure using anterior pelvic osteotomy of superior pubic rami. *J Fac Med Baghdad*, 2015, 57, 201-204.

[8] Varni, JW, Seid, M, Kurtin, PS. Pediatric health-related quality of life measurement technology: A guide for health care decision makers. *Jcom*, 1999, 6, 33-40.

[9] Stec, AA, Pannu, HK, Tadros, YE, Sponseller, PD, Fishman, EK, Gearhart, JP. Pelvic floor anatomy in classic bladder exstrophy using 3-dimensional computerized tomography: initial insights. *J Urol,* 2001, 4, 1444-1449.

[10] Grady, RW, Mitchell, ME. Complete primary repair of exstrophy. *J Urol*, 1999, 162, 1415-1420.

[11] Baird, AD, Nelson, CP, Gearhart, JP. Modern staged repair of bladder exstrophy: A contemporary series. *J Pediatr Urol,* 2007, 3, 311-315.

[12] Frey, P. Bilateral anterior pubic osteotomy in bladder exstrophy closure. *J Urol,* 1996, 156, 812-815.

[13] Gibbon, AJ, Maffulli, N, Fixsen, JA. Horizontal pelvic osteotomies for bladder exstrophy. *J Bone Jt Surg*, 1991, 73, 896-898.

[14] Riaz, S, Sarwar, S, Umar, M. Fixation of bilateral pelvic osteotomies with external fixator in exstrophy bladder complex. *J Pak Med Assoc,* 2005, 55, 537-539.

In: Case Reports in Surgery
Editors: Ahmad Jabir Rahyussalim et al.
ISBN: 978-1-53616-582-1

Chapter 23

Successful Treatment of Fracture at the Base of the Proximal Phalanx Using Extra-Articular Percutaneous K-Wiring with the Consideration of Safe Portals: A Case Report

Wahyu Widodo[1,*] and Andi Praja Wira Yudha Luthfi
[1]Orthopaedic Hand and Microsurgery, Faculty of Medicine,
RSUPN Dr. Cipto Mangunkusumo, Universitas Indonesia,
Jakarta, Indonesia

Abstract

Fracture of the phalanges can be caused by trauma under various circumstances. Most phalangeal fractures are unstable. The common treatment for unstable phalangeal fractures is Kirschner wire (K-wire) fixation using the most commonly used technique of extra-articular cross-pinning. Using this technique, a stable fracture can be fixed and early phalanx mobilization can be facilitated. To achieve these goals, the landmarks and safe portals for the insertion of the K-wire to the fracture site of the phalanges must be identified. Here we present the case of a 48-year-old woman with fracture at the base of the proximal phalanx of the left fourth finger. For 3 weeks, she underwent closed reduction and immobilization using the K-wire via the extra-articular cross-pinning technique. After 3 weeks of immobilization using the K-wire, no significant events were observed. After removal of the K-wire, we initiated the rehabilitation program. A desirable range of motion (ROM) was achieved at the metacarpophalangeal joint. The safe portals for the insertion of the K-wire for treating proximal phalanx fractures using the cross-pinning technique

* Corresponding Author's E-mail: wawidfkui@yahoo.com.

must be identified to achieve a desirable ROM. Thus, the extra-articular cross-pinning technique along with the safe portals must be used for treating fractures of the proximal phalanges.

Keywords: fractures, K-wire, phalanges

INTRODUCTION

Metacarpals and phalanges are the most common sites of fracture in the upper extremity, and such fractures can result from trauma under various circumstances [1]. Emmet and Breck have reported that 10% of 11,000 fractures were metacarpal or phalange fractures. Moreover, Faraqui et al. [2] have shown that fractures at these sites account for 23% of all below-the-elbow fractures in the United States. Proximal phalanx fractures occur more often than middle and distal phalangeal fractures [3]. Phalangeal fractures usually lead to undesirable outcomes because they are frequently neglected or considered insignificant [4].

The treatment of phalangeal fractures is based on several factors, such as location of intra-articular or extra-articular fracture, deformity, pattern of fractures, open or closed fractures, and correlated injuries adjacent to the fracture site. Age, preference of the surgeon, injury mechanism, and occupational need of the patient must also be considered [1, 5]. Treatment of phalangeal fractures, particularly in the extra-articular middle and proximalphalanx, aims to accomplish satisfactory anatomical reduction, maintenance of stability, and early controlled mobilization. Different treatment methods have been presented, which include buddy strapping, closed reduction internal fixation (CRIF) with Kirschner wires (K-wires), splinting, and open reduction internal fixation with plates and/or screws [3, 6].

Despite the availability of novel materials and techniques, the most commonly used tool for stabilization and fixation in phalangeal fractures is the steel pin, which was first introduced by Martin Kirschner in 1909 [7]. In the CRIF method, the safe portals for percutaneous K-wire insertion must be identified for successful treatment. A safe portal is defined as an area where entry of the K-wire will cause minimal soft tissue damage and will not damage major soft tissues, including those in the extensor tendon, nerve, vascular, and flexor tendon, there by treating pain and promoting active range of motion (ROM).

CASE ILLUSTRATION

A 48-year-old woman was admitted to our emergency department owing to pain and difficulty in moving the metacarpophalangeal (MCP) joint of her left ring finger. Six hours prior to admission, she slipped and fell on the floor, and her body fell on her left hand. She was wearing a ring on her left ring finger at that time. She felt extreme pain on her left ring finger. The patient was right-handed and worked as a nurse. Her general health condition was good, and she did not present with any comorbidities.

Upon examination, swelling and minimal deformity were observed on her left ring finger (Figure 1). Sensation at the distal part was good, and there was no disruption of blood flow to the distal part of the finger. However, she could not move the MCP joint due to extreme pain and swelling.

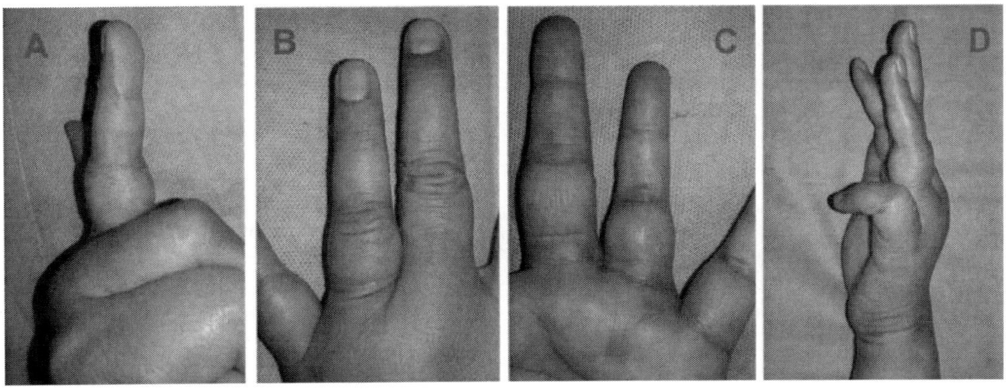

Figure 1. Clinical condition of the left fourth finger.

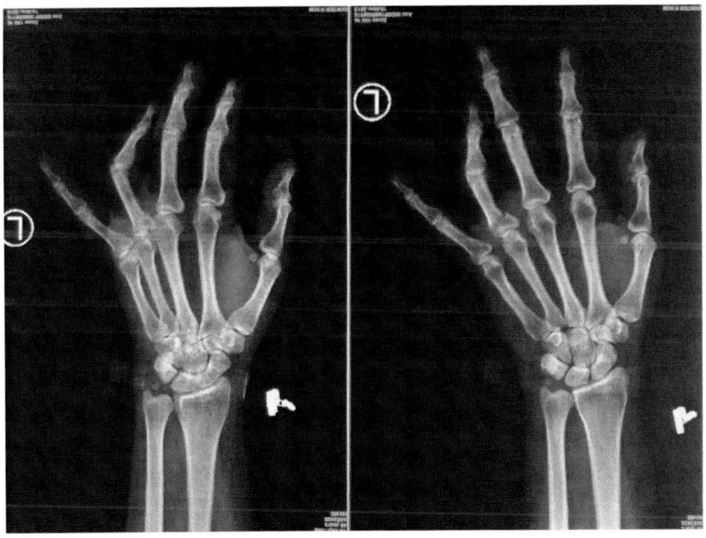

Figure 2. First radiography image of the left hand showing a fracture with a slight displacement at the base of the fourth finger.

Based on the radiological findings, an extra-articular fracture was observed at the base of the left proximal phalanx. At the emergency room, we performed closed reduction and immobilized her fingers using ulnar gutter splint and waited for 5 days until swelling in the soft tissue subsided. Treatment with percutaneous K-wiring was recommended, and the risk of joint stiffness and malunion was explained to the patient.

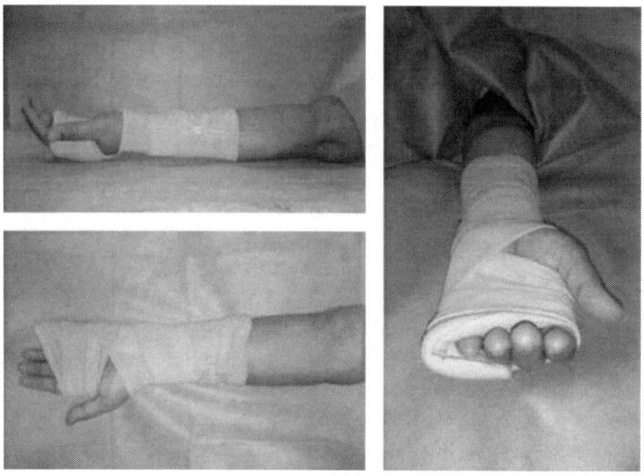

Figure 3. Ulnar gutter splint application was performed in the emergency room.

After 5 days, closed reduction was performed, and we inserted 2 K-wires with extra-articular cross-pinning technique percutaneously under C-arm guidance in the operating room. Regional anesthesia (axillary block) was administered prior to the procedure. First, we flexed the left proximal interphalangeal (PIP) joint of the fourth finger at 90°, and the K-wire was inserted percutaneously, dorsomedially, and dorsolaterally alongside the extensor tendon. Then, C-arm imaging was performed to identify the exact location of the wires. Results showed that the wires were placed properly. The fracture site was stable, and we flexed the MCP joint to ensure that the wire was not placed intra-articularly. The ring and middle fingers were protected with buddy tapping, and the patient was discharged from the hospital after the surgery.

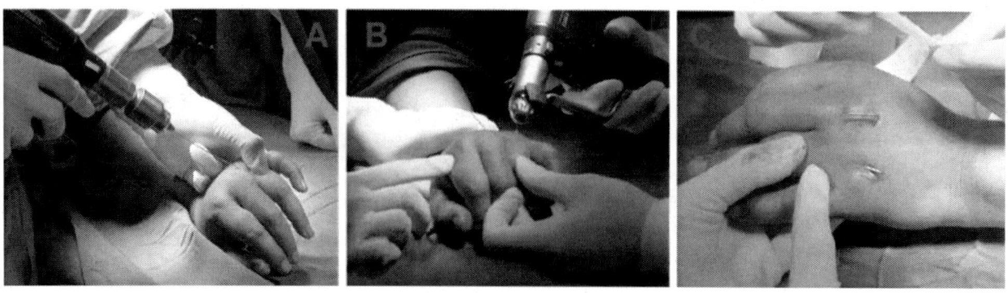

Figure 4. Insertion of the K-wire in the operating room. (a) The metacarpophalangeal joint was flexed; and (b) K-wires were inserted percutaneously; (c) After insertion, the tip of the wire was bended to immobilize the wires.

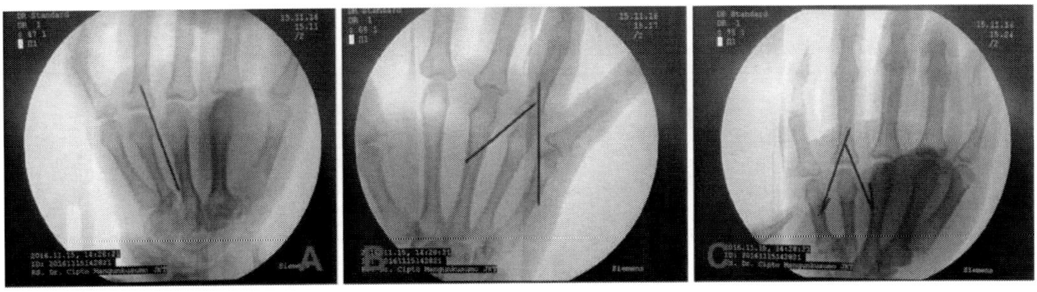

Figure 5. C-arm imaging confirmed the location of the wires in the operating room.

The patient was followed-up in the clinic after 1 week for wound inspection. The K-wire was removed 3 weeks after surgery, and the patient underwent further intensive physiotherapy with active and passive flexion and extension of the PIP joint. She regained full ROM of the MCP joint after 6 weeks. She was then discharged from the outpatient clinic. During follow-up after 3 months, the flexion and extension of the MCP joint were found to be satisfactory, and deformities were not observed.

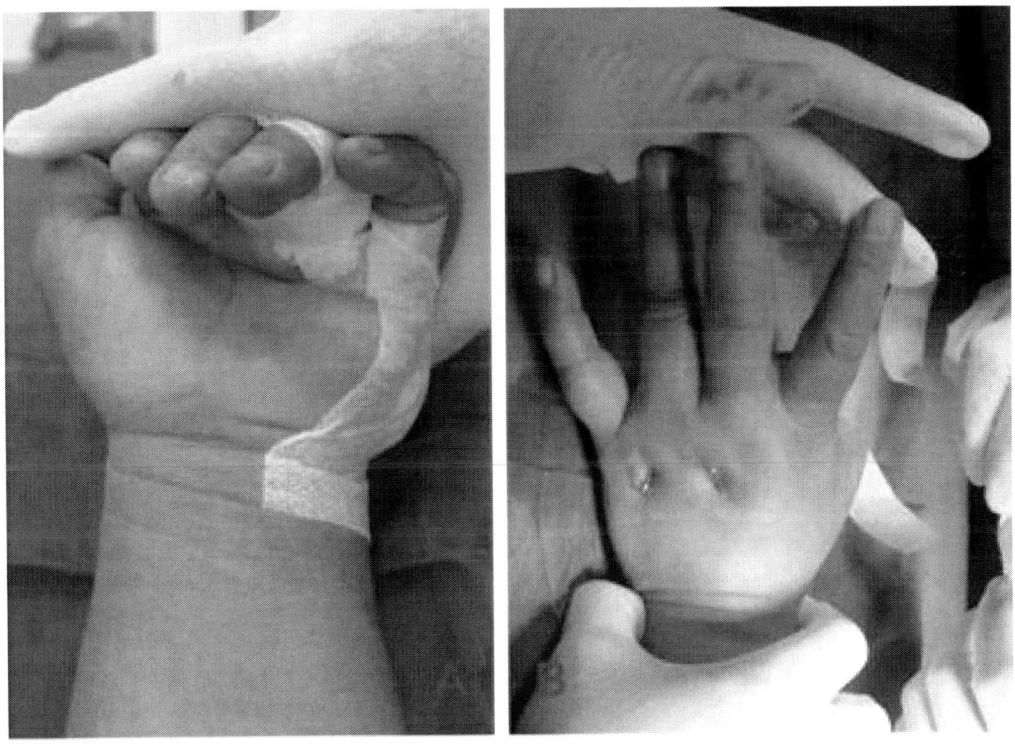

Figure 6. Range of motion of the metacarpophalangeal joint was assessed after operation by performing flexion (a) and extension (b) to ensure that the wires were inserted extra-articularly.

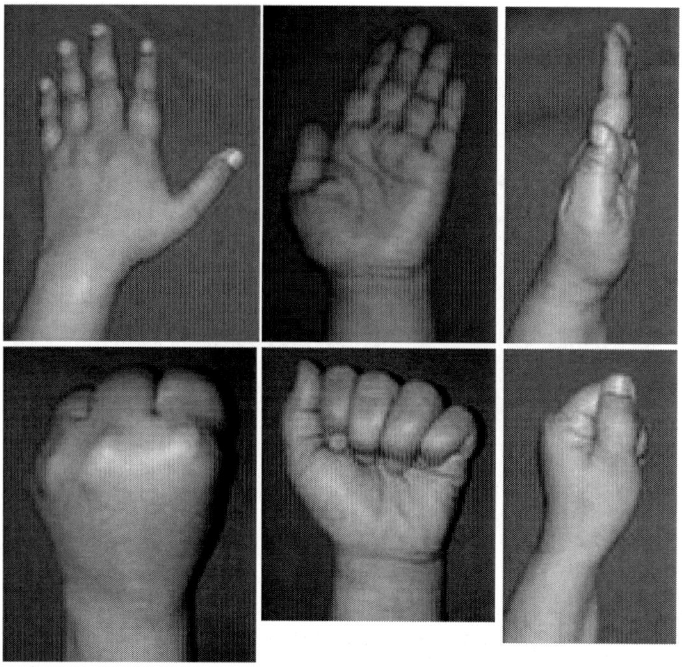

Figure 7. Range of motion of the metacarpophalangeal (MCP) joint during follow-up after 3 months. Image shows that flexion and extension of the MCP joint were satisfactory, and no deformities were observed.

DISCUSSION

Metacarpal and phalangeal fractures are more commonly observed in men than in women. The incidence is highest in the younger group due to road accidents, sports injuries, and industrial accidents [4]After reduction of a displaced or unstable proximal phalanx fracture, fixation must be performed with the use of the following implants: K-wires, cerclage wires, screws, plates, tension band wiring, intramedullar devices, external fixator, or staples. The use of the K-wires is the most common fixation method. Such method has several advantages, which include low cost, simple percutaneous application, and minimal disruption of soft tissues, which results in minimal soft tissue damage and preservation of soft tissues and periosteal stability. The removal of pins after fracture healing is not challenging. However, this method also has several disadvantages, which include susceptibility to infections in the pin tract, requirement of additional immobilization over the early healing process, and possible migration of the pin. The K-wires do not offer compression, and they can occasionally distract the fracture site. Although K-wires do not produce rigid fixation, they still provide enough fixation for restricted mobilization. A variety of configurations are commonly used. Each has different degrees of stability. The configurations include crossed-pinning K-wires, parallel K-wires across the fracture site, fixation of intramedullar wire, fixation of transarticular pin or along with wiring to generate a tension band construct, and combination of several types of fixation. The key goal is to achieve stable fixation and early mobilization [8, 9].

Safe corridor can be transcutaneously recognized in the base of the proximal phalanx through the identification of the central tendon at the MCP joint dorsally. It is safe corridor for the insertion of the K-wire on whichever side of the tendon, which has a wide triangular safe cone dorsolaterally and dorsomedially [4]. In our case, after the identification of the extensor tendon, which was located at the middle dorsal part of the MCP joint, the wires were inserted. By flexing the joint, the fracture was reduced. Then, an anterograde pin was placed through the metacarpal head, crossing the MCP joint and the fracture. Fracture immobilization was held for 3 weeks. Next, the pin was removed. Within the first week, the PIP joint motion was initiated. In a previous study, satisfactory results were achieved in 90% of fractures, which were treated within 5 days after injury [1].

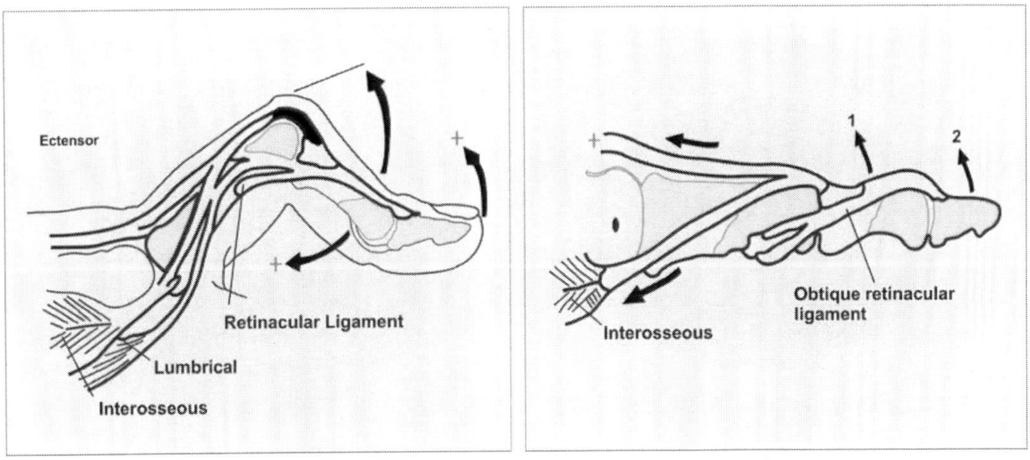

(A) (B)

Figure 8. (a) Safe corridors are distinct in each phalanx in flexed position (yellow). (b) Safe corridors are distinct in the interphalangeal joint in extended position (yellow) [4].

Stiffness is one of the most common issues in phalangeal fractures. Finger immobilization for 3 weeks leads to undesirable clinical results [2]. Therefore, in our case, we pulled out the wires after 3 weeks to prevent joint stiffness or other undesirable results. Passive flexion and extension of the MCP joint were achieved after the entry of the K-wire. Further active and passive MCP joint flexion and extension were continued through physiotherapy after the wire was pulled out.

This systematic review presented conflicting results about CRIF with transarticular or extra-articular K-wire entry [3, 10]. We used the extra-articular percutaneous cross-pinning technique for fixation, attributing to our goal of preserving the ROM of the MCP joint and preventing extensive soft tissue damage, which can result in fibrosis and adhesion adjacent to the extensor mechanism. Joshi [2] hare trospective series of 62 proximal phalanx fractures in 53 patients. The patients were treated with closed reduction and extra-articular percutaneous pinning technique. They had an overall satisfaction rate of 90%. Green and Anderson [2] have retrospectively evaluated 26 fractures in 21 patients and conducted closed reduction and extra-articular percutaneous pinning. An early motion program was initiated, and 18 of 21 patients achieved full ROM. Overall, there are no obvious differences in functional outcomes between percutaneous K-wire fixation and open reduction internal fixation of proximal phalangeal fractures [11].

CONCLUSION

Treatment of fractures at the base of the proximal phalanx using K-wires with the extra-articular percutaneous cross-pinning technique can have desirable clinical outcomes, which include restoration of full ROM. The safe portals for the insertion of the K-wire in treating proximal phalanx fractures with the cross-pinning technique must be identified to prevent soft tissue damage, which could result in unfavorable outcomes, including adhesion and joint stiffness.

CONFLICT OF INTEREST

The authors declare that there is no conflict of interests regarding the publication of this paper.

REFERENCES

[1] Day, C. S., Stern, P. J. (2011). Fractures of the metacarpals and phalanges. In: Wolfe SW, Hotchkiss RN, Pederson WC, Kozin SH (Eds.), *Green's Operative Hand Surgery* (6th edition, pp. 258-282). Philadelphia: Elsevier Inc.

[2] Faruqui, S., Stern, P. J., Kiefhaber, T. R. (2012). Percutaneous pinning of fractures in the proximal third of the proximal phalanx: complications and outcomes. *J. Hand Surg*.37, 1342-1348.

[3] Verver, D., Timmermans, L., Klaassen, C. H., van der Vlies, D. I., Vos, Schep, N. W. L. (2017). Treatment of extra-articular proximal and middle phalangeal fractures of the hand: a systematic review. Strateg. *Trauma Limb Reconstr*.12, 63-76.

[4] Rex, C., Vignesh, R., Javed, M., Balaji, S. C., Premanand, C., Zakki, S. A. (2015). Safe corridors for K-wiring in phalangeal fractures. *Indian J. Orthop.* 49, 388-392.

[5] Carpenter, S., Rohde, R. S. (2013). Treatment of phalangeal fractures phalanx phalangeal fracture treatment hand fracture. *Hand Clin*.29, 519-534.

[6] Haughton, D. N., Jordan, D., Malahias, M., Hindocha, S., Khan, W. (2012). Principles of hand fracture management. *Open Orthop*. J.6, 43.

[7] Edwards, G. S., O'Brien, E. T., Heckman, M. M. (1982). Retrograde cross-pinning of transverse metacarpal and phalangeal fractures. *Brit. Soc. Surg. Hand*.14, 141-148.

[8] Adams, J. E., Miller, T., Rizzo, M. (2013). The biomechanics of fixation techniques for hand fractures. *Hand Clin*.29, 493-500.

[9] Le Nen, D. (2014). Extra-articular fractures of the digital metacarpals and phalanges of the long fingers. *Chir. Main*.33, 1-12.

[10] Al-Qattan, M. M. (2011). Displaced unstable transverse fractures of the shaft of the proximal phalanx of the fingers in industrial workers: reduction and K-wire fixation leaving the metacarpophalangeal and proximal interphalangeal joints free. *J. Hand Surg. Eur*. Vol.36, 577-583.

[11] Gregory S., Lalonde D. H. (2014). Minimally Invasive Finger Fracture Management Wide-awake Closed Reduction, K-wire Fixation, and Early Protected Movement. *Hand Clin* 30. 7-15.

SECTION 4. ONCOLOGY AND ANATOMICAL PATHOLOGY

In: Case Reports in Surgery
Editors: Ahmad Jabir Rahyussalim et al.
ISBN: 978-1-53616-582-1

Chapter 24

THE ROLE OF ACUPUNCTURE IN A BREAST CANCER PATIENT WITH CANCER-INDUCED BONE PAIN

Kemas Abdurrohim, Irma Nareswari, and Diana Oei*
Department of Medical Acupuncture, RSUPN Dr. Cipto Mangunkusumo,
Universitas Indonesia, Jakarta, Indonesia

ABSTRACT

Bone pain is the most common type of cancer-related pain; it often occurs in cases of advanced cancer that have metastasized to bone, particularly prostate cancer, breast cancer, lung cancer, and multiple myeloma. This type of pain is usually severe, persistent, and hard to manage. Current pain-relieving strategies include the use of strong opioids, bisphosphonates, and radiotherapy. However, these approaches may cause unwanted side effects that affect a patient's quality of life. Acupuncture is an adjuvant therapy for pain relief; it has minimal side effects and may improve a patient's quality of life. This paper discusses a 42-year-old female with cancer-induced bone pain who underwent 10 acupuncture treatments at the LI4 Hegu, SP6 Sanyinjiao, SP9 Yinlingquan, ST36 Zusanli, GB34 Yanglingquan, LR3 Taichong, BL23 Shenshu, and GB30 Huantiao acupoints and experienced improvement in pain.

Keywords: Acupuncture, bone pain, cancer, non-pharmacological treatment

---

* Corresponding Author's E-mail: diana.oei@hotmail.com.

INTRODUCTION

Cancer pain is common in cancer patients. However, management of this type of pain is often not optimal. About 40–85% of cancer patients suffer from pain. Cancer pain can be seen in all stages of cancer: 25% of newly diagnosed patients, 33% of patients undergoing treatment, and about 75% of patients with advanced cancer [1].

Cancer-induced bone pain (CIBP) is often found in patients with prostate cancer, breast cancer, lung cancer, and multiple myeloma [2-4]. Approximately 50% of patients with bone metastases suffer from bone pain. CIBP is often felt in the lower back, pelvic area, long bones, and ribs [5]. The pain generally worsens as the disease progresses and can be divided into ongoing pain and breakthrough pain [2]. Several studies have suggested that CIBP is a unique and complex type of pain since it is caused by the hyperexcitation of cells in the dorsal horn and involves both neuropathic and inflammatory pathways [6-10].

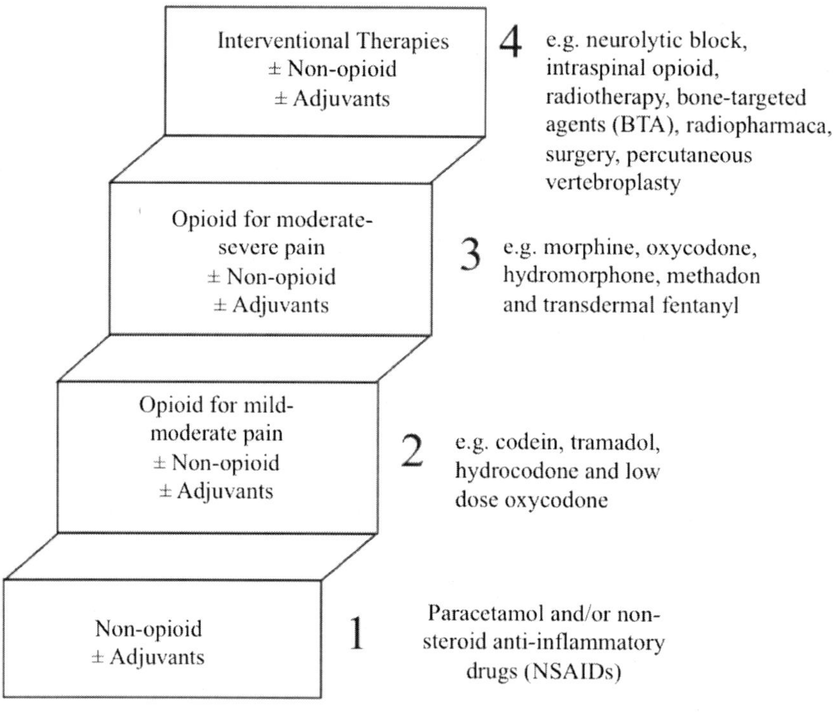

Figure 1. Modified World Health Organization analgesic ladder.

The modified World Health Organization analgesic ladder (Figure 1) [13] describes the mainstream therapies for CIBP [11-14]. However, these approaches are often accompanied by adverse effects, including constipation, nausea and vomiting, drowsiness, urinary retention, itch, myoclonus, loss of consciousness, respiratory depression, opioid-induced hyperalgesia, and pain flare, which can decrease the quality of life in such patients

[11, 12, 15]. In addition to conventional therapies, acupuncture has been used to manage cancer pain and improve quality of life in cancer patients with minimal side effects [16].

In this report, we present a case of CIBP treated with manual acupuncture as an adjunct treatment to conventional therapies in a patient with breast cancer.

Case Illustration

A 42-year-old female complained of persistent pain (5 months duration) that radiated from the right hip toward the lateral malleolus. The pain was evident upon sitting or lying down and relieved when walking. At a follow-up 2 months later, she reported worsening of the pain when walking and sleeping. There were no complaints regarding micturition or passing stool.

The patient had a history of breast cancer that had metastasized to the bone 2 years prior. She had undergone six sessions of chemotherapy and was given an aromatase inhibitor (Aromasin) to limit metastases.

The patient went to Cipto Mangunkusumo Hospital for pain management and was suggested to undergo a bone scan. The resulting bone scan showed an increase in bone metastases, which was deemed responsible for the pain. The metastases were seen in the seventh posterior rib (left), seventh thoracic vertebra, second lumbar vertebra, sacrum, right ilium, right ischium, right acetabulum, and right proximal femur.

Pain was measured using the numeric analog scale (NAS). The patient reported a NAS score of 7, even after treatment with pain medication and radiotherapy.

On physical examination, multiple small masses were seen in her right breast; there were scar tissues under her umbilicus and in the inguinal region as the result of ovariectomy, which was part of her cancer treatment. A positive straight leg raise test and Patrick's test were found in this patient indicating the possibility of nerve root involvement in this patient. There was also pain due to pressure around the GB30 Huantiao acupoint.

Manual acupuncture was then administered to this patient twice per week for 5 weeks using a Huanqiu acupuncture needle (0.25×25 mm and 0.25×60 mm). The chosen acupoints were bilateral LI4 Hegu, SP6 Sanyinjiao, SP9 Yinlingquan, ST36 Zusanli, GB34 Yanglingquan, LR3 Taichong, BL23 Shenshu, and right GB30 Huantiao. Manipulation of the needle was performed until a needling sensation (*deqi*) was achieved; the needle was then left in place for 30 min. Thermal stimulation was also applied to the hip using a TDP lamp.

After the first acupuncture treatment, the patients's pain was reduced to a NAS score of 3. She continued taking pain medication between acupuncture treatments. After the third session, the pain NAS score was 0, and the pain was only felt occasionally at night. However, by the fifth session, the pain had returned at a NAS score of 3 but had migrated to her left hip. After the 10th treatment, the NAS score again returned to 0.

DISCUSSION

The pain suffered by this patient is consistent with the results of the bone scan, which revealed metastases in the hip and lower back regions. Although the physiological mechanisms of bone pain are not fully known, several factors may play a role in the mechanism of CIBP, including the release of proinflammatory mediators causing peripheral sensitization, damage to the periosteum from an increase in osteoclastic activity, microfractures, increased pressure within the bone, periosteal stretching, muscle spasms, nerve root infiltration, and nerve compression due to vertebral collapse. CIBP is likely due to a combination of peripheral and central mechanisms involving both neuropathic and inflammatory pathways [12, 16].

In bone metastases, an increase in levels of receptor activator of nuclear factor kappa-B ligand upsets the balance between bone resorption and formation, causing an increase in osteoclastic activity and destruction of the bone. Such bone destruction may lead to pain via the stimulation of mechanoreceptors in the periosteum; excessive osteoclastic activity may also damage sensory nerve fibers, causing neuropathic-type of pain. Sensory neurons in the periosteum may also be affected by an increase in mechanical stress within the bone that causes pain and increased sensitization [2, 11].

Tumors are known to contain many inflammatory cells. Local inflammatory cells and tumor cells produce various chemical mediators [prostaglandin, endothelin, tumor necrosis factor (TNF)], interleukin-1 (IL-1)] that can stimulate sensory nerve fibers in bones and cause localized acidosis, in turn sensitizing acid-sensing ion channels such as the transient receptor potential vanilloid receptor 1 (TRPV1). Previous studies have shown the importance of TRPV1 in modulating CIBP [2, 11, 12, 15].

CIBP is a unique type of pain in which increases in dynorphin regulation and c-fos expression are seen in the deep dorsal horn. In rat models of CIBP, repeated activation of primary C-fiber afferents by noxious stimulants resulted in a “wind-up” phenomenon, which is characterized by an escalation of nociception by cells in the dorsal horn. This phenomenon causes central sensitization via the stimulation of wide-dynamic range (WDR) cells, which results in the amplification and prolongation of nociception in the central nervous system. This sensitization causes allodynia and hyperalgesia. CIBP also causes central sensitization via the activation of N-methyl-D-aspartate (NMDA)-type glutamate receptors, which is a feature of chronic pain [12].

Changes in the phenotype of dorsal horn neurons, characterized by an increase in WDR neurons, were also seen in CIBP. These changes result in hypersensitivity to mechanical input and movement-related CIBP [16].

Hu et al., (2012) reported that expression of monocyte chemoattractant protein-1 (MCP-1) and CCR2 increases in the spinal cord as the result of neuronal damage in CIBP. MCP-1 is expressed in primary afferent neurons in the spinal cord and is co-expressed with other noxious neuropeptides, such as substance P, calcitonin gene-related peptide, and

TRPV1, causing the release of various proinflammatory cytokines and chemokines that can induce central sensitization and worsen CIBP [17, 18].

In traditional Chinese medicine (TCM), the etiology and mechanism of cancer pain can be categorized into stagnation and cachexia, which are characterized by excess and deficiency, respectively. As a general rule, CIBP in the early and middle stages of cancer is considered excess pain, whereas CIBP in advanced cancer is considered deficient or mixed pain. According to TCM, the key to pain relief is to "unblock" the meridian/channel and regulate the qi/blood [19].

The acupuncture points chosen for this patient were gathered from several case reports and studies of CIBP management [6, 20-23]. Local and segmental points, such as GB30 Huantiao, BL23 Shenshu, ST36 Zusanli, and GB34 Yanglingquan, were used to modulate nociception. The activation of type A and type C nerve fibers during acupuncture manipulation stimulates inhibitory mediators and negative feedback mechanisms related to certain autoreceptors, causing the attenuation of afferent signal transmission distal from the acupuncture points [24]. Segmental points also stimulate Aδ fibers in the muscle and skin that synapse with interneurons in the substantia gelatinosa, causing the release of inhibitory neuromodulators, such as enkephalin. This process can decrease the activity of WDR and nociceptive-specific cells, inducing analgesia along the dermatome and its proximal spinal segments [12].

A previous study showed that needling at acupoint GB30 Huantiao decreases the expression of IL-1β [25]. IL-1β is known to facilitate nociception in neuropathic and inflammatory pain via several distinct signal transduction pathways. For example, IL-1β can activate the p38 mitogen-activated protein kinase (MAPK) pathway to cause hyperalgesia; it can also induce the phosphorylation of NR1, a subunit of the NMDA receptor, [25] which plays a role in the transmission of pain in the spinal cord. As previously mentioned, the activation of the NMDA receptor is a feature of chronic pain. Thus, attenuating NMDA receptor activity using acupuncture can help relieve CIBP. A study by Zhang et al., (2008) showed that electroacupuncture at acupoint GB30 Huantiao attenuates the upregulation of preprodynorphin mRNA and dynorphin, resulting in a lessening of hyperalgesia [21].

Several studies have also shown that needling at acupoint ST36 Zusanli along with other acupuncture points can lead to a decrease in the levels of proinflammatory mediators, such as TNF-α, MCP-1, and IL-6, and an attenuation of the expression of Toll-likereceptor 4 (TLR4), myeloid differentiation factor 88, and NF-κB, resulting in CIBP relief [26-28]. A study of adjuvant-induced arthritis showed that needling the ST36 Zusanli, BL23 Shenshu, and GB39 Xuanzhong acupoints increased the expression of vasoactive intestinal peptide, whichis negatively correlated with TLR4 signaling [29]. Both TLR4-p38 MAPK and MCP-1 (with CCR2 in the dorsal horn) play roles in nociception in CIBP [17, 18]. Therefore, attenuating such proinflammatory mediators may improve CIBP. A study conducted in a mouse inflammatory pain model showed that low-frequency electroacupuncture at acupoint ST36 Zusanli attenuated the expression of TRPV1 and TRPV4, which are crucial receptors involved in nerve excitation [30].

Li et al., (2017) showed that acupuncture at the GB34 Yanglingquan acupoint increased progranulin (PGRN) levels. PGRN is a multi-functional growth factor expressed by various cells thatplays a role in wound healing, cancer, and inflammation. An increase in PGRN during acupuncture can attenuate the activation of NF-κB, which is mediated by the competitive binding of TNF-α to TNFR1 and TNFR2 [31]. Chang et al., (2014) showed that needling both SP9 Yinlingquan and ST36 Zusanli acupoints decreased c-Fos expression in laminae II and V in the dorsal horn of the spinal cord. This decrease in c-Fos improves pain caused by inflammation. Acupoint SP6 Sanyinjiao, which decreases proinflammatory macrophages while increasing anti-inflammatory macrophages and IL-10 levels, was chosen for this patient due to its antinociception and anti-inflammatory effects [32]. The combination of the LI4 Hegu, LR3 Taichong, ST36 Zusanli, and SP9 Yinlingquan acupointscan effectively decrease nociceptive pain due to inflammation [33].

As it is known that a decrease in nociception in the dorsal horn via Aδ inputs can be maintained via regular acupuncture sessions [12, 34]. Our patient was advised to undergo acupuncture twice per week for 5 weeks to achieve optimal outcomes.

Conclusion

This report describes the benefits of acupuncture as a complementary therapy for CIBP management in a patient who suffers from CIBP despite administration of pain medication and radiotherapy.

References

[1] Lu, W; Rosenthal, DS. Acupuncture for cancer pain and related symptoms. *Current Pain and Headache Reports,* 2013, 17, 321.

[2] Luger, NM; Mach, DB; Sevcik, MA; Mantyh, PW. Bone cancer pain: From model to mechanism to therapy. *Journal of Pain and Symptom Management* 2005, 29(*5 Suppl*), S32-S46.

[3] Lipton, A. Pathophysiology of bone metastases: how this knowledge may lead to therapeutic intervention. *Journal of Supportive Oncology,* 2004, 2, 205-213.

[4] Diel, IJ. What do patients with metastatic bone pain need? *European Journal of Cancer Supplements,* 2006, 4, 1-3.

[5] Coleman, RE. Clinical features of metastatic bone disease and risk of skeletal morbidity. *Clinical Cancer Research,* 2006, 12, 6243s–6249s.

[6] Paley, CA; Johnson, MI. Acupuncture for cancer-induced bone pain: a pilot study. *Acupuncture in Medicine,*2011, 29, 71-73.

[7] Urch, CE; Donovan-Rodriguez, T; Dickenson, AH. Alterations in dorsal horn neurones in a rat model of cancer-induced bone pain. *Pain,* 2003, 106, 347-356.

[8] Donovan-Rodriguez, T; Dickenson, AH; Urch, CE. Gabapentin normalizes spinal neuronal responses that correlate with behavior in a rat model of cancer-induced bone pain. *Anesthesiology,* 2005, 102, 132-140.

[9] Urch, CE; Donovan-Rodriguez, T; Gordon-Williams, R; Bee, LA; Dickenson, AH. Efficacy of chronic morphine in a rat model of cancer-induced bone pain: behavior and in dorsal horn pathophysiology. *Journal of Pain,* 2005, 6, 837-845.

[10] Sevcik, MA; Ghilardi, JR; Peters, CM; Lindsay, TH; Halvorson, KG; Jonas, BM; Kubota, K; Kuskowski, MA; Boustany, L; Shelton, DL; Mantyh, PW. Anti-NGF therapy profoundly reduces bone cancer pain and the accompanying increase in markers of peripheral and central sensitization. *Pain,* 2005, 115, 128-141.

[11] Kane, CM; Hoskin, P; Bennett, MI. Cancer induced bone pain. *BMJ,* 2015, 350, h315.

[12] Paley, CA; Bennett, MI, Johnson, MI. Acupuncture for cancer-induced bone pain? *Evidence-Based Complementary and Alternative Medicine,* 2011, 2011, 671043.

[13] Tay, W; Ho, KY. The role of interventional therapies in cancer pain management. *Annals of the Academy of Medicine, Singapore,* 2009, 38, 989-997.

[14] Miguel, R. Interventional treatment of cancer pain: the fourth step in the World Health Organization analgesic ladder? *Cancer Control,* 2000, 7, 149-156.

[15] Costa, L; Ripamonti, CI; Niepel, D; Santini, D Improving quality of life in patients with advanced cancer: Targeting metastatic bone pain. *European Journal of Cancer,* 2017, 71, 80-94.

[16] Paley, CA; Johnson, MI; Bennett, MI. Should physiotherapists use acupuncture for treating patients with cancer-induced bone pain? A discussion paper. *Physiotherapy,* 2011, 97, 256-263.

[17] Hu, JH; Zheng, XY; Yang, JP; Wang, LN; Ji, FH. Involvement of spinal monocyte chemoattractant protein-1 (MCP-1) in cancer-induced bone pain in rats. *Neuroscience Letters,* 2012, 517, 60-63.

[18] Jin, D; Yang, JP; Hu, JH; Wang, LN; Zuo, JL. MCP-1 stimulates spinal microglia via PI3K/Akt pathway in bone cancer pain. *Brain Research,* 2015, 1599, 158-167.

[19] Ling, Y. Traditional Chinese medicine in the treatment of symptoms in patients with advanced cancer. *Annals of Palliative Medicine,* 2013, 2, 141-152.

[20] Zhang, RX; Li, A; Liu, B; Wang, L; Ren, K; Qiao, JT; Berman, BM; Lao, L. Electroacupuncture attenuates bone cancer pain and inhibits spinal interleukin-1 beta expression in a rat model. *Anesthesia and Analgesia,* 2007, 105, 1482-1488.

[21] Zhang, RX; Li, A; Liu, B; Wang, L; Xin, J; Ren, K; Qiao, JT; Berman, BM; Lao, L. Electroacupuncture attenuates bone cancer-induced hyperalgesia and inhibits spinal

preprodynorphin expression in a rat model. *European Journal of Pain,* 2008, 12, 870-878.

[22] Su, CF. Home care with acupuncture increased the quality of life in patient with advanced cancer with neuropathic pain induced by bone metastasis: a case report. *Journal of Integrative Medicine,* 2018, 16, 208-210.

[23] Lee, HJ; Lee, JH; Lee, EO; Lee, HJ; Kim, KH; Kim, SH; Lee, KS; Jung, HJ; Kim, SH. Substance P and beta-endorphin mediate electro-acupuncture induced analgesia in mouse cancer pain model. *Journal of Experimental and Clinical Cancer Research,*2009, 28, 102.

[24] Zhang, ZJ; Wang, XM; McAlonan, GM. Neural acupuncture unit: A new concept for interpreting effects and mechanisms of acupuncture. *Evidence-Based Complementary and Alternative Medicine,* 2012, 2012, 429412.

[25] Zhang, RX; Liu, B; Li, A; Wang, L; Ren, K; Qiao, JT; Berman, BM; Lao, L. Interleukin 1β facilitates bone cancer pain in rats by enhancing NMDA receptor NR-1 subunit phosphorylation. *Neuroscience,* 2008, 154, 1533-1538.

[26] Xu, Y; Hong, S; Zhao, X; Wang, S; Xu, Z; Ding, S; Zhang, K; Zhang, Y; Xu, L; Yu, N; Zhao, T; Yan, Y; Yang, F; Liu, Y; Yu, K; Liu, B; Guo, Y; Pang, G. Acupuncture alleviates rheumatoid arthritis by immune-network modulation. *American Journal of Chinese Medicine,* 2018, 46, 997-1019.

[27] Dong, Z-Q; Zhu, J; Lu, D-z; Chen, Q; Xu, Y-l. Effect of electroacupuncture in "Zusanli" and "Kunlun" acupoints on TLR4 signaling pathway of adjuvant arthritis rats. *American Journal of Therapeutics,* 2016, 0, 1-6.

[28] Wen, CK; Lee, TY. Electroacupuncture decreases the leukocyte infiltration to white adipose tissue and attenuates inflammatory response in high fat diet-induced obesity rats. *Evidence-Based Complementary and Alternative Medicine,* 2014, 2014, 473978.

[29] He, TF; Yang, WJ; Zhang, SH; Zhang, CY; Li, LB; Chen, YF. Electroacupuncture inhibits inflammation reaction by upregulating vasoactive intestinal peptide in rats with adjuvant-induced arthritis. *Evidence-Based Complementary and Alternative Medicine,* 2011, 2011.

[30] Chen, WH; Tzen, JTC; Hsieh, CL; Chen, YH; Lin, TJ; Chen, SY; Lin, YW. Attenuation of TRPV1 and TRPV4 expression and function in mouse inflammatory pain models using electroacupuncture. *Evidence-Based Complementary and Alternative Medicine,* 2012, 2012, 636848.

[31] Li, Y; Fan, X; Liu, J; Wu, Y; Zhang, R. Acupuncture at Yanglingquan (GB34) acupoint alleviates lumbar intervertebral disc degeneration in rats. *International Journal of Clinical and Experimental Medicine,* 2017, 10, 2746-2754.

[32] Silva, MDd; Bobinski, F; Sato, KL; Kolker, SJ; Sluka, KA; Santos, ARS. IL-10 cytokine Released from M2 Macrophages is Crucial for analgesic and anti-inflammatory effects of Acupuncture in a Model of inflammatory Muscle Pain. *Molecular Neurobiology,* 2014, 51, 19-31.

[33] Oh, JH; Bai, SJ; Cho, ZH; Han, HC; Min, SS; Shim, I; Lee, HJ; Lee, H; Lee, BH. Pain-relieving effects of acupuncture and electroacupuncture in an animal model of arthritic pain. *International Journal of Neuroscience,* 2006, 116, 1139-1156.
[34] Filshie, J. Acupuncture for malignant pain. *Acupuncture in Medicine,* 1990, 8, 38-39.

In: Case Reports in Surgery
Editors: Ahmad Jabir Rahyussalim et al.
ISBN: 978-1-53616-582-1

Chapter 25

A Rare Case of CD8-Negative Monomorphic Epitheliotropic Intestinal T-Cell Lymphoma

Agnes Stephanie Harahap*, Lydia Kencana, Maria Francisca Ham, Budiana Tanurahardja and Endang S. R. Hardjolukito
Department of Anatomical Pathology, RSUPN Dr. Cipto Mangunkusumo, Universitas Indonesia, Jakarta, Indonesia

Abstract

Monomorphic epitheliotropic intestinal T-cell lymphoma (MEITL) is an uncommon subtype of intestinal lymphoma that is usually found in Asian populations. MEITL causes non-specific gastrointestinal-related symptoms; thus, it is often overlooked and misdiagnosed, resulting in complications and improper therapeutic approaches. A 75-year-old Asian female was admitted to the emergency room with signs and symptoms of ileal obstruction. She had no history of celiac disease. Surgical resection was performed; the tumor consisted of small- to medium-sized tumor cells arranged in a monomorphic and diffuse pattern. The tumor was positive for CD3 and CD56 but negative for CD8. She was diagnosed with MEITL. Although most MEITL tumors are positive for CD3, CD56, and CD8, CD8-negative MEITL has been reported in some studies and is thought to originate from double-negative intraepithelial lymphocytes. We described a rare case of MEITL with an unusual negative CD8 expression.

Keywords: Intestinal lymphoma, monomorphic epitheliotropic intestinal T-cell lymphoma (MEITL)

* Corresponding Author's E-mail: agnharahap@gmail.com.

INTRODUCTION

Monomorphic epitheliotropic intestinal T-cell lymphoma (MEITL) is a rare type of intestinal lymphoma that arises from intraepithelial lymphocytes (IELs). MEITL was formerly designated as a subtype of enteropathy-associated T-cell lymphoma (EATL) type II. It was recognized as a different entity in the latest WHO classification because of its apparent morphological and immunophenotypic features [1, 2].

Despite its rarity, MEITL occurs worldwide and is the most common type of primary intestinal T-cell lymphoma in Asian populations. MEITL usually manifests with non-specific signs and symptoms, which makes it difficult to diagnose, leading to a higher risk of misdiagnosis and complications as a result of inaccurate therapeutic approaches and procedures. Symptoms range from abdominal pain, weight loss, and diarrhea to intestinal obstruction, which can lead to perforation and bleeding. MEITL is clinically aggressive and generally diagnosed late, with poor prognosis at the time of diagnosis. Therefore, MEITL should always be considered as a differential diagnosis in intestinal tumors, particularly in tumors present in the small intestine [1, 3–5].

MEITL has distinct morphologic and immunophenotypic features. It is composed of monomorphic small- to medium-sized tumor cells that are positive for CD3, CD56, and CD8. However, these expressions vary in some cases, making diagnosis even more difficult. Variations in marker expressions depend on the diverse cellular origin of the tumor.

We present a case of a 75-year-old female with intestinal obstruction due to MEITL with unusual negative CD8 expression.

CASE

A 75-year-old Asian female admitted to the emergency room presented with fever, weakness, nausea and vomiting, abdominal distention, pain, and diarrhea. She had been experiencing abdominal discomfort for approximately 2 months before admission and was assessed as having gastritis. She also had difficulty eating but had no history of celiac disease. A physical examination did not identify any masses or lymphadenopathy at other sites. The laboratory examination showed leukocytosis (14,300/μl) and increased serum Ca125 (185.5 U/mL) levels. Her LDH level was within the normal range (308 U/L). HLA typing was not performed. Chest X-ray showed no mediastinal or lymph node enlargement (Figure 1).

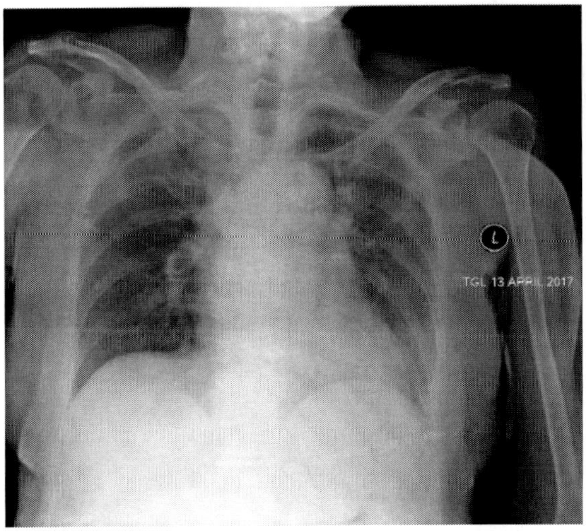

Figure 1. Chest X-ray. No mediastinal orlymph node enlargement was observed.

An abdominal ultrasound showed intestinal inflammation with segmental dilatation and a heterogenous lesion in the lower abdomen compatible with either a fecal mass or tumor. Abdominal computed tomography showed intestinal wall thickening and an ileal mass responsible for obstruction, with dilatation of the proximal segments (Figure 2).

A small intestinal resection was performed. Macroscopically, the tumor measured 4×4×2 cm; it bulged into the serous layer and was whitish and rubbery in consistency. The non-tumorous mucosa showed no marked abnormalities (Figure 3).

Histopathologic examination of the ileal tissue resection showed diffuse transmural proliferation of monotonous medium-sized lymphoid cells with dispersed chromatin, inconspicuous nucleoli, and clear cytoplasm. The tumor lacked inflammatory infiltrates. The adjacent mucosa showed blunting villi and ulcerations. There was also evidence of epitheliotropism characterized by infiltration of lymphocytes in the epithelium. No enteropathy changes (crypt hyperplasia and villous atrophy) or necrosis were found (Figure 4).

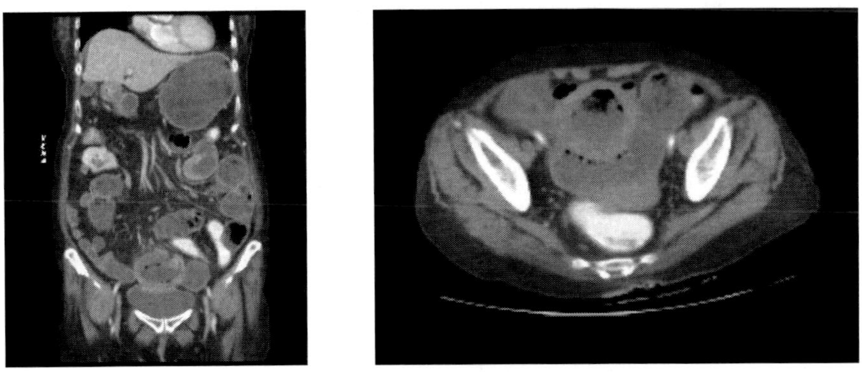

Figure 2. Abdominal CT scan showing intestinal wall thickening and an obstructing mass in the ileum, with proximal intestinal and gastric dilatation.

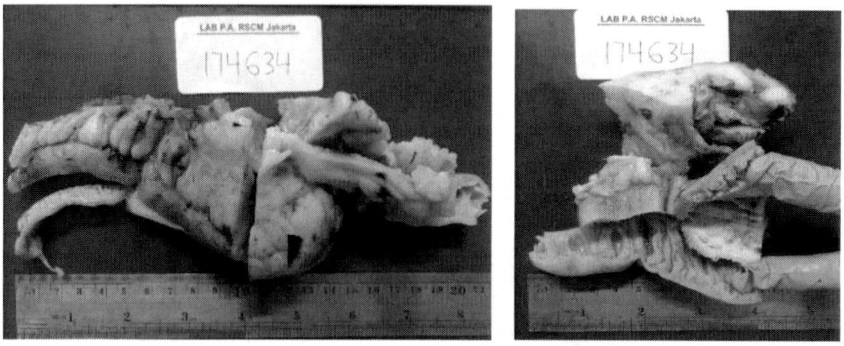

Figure 3. The tumor appeared as a bulging, whitish, and rubbery mass in the ileal wall (formalin fixed tissue).

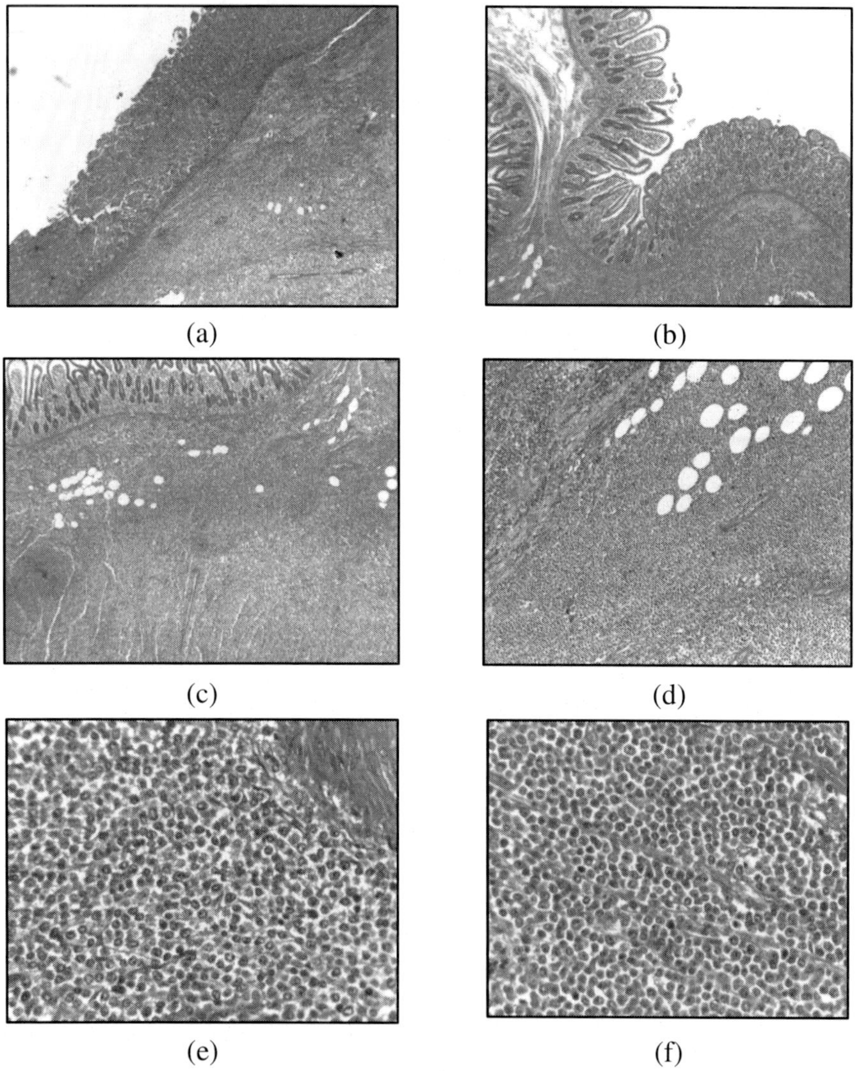

Figure 4. Histopathological features. (a, b) The affected intestinal mucosa showed blunting of the villi and ulceration, H&E 40×. (c) There was a diffuse transmural proliferation of lymphoid cells, H&E 40×. (d) The tumor cells are arranged in a monotonous and diffuse pattern, H&E 100×. (e, f) The tumor consists of medium-sized lymphoid cells with dispersed chromatin, inconspicuous nucleoli, and clear cytoplasm, H&E 400×.

The tumor cells were positive for CD3, CD7, CD56, T-cell intracytoplasmic antigen (TIA)-1, and perforin. The Ki67 proliferation index was 70–80%. Other markers such as CD8, CD4, CD30, CD5, CD20, CD79a, CD10, granzyme B, and Epstein–Barr virus-encoded small RNA (EBER) *in situ* hybridization were all negative. Several important markers (megakaryocyte-associated tyrosine kinase (MATK), CD103, TCRαβ, and TCRγδ) were not available (Figure 5 and 6).

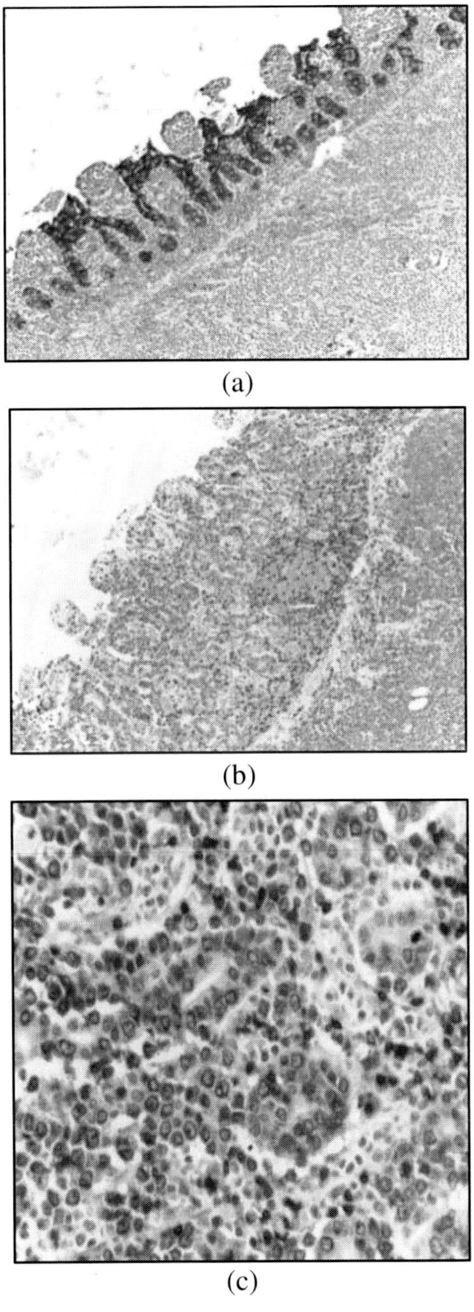

Figure 5. (Continued).

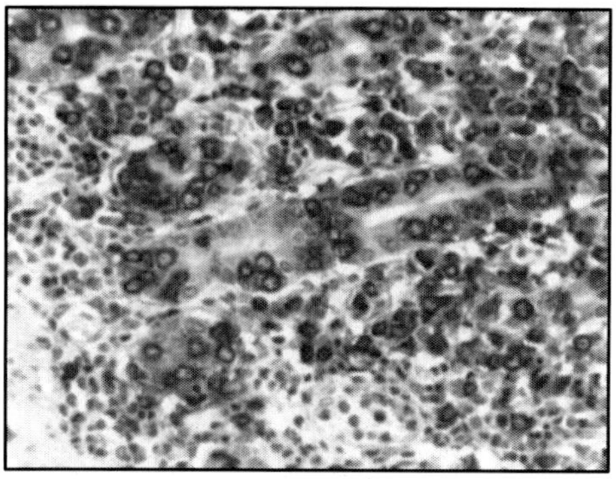

(d)

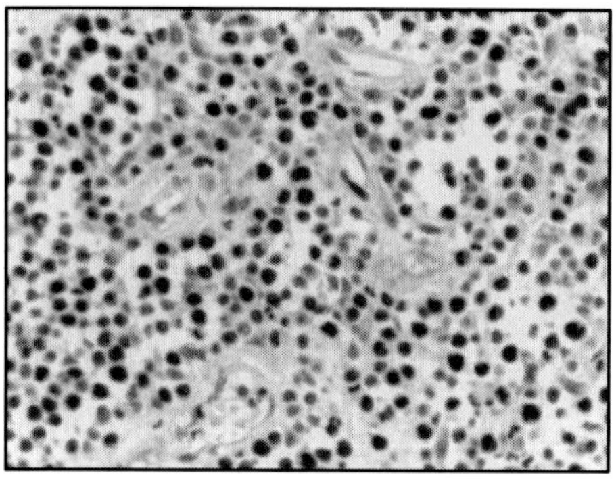

(e)

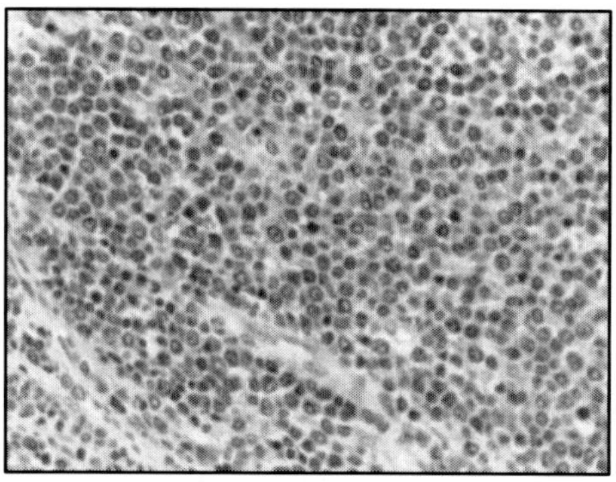

(f)

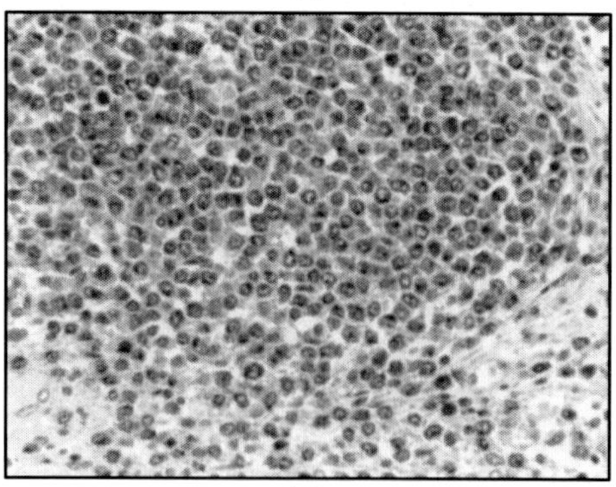

(g)

Figure 5. (Continued).

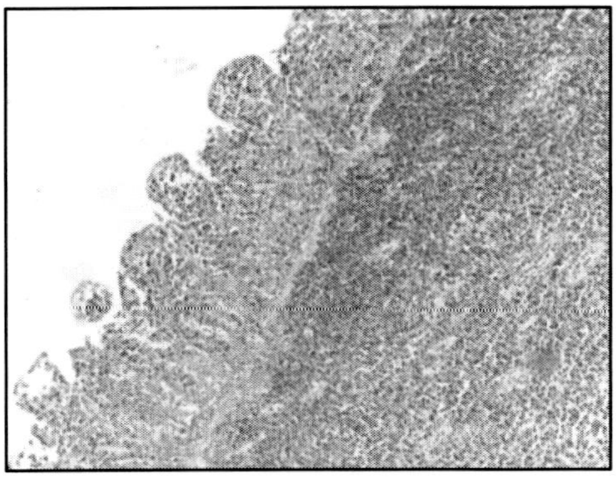

(h)

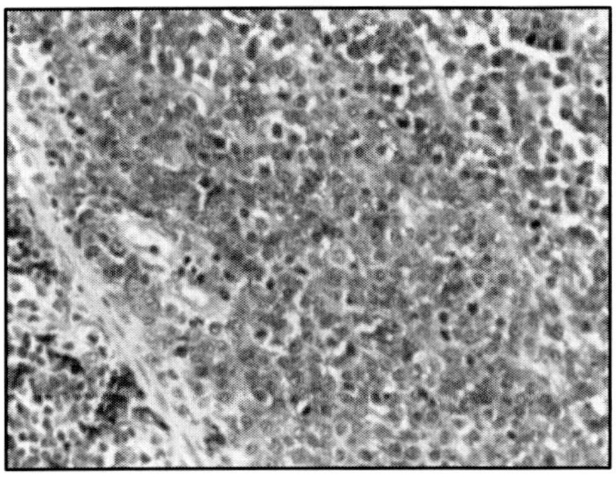

(i)

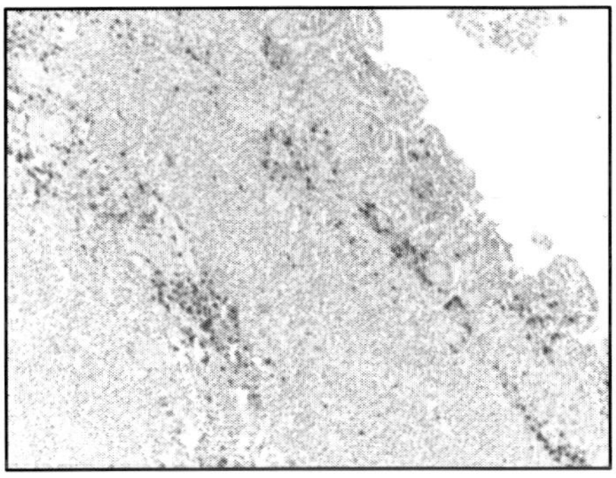

(j)

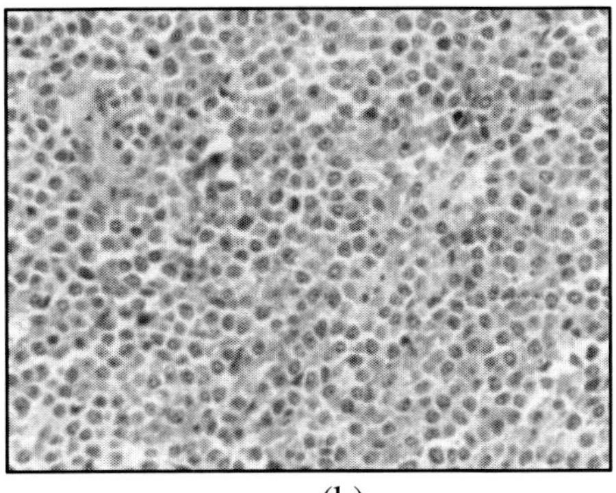

(k)

Figure 5. (Continued).

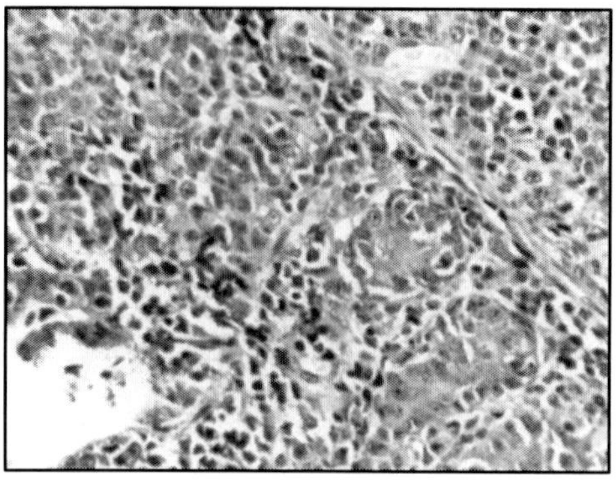

(l)

Figure 5. Immunohistochemistry profile. (a) AE 1/3, negative, 100×; (b, c) CD3, diffusely positive, 100× and 400×; (d) CD7, diffusely positive, 400×; (e) Ki67, positive in 70–80% of tumor cells, 400×; (f) Bcl-2, positive, 400×; (g) TIA1, positive, 400×; (h) perforin, positive, 100×; (i) CD56, positive, 400×; (j) CD20, negative, 100×; (k) CD4, negative, 400×; and (l) CD8, negative, 400×.

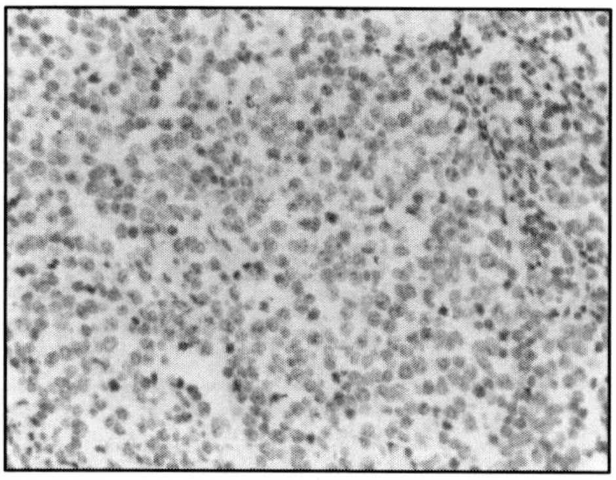

Figure 6. EBER, *in situ* hybridization, 400×.

The immunohistochemistry features are more identical to those of extranodal NK/T-cell lymphoma, nasal type (ENKTL). However, due to the negative EBER test and no manifestation in nasal, the patient was diagnosed with MEITL. The patient gave up treatment and died within 1 month after surgery.

Discussion

The gastrointestinal tract is the most common extranodal site of lymphoma; 30–40% of all extranodal lymphomas occur here. However, primary lymphoma of the gastrointestinal tract is very rare and constitutes only approximately 1–4% of gastrointestinal malignancies. Most cases of gastrointestinal lymphoma belong to the non-Hodgkin lymphoma (NHL) subtype, such as diffuse large B-cell lymphoma, mucosa-associated lymphoid tissue lymphoma, follicular lymphoma, Burkitt lymphoma, mantle cell lymphoma, peripheral T-cell lymphoma (PTCL), ENKTL, adult T-cell leukemia/lymphoma (ATLL), EATL, and MEITL [6–10].

The current patient presented with gastrointestinal-related signs and symptoms due to intestinal obstruction from an ileal tumor, which can be caused by intestinal lymphoma. According to Dawson [11], intestinal lymphoma is considered primary if it has the following clinical characteristics: (1) no palpable superficial lymphadenopathy, (2) no obvious enlargement of mediastinal lymph nodes due to chest radiographs, (3) normal white blood cell counts (total and differential), (4) predominating bowel lesions in laparotomy, with the affected lymph nodes being in its immediate neighborhood, and (5) no lymphoid tumor involvement in the liver or spleen. The physical, laboratory, and radiologic examination of our patient showed neither lymphadenopathy nor tumor in the liver and spleen. Although the leukocyte count was above normal levels, the signs and symptoms fit four of Dawson's five criteria for primary gastrointestinal lymphoma. The high leukocyte count was likely due to infection because the patient also presented with fever.

The histopathologic features showed medium-sized, monomorphic tumor cells with round nuclei that were arranged in a diffuse pattern, suggesting NHL. Although most primary gastrointestinal lymphomas are of B-cell lineage, the immunophenotype of this patient was CD3-positive and CD20-negative, suggesting that the tumors were of T-cell origin, which occurs in only 9% of primary gastrointestinal lymphomas [8, 11].

The differential diagnosis of T-cell lymphoma in the intestine includes MEITL, EATL, ENKTL, PTCL, ATLL, and gamma delta T-cell lymphoma. The clinical, histopathological, and immunohistochemistry findings of this patient displayed tendencies associated with primary intestinal T-cell lymphoma. However, considering its rarity, we could not yet exclude the possibility of the tumor representing the extranodal involvement of other T-cell lymphomas [1, 3, 4, 12].

In this case, the immunophenotype of the tumor fit that of MEITLand ENKTL the best. The clinical features, morphology, and immunophenotype of MEITL and ENKTL are described in Table 1.

Our patient was an Asian female in her 70s; therefore, she had a supporting demographic background for both MEITL and ENKTL. The tumor was present as a mass in the ileum and thickening of the intestinal wall with no involvement of other areas was noted; this manifestation is more commonly found in MEITL.

MEITL is composed of monomorphic small- to medium-sized tumor cells, with round and regular nuclei, finely dispersed chromatin, inconspicuous nucleoli, and clear cytoplasm. The tumor cells also show prominent epitheliotropism. MEITL has no known association with celiac disease; thus, the non-neoplastic areas are absent of the features found in celiac disease. The villous architecture is distorted with broad villi as a result of tumor cell expansion in the lamina propria, but no inflammatory background is present. The morphologic features in our case fit those of MEITL [1, 3–5].

The MEITL immunophenotype is quite distinctive: CD3, CD8, and CD56 are positive in most cases, with CD8 and CD56 being highly specific markers. MEITL is negative for CD4 and CD30 and is often negative for CD5 since most MEITL cases express gamma delta T-cell receptor (TCR). The most frequently expressed TCR in MEITL is of the gamma subtype, but some cases express TCR beta, TCR gamma and beta, and CD8 alpha homodimers. Some studies have also reported silent TCR tumor cells. TIA1 is usually positive, whereas the expressions of perforin and granzyme are inconsistent. MATK is expressed in more than 80% of tumor cells in most cases and is a helpful marker to differentiate MEITL from EATL [1, 16, 17].

The tumor cells in our case were positive for CD7, CD56, TIA1, and perforin and negative for CD5, CD4, CD30, and granzyme B, which is in line with the MEITL immunophenotype according to the literature. Intriguingly, CD8 was not expressed. There are, however, some previous reports of CD8-negative MEITL [16, 18–20].

MEITL arises from several subtypes of intestinal IELs that express different types of surface receptors, which is resembled in the immunophenotype. Most IELs express TCR; however, some studies have recently reported TCR-negative IELs. In addition to TCR expression, there are also variations in CD4 and CD8 expressions. During the differentiation process, most lymphocytes undergo positive selection in the thymus before differentiating into single-positive T-cells and migrating into the intestine. By contrast, the remaining lymphocytes are double negative when transferred into the intestine. The latter then differentiate into single-positive T-cells following antigenic stimulation. Both the TCR-positive and TCR-negative and single-positive and double-negative T-cells have the potential to transform into MEITL and affect its immunophenotype.

MEITL originating from the double-negative T-cells presents with CD3+ CD8− tumor cells, as in our case. Perforin was positive in this case, which is an uncommon feature in double-negative T-cells and is thus considered aberrant. However, perforin transcription process starts in the stage of double-negative, making it possible to be detected in unusual cases [16, 18, 19].

ENKTL was considered as a differential diagnosis in this case because of the more identical immunophenotype and higher prevalence compared with MEITL. However, when found in the gastrointestinal tract, ENKTL most commonly manifests as an extranodal spread rather than as a primary lesion. According to Dawson's criteria [11], the tumor in our case was more likely a primary intestinal lymphoma. ENKTL consists of small, medium, large, or anaplastic tumor cells and is usually accompanied by coagulative necrosis admixed apoptotic bodies and inflammatory infiltrate. These morphologic features are not in line with those of our case since there was no inflammatory infiltrate or necrosis. The immunophenotype of ENKTL is CD3+, CD56+, and CD8−, which is identical with the patient's immunophenotype. However, ENKTL is strongly associated with Epstein–Barr virus infection. Although the immunohistochemistry profile might be compatible, the clinical and morphologic features and the negative EBER ruled out ENKTL.

Table 1. Clinical, morphologic, and immunophenotypic features of MEITL and ENKTL [1,4,13–15]

	MEITL	ENKTL
Clinical features	Abdominal pain, obstruction or perforation, weight loss, diarrhea, gastrointestinal bleeding.	Nasal obstruction-related signs and symptoms in most cases. Intestinal lesions manifest as perforation or gastrointestinal bleeding.
Median age	60 years old	44-54 years old
Male:female ratio	2:1	2:1
Epidemiology	Asia, Hispanic	Asia, Mexico, Central and South America
Frequency	1% of NHL	10% of NHL
Localization	Small intestine, jejunum more often involved than the ileum. It can disseminate to extranodal sites (stomach, large bowel) and regional lymph nodes.	Most commonly involves the nasal cavity. Other sites of involvement include upper aerodigestive tract, skin, soft tissue, gastrointestinal tract, and testes.
Primary/secondary intestinal lesion	Primary	Secondary involvement is more common than primary
Gross appearance	Plaques and nodules	Mass and perforation
Cytological features	Small to medium-sized tumor cells, monomorphic	Broad cytological spectrum. Most tumors consist of medium-sized cells or a mixture of small and large cells.
Necrosis	Uncommon	Common
Inflammatory background	Uncommon	Heavy, can mimic inflammatory process
Mucosa away from tumor	Normal	Normal
CD3	+	+
CD5	−	−
CD56	+	+
CD4	−	−
CD8	+	−
CD7	+	+
CD30	−	±
TIA1	+	+
Granzyme B, perforin	variable	+
HLA-DR	−	+
MATK	+	+
EBV infection	No known association	Very strong association

Another possible differential diagnosis of this patient was EATL. EATL is commonly found in Northern Europe, usually occurs in the small intestine, and is associated with celiac disease. The tumor cells are polymorphic and are composed of pleomorphic medium to large cells with prominent nucleoli. EATL is accompanied by an inflammatory background and often necrosis. The features of celiac disease can be found in the adjacent mucosa, particularly in the jejunum. The tumor cells are usually CD3+, CD5−, CD7+, CD4−, CD8−, and CD103+. They also express cytotoxic granule-associated proteins, e.g., TIA1, granzyme B, and perforin. CD30 expression differs according to the cytomorphology, but almost all large-cell EATL are CD30+. In this case, EATL was unlikely because of the demographic background of the patient, no history of celiac disease, and the irrelevant morphologic features. CD103 and MATK immunostaining was necessary to confirm the diagnosis, but these procedures were not available in our country [1, 21].

The patient underwent surgical resection and then stopped treatment and died 1 month later. There is currently no established treatment for MEITL. In most cases, patients undergo surgical resection due to the emergency presentation or the need for a histopathological examination. In our case, the surgery was performed because of the ileal obstruction and to prevent perforation. Surgery followed by chemotherapy tends to have a better outcome than surgery alone. However, the most efficient chemotherapy regimen has yet to be discovered. The most commonly used chemotherapy regimens are CHOP (cyclophosphamide, doxorubicin, vincristine, and prednisone), SMILE (dexamethasone, methotrexate, ifosfamide, L-asparaginase, and etoposide), and IVEMTX (ifosfamide, vincristine, and etoposide/methotrexate). MEITL is considered aggressive and has a poor prognosis, even when treated using chemotherapy, with a median overall survival of 7 months. Nonetheless, some studies showed that early detection and treatment result in better therapy response and even long-term survival. Some studies also reported the use of hematopoietic stem cells [16, 18, 20].

CONCLUSION

Primary intestinal lymphoma is very rare and often misdiagnosed. Various subtypes of lymphomas can occur in the gastrointestinal tract, with diverse morphology and immunophenotypes. We reported a rare case of primary lymphoma of the gastrointestinal tract, with the immunophenotype suggesting ENKTL. However, because of its clinical and morphologic features and negative EBER test, the patient was diagnosed with CD8-negative MEITL. CD8 and CD56 are the highly specific markers for MEITL, but they might not be expressed in particular cases. The expression of T-cell markers depends on the cellular origin of the tumor. MEITL arises from IELs residing in the intestine, which have diverse phenotypes and are present in various stages of differentiation. Therefore, it is possible for MEITL to have uncommon and aberrant marker expressions that should not be overlooked.

Conflicts of Interest

The authors declare no conflicts of interest.

References

[1] Swerdlow SH, Campo E, Harris NL, Jaffe ES, Pileri SA, Stein H, et al. WHO classification of tumors of haemopoietic and lymphoid tissues. Revised 4th edition. *Lyon: International Agency for Research on Cancer*; 2017.

[2] Skinnider BF. Lymphoproliferative disorders of the gastrointestinal tract. *Arch. Pathol. Lab. Med.* 2018;142:44-52.

[3] Weindorf SC, Smith LB, Owens SR. Update on gastrointestinal lymphomas. *Arch. Pathol. Lab. Med.* 2018;142:1347-51.

[4] Medeiros LJ, Miranda RN. *Diagnostic pathology: Lymph nodes and extranodal lymphomas.* 2nd edition. Canada: Elsevier; 2018.

[5] Sun ZH, Zhou HM, Song GX, Zhou ZX, Bai L. Intestinal T-cell lymphomas: A retrospective analysis of 68 cases in China. *World J. Gastroenterol.* 2014; 20:296-302.

[6] Arora N, Manipadam MT, Pulimood A, Ramakrishna BS, Chacko A, Kurian SS, et al. Gastrointestinal lymphomas: pattern of distribution and histological subtypes: 10 years experience in a tertiary centre in South India. *Indian J. Pathol. Microbiol.* 2011;54:712-9.

[7] Freedman AS. Clinical presentation and diagnosis of primary gastrointestinal lymphomas [Internet]; 2019 [cited 2019 Feb 17]. Available from: https://www.uptodate.com/contents/clinical-presentation-and-diagnosis-of-primary-gastrointestinal-lymphomas.

[8] Ghimire P, Wu GY, Zhu L. Primary gastrointestinal lymphoma. *World J. Gastroenterol.* 2011;17:697-707.

[9] Cardona D, Layne A, Lagoo A. Lymphomas of the gastro-intestinal tract - pathophysiology, pathology, and differential diagnosis. *Indian J. Pathol. Microbiol.* 2012;55:1-16.

[10] Wang G, Xu G, Luo G, Shan H, Li Y, Gao X, et al. Primary intestinal non-Hodgkin's lymphoma: a clinicopathologic analysis of 81 patients. *World J. Gastroenterol.* 2011;17:4625-31.

[11] Dawson IM, Cornes JS, Morson BC.Primary malignant lymphoid tumours of the intestinal tract. Report of 37 cases with a study of factors influencing prognosis. *Br. J. Surg.* 1961;49:80-9.

[12] Zing NPC, Fischer T, Zain J, Federico M, Rosen ST. Peripheral T-cell lymphomas: incorporating new developments in diagnostics, prognostication, and treatment into clinical practice-part 2: ENKTL, EATL, indolent T-Cell LDP of the GI tract, ATLL, and hepatosplenic T-Cell lymphoma.*Oncology* 2018;32:e83-9.

[13] Makruasi N, Makruasi S, Trongwongsa T. Enteropathy type II associated T-cell non-Hodgkin lymphoma: a case report. *J. Hematol.* 2015;4:144-7.

[14] Geetha V, Kudva R, Amprayil AJ. Enteropathy associated T cell lymphoma—a case report of an uncommon extranodal T cell lymphoma. *J. Clin. Diagn. Res.* 2014;8:FD10-2.

[15] Haverkos BM, Pan Z, Gru AA, Freud AG, Rabinovitch R, Xu-Welliver M, et al. Extranodal NK/T cell lymphoma, nasal type (ENKTL-NT): an update on epidemiology, clinical presentation, and natural history in North American and European cases. *CurrHematol.vMalig. Rep.* 2016;11:514-27.

[16] Aoyama Y, Tsunemine H, Zushi Y, Maruoka H, Goto Y, Kodaka T, et al. Colonal monomorphic epitheliotropic intestinal T-cell lymphoma with novel phenotype of cytoplasmic CD3 expression. *J. Clin. Exp. Hematop.* 2018;58:102-6.

[17] Tan SY, Chuang SS, Tang T, Tan L, Ko YH, Chuah KL, et al. Type II EATL (epitheliotropic intestinal T-cell lymphoma): a neoplasm of intra-epithelial T-cells with predominant CD8αα phenotype. *Leukemia* 2013;27:1688-96.

[18] Kikuma K, Yamada K, Nakamura S, Ogami A, Nimura S, Hirahashi M, et al. Detailed clinicopathological characteristics and possible lymphomagenesis of type II intestinal enteropathy-associated T-cell lymphoma in Japan. *Hum. Pathol.* 2014;45:1276-84.

[19] Olivares-Villagómez D, Van Kaer L. Intestinal intraepithelial lymphocytes: sentinels of the mucosal barrier. *Trends Immunol.* 2018;39:264-75.

[20] Tse E, Gill H, Loong F, Kim SJ, Ng SB, Tang T, et al.Type II enteropathy-associated T-cell lymphoma: a multicenter analysis from the Asia Lymphoma Study Group. *Am. J. Hematol.* 2012;87:663-8.

[21] Ishibashi H, Nimura S, Kayashima Y, Takamatsu Y, Aoyagi K, Harada N, et al. Multiple lesions of gastrointestinal tract invasion by monomorphic epitheliotropic intestinal T-cell lymphoma, accompanied by duodenal and intestinal enteropathy-like lesions and microscopic lymphocytic proctocolitis: a case series. *Diagn. Pathol.* 2016;11:66.

In: Case Reports in Surgery
Editors: Ahmad Jabir Rahyussalim et al.
ISBN: 978-1-53616-582-1

Chapter 26

A RARE CASE OF CLEAR CELL PAPILLARY RENAL CELL CARCINOMA

***Fili Sufangga*[1] *and Budiana Tanurahardja*[2,*]**
[1]Anatomical Pathology Residency Program, Faculty of Medicine, Universitas Indonesia, Jakarta, Indonesia
[2]Department of Anatomical Pathology, Faculty of Medicine, Universitas Indonesia, Jakarta, Indonesia

ABSTRACT

Clear cell papillary renal cell carcinoma is an indolent neoplasm composed of clear epithelial cells arranged in tubules and a papillary structure, with predominantly linear nuclear alignment away from the basement membrane. In this paper, we report our experience of diagnosing a rare case of clear cell papillary renal cell carcinoma. The patient was a 50-year-old male with a chief complaint of abdominal pain. A computed tomographic abdominal scan revealed a large heterogeneous multicystic mass on the left kidney. On the basis of the macroscopic examination, microscopy, and immunohistochemical staining, we diagnosed the tumor as a clear cell papillary renal cell carcinoma. This tumor is an uncommon variant of a renal cell neoplasm that has distinct histological and immunohistochemical characteristics. Pathologists should be aware of this entity because the biological behavior of this tumor is very different from that of conventional clear cell carcinoma.

Keywords: clear cell papillary renal cell carcinoma, renal cell carcinoma

* Corresponding Author's E-mail: budiana.t@gmail.com.

Introduction

Renal cell carcinoma (RCC) is the most common malignancy of the kidney, accounting for up to 90% of renal neoplasms in adults. The most common type is clear cell RCC, followed by papillary RCC. Clear cell RCC is a malignant tumor composed of cells with clear or eosinophilic cytoplasm. Papillary RCC has a papillary or tubulopapillary structure and is often circumscribed. The papillae are separated by delicate fibrovascular cores with foamy macrophages and hemosiderin. Other subtypesare Xp11.2 translocation-associated RCC and clear cell papillary RCC (CCPRCC) with papillary architectures and a clear cell morphology [1, 2].

CCPRCC is an indolent renal tumor composed of a single layer of cells with clear cytoplasm with tubules and a papillae structure. Tickoo et al. reported a lesion appearing in patients with end-stage kidney disease, but these tumors could be found in otherwise normal kidney. Aydin et al. in a large series reported similar tumors as clear cell tubulopapillary RCC (CCTPRCC) [1, 3-5].

Patients with CCPRCC usually are asymptomatic and sometimes present with abdominal pain. Some tumors are found in the follow-up after dialysis. This tumor accounts for 1%-4% of all resected renal neoplasms. The ages of patients range from 18 to 88 years, with a mean of 70 years. There is no sex predilection [1, 6]. The tumor sizes range from 0.2 to 7.5 cm (mean, 2.0; median, 1.8 cm). The tumor is commonly well defined and well encapsulated with cystic changes, and it sometimes presents as a solitary mass. CCPRCC is characterized by tubular papillary infoldings, and acinar cystic, ribbon-like, and solid patterns are seen in varying proportions. The tumor cells are cuboidal to low columnar, with clear cytoplasm or scant eosinophilic cytoplasm and uniform nuclei with inconspicuous nucleoli arranged linearly away from the basement membrane. Immunohistochemically, these tumors show positivity for cytokeratin 7 (CK7), carbonic anhydrase IX (CA9), and vimentin and negativity for CD10, RCC marker, and alpha-methylacyl-CoA racemase (AMACR). CCPRCC is different from conventional cell RCCsthat are CK7 negative and CD10 positive and from papillary cell carcinomas that are CK7, CD10, and racemase positive [6-9].

Because of its rarity, we report a case of CCPRCC that had overlapping features with those of papillary RCC and clear cell RCC but different genetic and immunohistochemical features and seemed to be indolent, with no detectable metastases.

Case Report

A 50-year-old male patient came to the Islamic Jakarta Hospital on December 20, 2014, with a chief complaint of flank pain and hematuria. He had experienced intermittent flank pain since 1 year prior to hospital admission. During that time, he had gone to a doctor and been told that he had muscle pain. He had a 4-year history of hypertension and was regularly taking captopril 2 × 25 mg. The patient also had experienced hematuria but had ignored it. A history of pain during urination was denied. He had experienced weight loss and felt a mass in his left abdomen 6 months prior to hospital admission. He had a smoking habit of 3-4 cigarettes per day.

On December 20, 2014, he felt severe flank pain and hematuria. He then felt nausea and experienced vomiting. In the Islamic Jakarta hospital, he underwent a computed tomography (CT) abdominal scan without contrast, which revealed a large heterogeneous 9.5 × 11 × 14-cm mass on the left kidney that had already passed through the capsule but not the Gerota fascia. A focus of calcification was also observed.

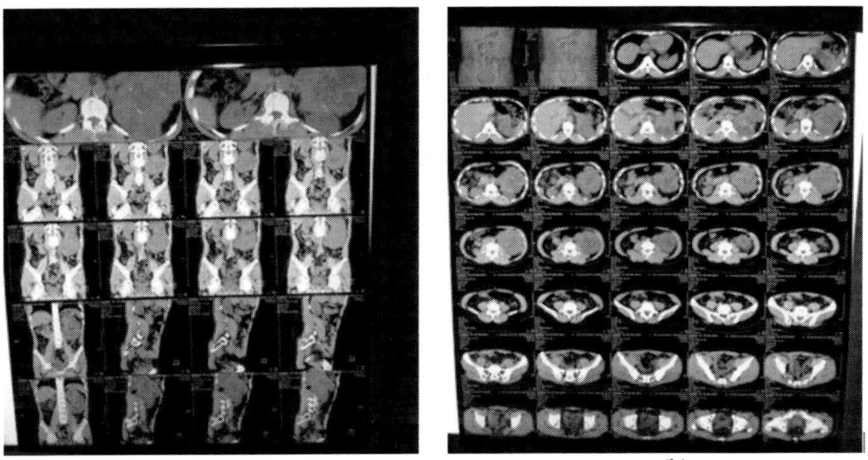

(a) (b)

Figure 1. A Coronal section of the abdomen CT Scan shows a large (9.5 × 11 × 14 cm) heterogeneous mass that has already passed through the capsule but has not yet invaded the Gerotafascia. Calcification is also shown. B. Axial section of the abdomen CT Scan.

Table 1. Patient's laboratory results

Type of examination	Result	Unit
Hemoglobin	13.9	g/dL
Hematocrit	41.6	%
Erythrocyte	4.72	10^6/μL
Leukocytes	7390	μL
Platelets	210.000	μL
Urea	35	mg/dL
Creatinine	1.6	mg/dL
Glomerular filtration rate	50,9	mL/min/1.73m^2
Sodium	143	mEq/L
Potassium	4.94	mEq/L
Chloride	100	mEq/L

The urologist suggested that the patient needed surgery in Dr. Cipto Mangunkusumo Hospital. On February 3, 2015, a nephrectomy was performed. The results of the laboratory testing performed on February 2, 2015, are presented in Table 1.

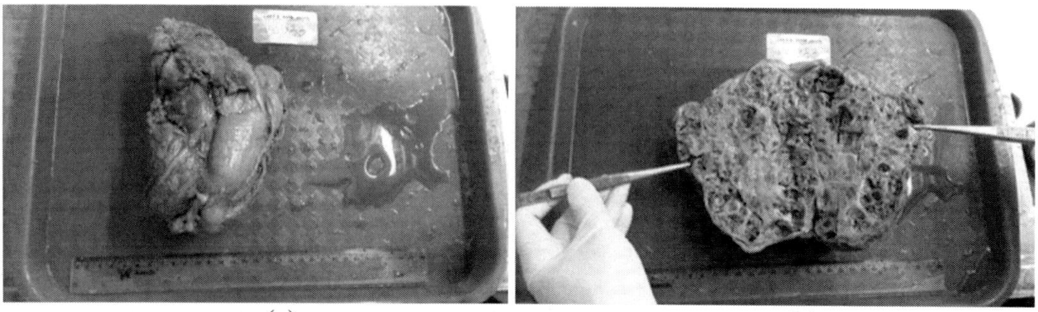

(a) (b)

Figure 2. Gross pathology. (a) The surface of the kidney; (b) Cut surface of the kidney, which shows a multicystic partially solid mass.

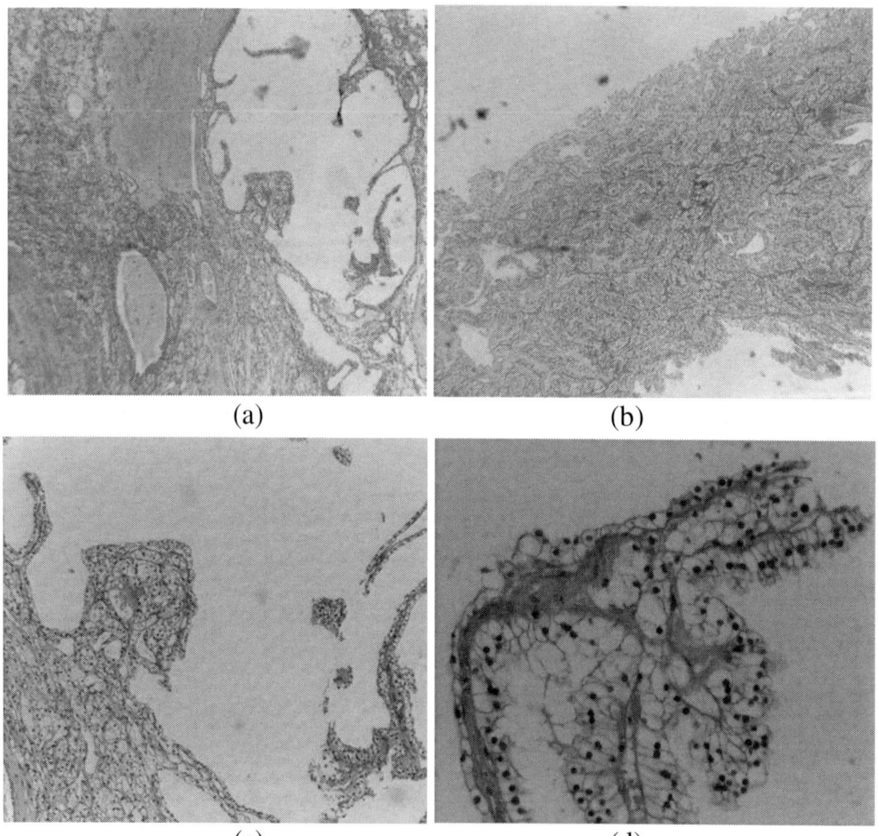

(a) (b)

(c) (d)

Figure 3. Microscopic image showing hematoxylin and eosin staining. A. Cystic and papillary structure (40×). B. Solid structure (40×). C. Papillary structure (100×). D. The nuclei is situated away from the basement membrane (400×).

The specimen was sent to the anatomical pathology laboratory. On macroscopic examination, the size of the left kidney was 18 × 11.5 × 8.5 cm, and the outer surface was smooth, brown in color, and rubbery in consistency. A cut surface showed a multicystic partially solid mass that filled almost all of the kidney parenchyma. The size of the tumor was 17 × 6 × 5 cm. The mass had infiltrated the pelviocalyceal system but had not penetrated the capsule. A microscopic examination showed that the epithelial tumor hadan acinar, multicystic, solid papillary structure. The tumor cells had small, hyperchromatic, vesicular nuclei located on the apical side of the cell. The cytoplasm was mostly clear. The stroma was fibrotic and had been infiltrated by inflammatory cells. The tumor had infiltrated the capsule but had not yet penetrated the perirenal fat. The tumor was diagnosed as a clear cell papillary RCC.

On April 19, 2016, we performed immunohistochemistry staining, including CK7, CD10, AMACR, vimentin, high molecular weight cytokeratin (HMWCK), CK8, CK18, epithelial membrane antigen (EMA), and Ki67 of the tumor to provide supporting results for the diagnosis. The results showed that the tumor was positive for CK8, CK18, EMA, CK7, CD10, HMWCK, and vimentin and negative for AMACR and Ki67 < 1%.

DISCUSSION

CCPRCC is a low-grade RCC that occurs in both end-stage kidney disease and normal kidneys and is usually located in the renal cortex. More than 95% of tumors are pT1 at presentation and are rarely multilocal or bilateral [6, 7]. Radiographically, CCPRCC is located mid-pole in the kidneys. Some studies have reported that CCPRCC showed frequent heterogeneity suggestive of a mixed solid-cystic nature, and homogeneous solid appearing tumors have also been seen [1, 2, 6].

These tumors are often small, well circumscribed, and well encapsulated. Surface coloration is variable and necrosis is absent. Histopathologically, CCPRCC commonly shows cystic, tubular, acini, papillary, ribbon-like, and solid patterns in varying proportions. The cells are cuboidal to low columnar, with clear or scant eosinophilic cytoplasm, round uniform nuclei and a low Fuhrman nuclear grade (1 or 2). The cells are arranged linearly away from the basement membrane or toward the apical surface. It is believed that CCPRCC has a better prognosis than those ofclear cell RCC and papillary RCC. Smooth muscle and fibrous stroma in varying amounts have been noted. There is no tumor necrosis, perirenal invasion, or lymphovascular invasion in CCPRCC [2, 3, 6].

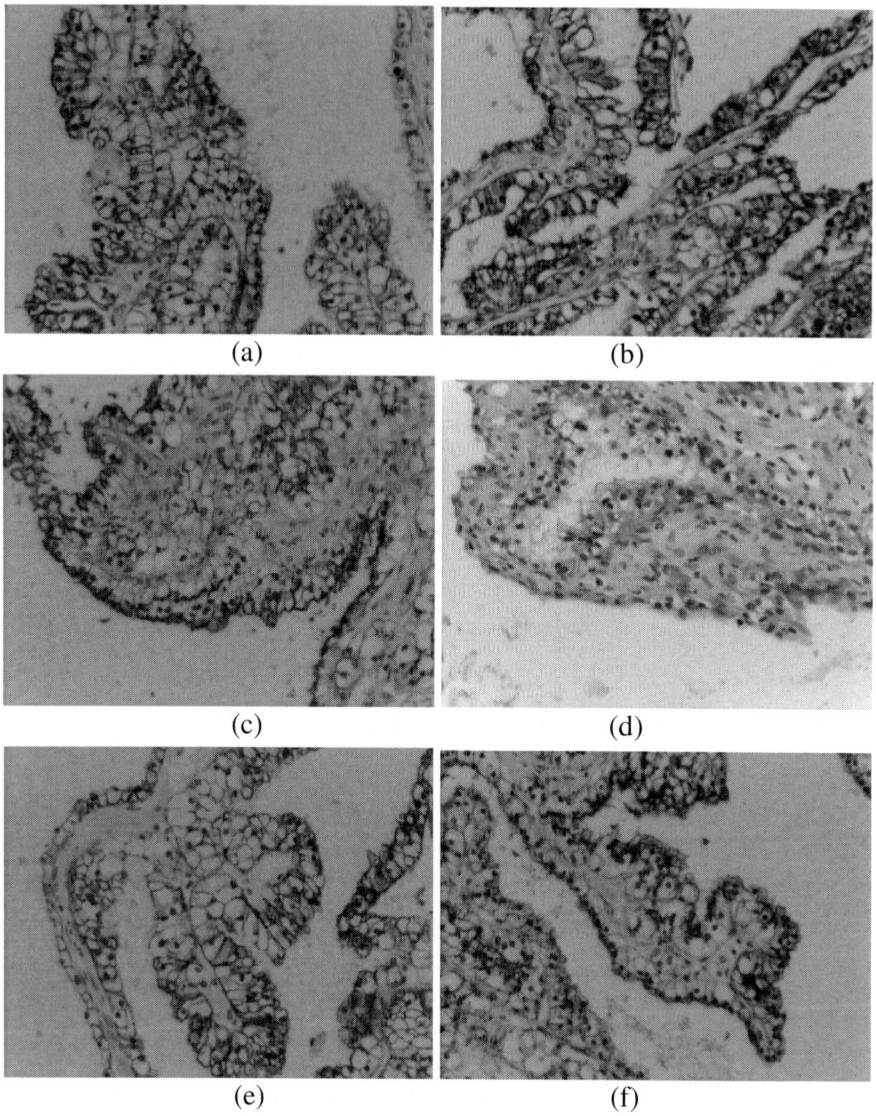

Figure 4. A. Positive staining for CK8 (400×). B. CK18 (400×). C. EMA (400×). D. HMWCK (400×). E. CK7 (400×). F. CD10 (400×).

Immunohistochemically, tumor cells usually show positive expression for cytokeratin 7, CA9, hypoxia-inducible factor-1, glucose transporter 1, HMWCK, paired box 2 (PAX2), PAX-8, and smooth muscle actin but negative for AMACR, RCC Ma, TFEB, TFE3, parvalbumin, vinculin, and cathepsin K. Most tumors are negative or focally positive for CD10 [1, 9-13]. In renal cell tumors, CK7 is often use to distinguish ccRCC and its differential diagnosis. PRCC and chromophobe RCC are positive for CK7. CCPRCC is diffusely positive in a membranous pattern, which is useful in distinguishing between conventional clear cell carcinoma CCPRCC. CA9 is a hypoxia-induced protein and predominantly positive in clear cell RCC. CA9 is expressed in cup-shaped distribution in CCPRCC. CA9 is useful in differentiating papillary RCC with clear cell changes from clear cell RCC and CCPRCC. CCRCC and CCPRCC are positive for CA9, whereas PRCC is completely negative or may be focally positive. AMACR is usually negative in CCPRCC and shows diffusely strong cytoplasmic staining in PRCC. CD10, a proximal tubule marker, is positive in conventional clear cell RCC with a membranous pattern [6, 9, 11, 14]. CD10 is variably expressed in most tumors and shows focal staining [15].

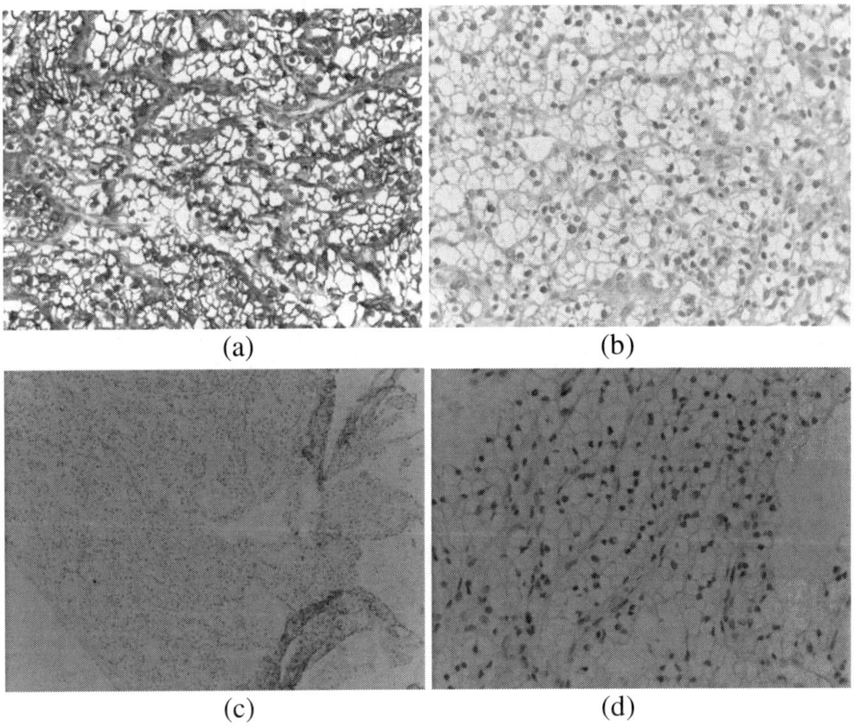

Figure 5. A. Vimentin (+) (400×). B. Negative for AMACR (400×). C and D. Ki67 < 1% (100× and 400×).

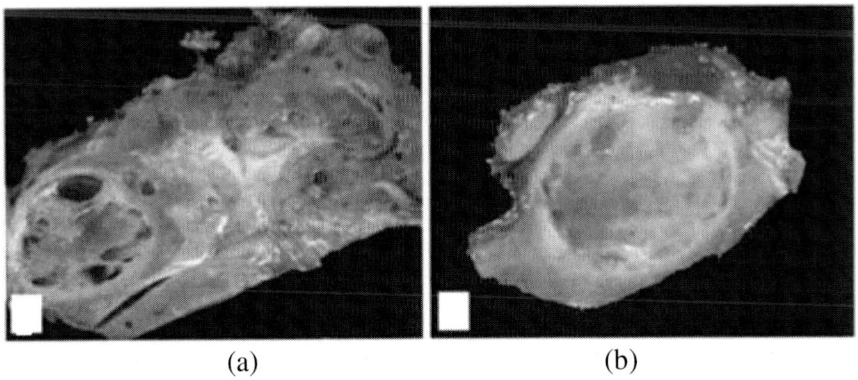

Figure 6. CCPRCC. A. Macroscopic view of the tumor showing a tan cut surface with a mixed cystic/solid appearance. B. Shown is a pink-tan cut surface with solid architecture and a thin capsule [8].

This tumor generally lacks genetic abnormalities observed in either conventional clear cell RCC or papillary RCC. CCPRCC does not harbor the chromosome 3p deletions that occur in clear cell RCC or demonstrate trisomies 7 and 17 or loss of Y in papillary RCC. Both mutations and methylation of the VHL gene promoters have not been reported to date [16-18].

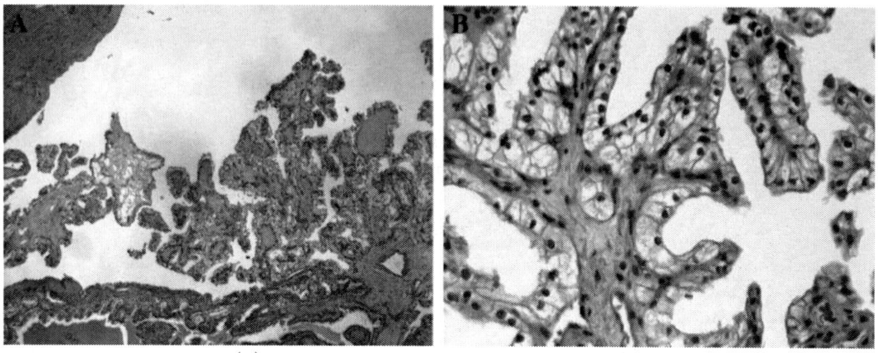

(a) (b)

Figure 7. (a) CCPRCC with papillary architecture (40×); (b) Nuclei situated away from the basement membrane (400×) [9].

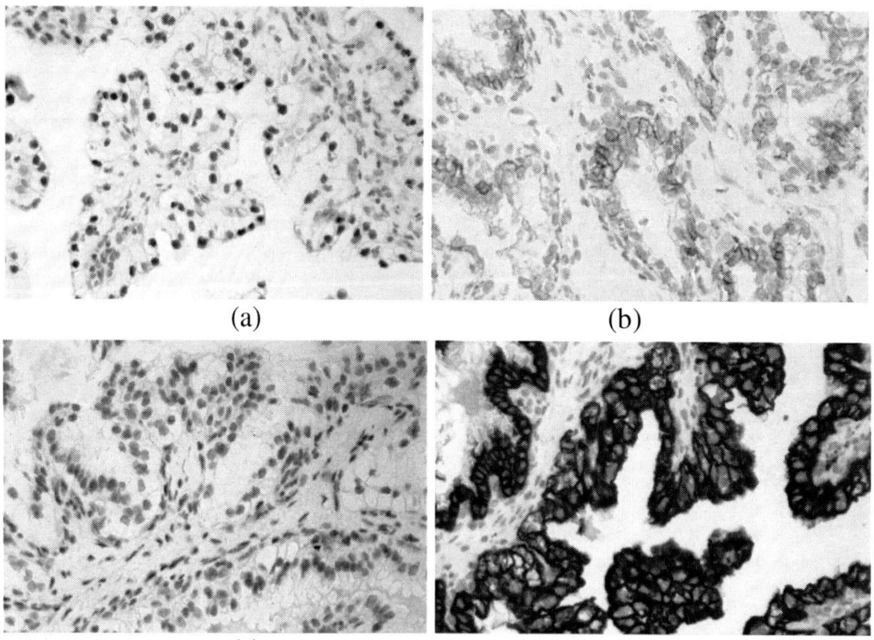

(c) (d)

Figure 8. Immunohistochemical staining results. (a) PAX-8, 400x; (b) CA9, 400x; (c) AMACR, 400x; (d) CK7, 400x [9].

The key to distinguishing between CCPRCC and CCRCC includes the pink-tan cut surface and nuclear positioning away from the basement membrane in CCPRCCand golden-yellow cut surface, mitoses, necrosis, vascular invasion, and network of small thin-walled blood vessels in CCRCC. Often, CCRCC is positive for CD10, PAX8, and CA9 and negative for CK7, with variable results for AMACR. Deletion of chromosome 3p and mutation of the VHL gene are seen in CCRCC [1, 15-19]. Macroscopically, papillary RCC is usually well circumscribed and surrounded by a fibrous pseudocapsule. Immunohistochemically, PRCC often shows positivity for CK7, HMWCK, AMACR, RCC marker, and CD10. CK7 expression is more common in type 1 PRCC than in the type 2 tumor [6, 9]. Multilocular cystic renal cell neoplasms of low malignant potential are indicated byseptated, variably sized, thin-walled cysts separated from the uninvolved renal tissue by a fibrous capsule. These clear cells show low-grade nuclear features lining the cystic spaces within afibrous septa, although solid areas are, by definition, absent. CCPRCC is strongly positive for cytokeratin 34 and betaE12 and negative for AMACR [1, 8, 9]. Multilocular cystic renal cell neoplasms of low malignant potential also show mutations of the VHL gene and deletion of chromosome 3p. Another differential diagnostic is an RCC with Xp11.2 translocations. The most distinctive and common pattern is the presence of a papillary architecture composed of clear cells with high-grade nuclei and some stromal hyaline nodules and psammomatous calcifications. The Xp11.2 translocation type shows the TFE3 protein in nuclear staining [8, 20].

Conclusion

In summary, CCPRCC is a relatively common renal cell neoplasm. Pathologists should be aware of the common incidence of this entity and its overlapping features with other RCCs to avoid the misclassification of CCPRCC as a CCRCC and vice versa. In equivocal cases, immunohistochemical stains such as CK7, AMACR, or CD10 are helpful in determining the correct diagnosis.

References

[1] Kuroda, N; Ohe, C; Kawakami, F; Mikami, S; Furuya, M; Matsuura, K; et al. (2014). Clear cell papillary renal cell carcinoma: a review. *International Journal of Clinical and Experimental Pathology,* 7: 7312-318.

[2] Gill, S; Kauffman, EC; Kandel, S; George, S; Schwaab, T; Xu B. (2016). Incidence of Clear Cell Papillary Renal Cell Carcinoma in Low-Grade Renal Cell Carcinoma Cases: A 12-Year Retrospective Clinicopathologic Study From a Single Cancer Center. *International Journal of Surgical Pathology*, 24: 207-12.

[3] Bing, Z; Tomaszewski, JE. (2011). Clear cell papillary renal cell carcinoma in the bilateral native kidneys after 2 years of renal transplantation: report of a case and review of the literature. *Case Reports in Transplantation*, 2011: 1-4.

[4] Shi, SS; Shen, Q; Xia, QY; Tu, P; Shi, QL; Zhou, XJ; et al.(2013). Clear cell papillary renal cell carcinoma: a clinicopathology study emphasizing ultrastructural features and cytogenetic heterogeneity. *International Journal of Clinical and Experimental Pathology*, 6: 2936-42.

[5] Liddell, H; Mare, A; Heywood, S; Bennet, G; Chan, HF. (2015). Clear cell papillary renal cell carcinoma: a potential mimic of conventioanal clear cell renal carcinoma on core biopsy. *Case Reports in Urology*, 1-4.

[6] Srigley, JR; Cheng, L; Grignon, DJ; Tickoo, SK. Clear cell papillary renal cell carcinoma. (2016). In: Moch H, Humphrey PA, Ulbright TM, Reuter VE editors. *World Health Organization Classification of Tumors. Pathology and genetic of tumor of the urinary system and male genital organ.* Lyon: IARC Press; 40-1.

[7] Park, JH; Lee, C; Suh, JH; Moon, KC. (2012). Clear cell papillary renal cell carcinoma: a report of 15 cases including three cases of concurrent other-type renal cell carcinomas. *Korean Journal of Pathology,* 46: 541-47.

[8] Alexiev, BA; Drachenberg, CB. (2014). Clear cell papillary renal cell carcinoma: Incidence, morphological features, immunohistochemical profile, and biologic behavior: A single institution study. *Pathology-Research and Practice*, 210: 234-41.

[9] Pramick, M; Zobier, A; Bing, Z. (2013). Useful immunohistochemical panel for differentiating clear cell papillary renal cell carcinoma from its mimics. *Annals of Diagnostic Pathology*, 17: 437-40.

[10] Zhou, H; Zheng, S; Troung, LD; Ro, JY; Alaya, AG; Shen, SS. (2014). Clear cell papillary renal cell carcinoma is the fourth most common histologic type of renal cell carcinoma in 290 consecutive nephrectomies for renal cell carcinoma. *Human Pathology*, 45: 59-64.

[11] Williamson, SR; Eble, JN; Cheng, L; Grignon, DJ. (2013). Clear cell papillary renal cell carcinoma differential diagnosis and extended immunohistochemical profile. *Modern Pathology*, 26: 697-708.

[12] Alexiev, BA. (2012). Clear cell papillary renal cell carcinoma: A novel category of renal cell neoplasm. *Journal of Cytology and Histology*,3: 1-2.

[13] Yan, WX; Cao, WR; Zhao, J; Zhang, W; Wang, XL; Yuan, Q; et al. (2015). Original Article Clear cell papillary renal cell carcinoma: a clinicopathologic analysis of 6 cases. *Internatinal Journal of Clinical and Experimental Pathology*, 8: 4595-99.

[14] Deml, KF; Schildhaus, HU; Comperat, E; Teichman, AV; Storz, M; Schraml, P; et al. (2015). Clear cell papillary renal cell carcinoma and renal angiomyo adenomatous tumor-two variants of a morphologic, immunohistochemical and genetic distinct entity of renal cell carcinoma. *The American Journal of Surgical Pathology,* 39: 889-901.

[15] Rao, P; Monzon, F; Jonasch, E; Matin, SF; Tamboli, P. (2014). Clear cell papillary renal cell carcinoma in patients with von Hippel-Lindau syndrome—clinicopathological features and comparative genomic analysis of 3 cases. *Human Pathology*, 45: 1966-72.

[16] Rohan, SM; Xiao, Y; Liang, Y; Dudas, ME; Al-Ahmadie, HA; Fine, SW; et al. (2011). Clear-cell papillary renal cell carcinoma: molecular and immunohistochemical analysis with emphasis on the von Hippel–Lindau gene and hypoxia-inducible factor pathway-related proteins. *Modern Pathology*, 24: 1207-20.

[17] Shazad, H; Kehar, SI; Ali, S; Tariq, N. (2014). Expression of Von Hippel-Lindau (VHL) gene mutation in diagnosed cases of renal cell carcinoma. *Pakistan Journal of Medical Sciences*, 30: 880-5.

[18] Petersson, F; Grossmann, P; Hora, M; Sperga, M; Montiel, DP; Martinek, P; et al. (2013). Renal cell carcinoma with areas mimicking renal angiomy oadenomatous tumor/clear cell papillary renal cell carcinoma. *Human Pathology*, 44: 1412-20.

[19] Moch, H; Bonsib, SM; Delahunt, B; Eble, J; Egevad, L; Grignon, DJ; et al. (2016). Clear cell renal cell carcinoma. In: Moch H, Humphrey PA, Ulbright TM, Reuter VE editors. *World Health Organization Classification of Tumors. Pathology and genetic of tumor of the urinary system and male genital organ*. Lyon: IARC Press; 18-21.

[20] Parihar, A; Tickoo, SK; Kumar, S; Arora, VK. (2015). Xp11 translocation renal cell carcinoma morphologically mimicking clear cell-papillary renal cell carcinoma in an Adult Patient: Report of a Case Expanding the morphologic Spectrum of Xp11 Translocation Renal Cell Carcinomas. *International Journal of Surgical Pathology*, 23: 234-7.

In: Case Reports in Surgery
Editors: Ahmad Jabir Rahyussalim et al.
ISBN: 978-1-53616-582-1

Chapter 27

RARE CASE OF MYELOLIPOMATOUS METAPLASIA WITHIN AN ADRENOCORTICAL ADENOMA

Monik Ediana Miranda[1,*], Maria Francisca Ham[2], Agnes Stephanie Harahap[2], and Benyamin Makes[2]

[1]Anatomical Pathology Residency Program, Faculty of Medicine, Universitas Indonesia, Jakarta, Indonesia

[2] Department of Anatomical Pathology, Faculty of Medicine, Universitas Indonesia, Jakarta, Indonesia

ABSTRACT

The actual incidence of adrenocortical adenoma (ACA) remains unknown. Data obtained from 2011 to 2015 in Cipto Mangunkusumo Hospital have revealed that only 14 patients presented with adrenal neoplasms; of these patients, 11 were diagnosed with ACA. Myelolipomatous metaplasia is characterized by the presence of foci of hematopoietic cells comprising erythroids, myeloids, and megakaryocytes within a tumor. This metaplasia is an extremely rare finding in adrenal tumors, particularly in ACA. The pathogenesis of myelolipomatous metaplasia remains unclear. Herein, we report the case of a 40-year-old man who presented with a mass in his abdomen. Without any contributory signs and symptoms, the size of the mass increased within 4 months of diagnosis. Computed tomography of the abdomen showed a heterogenous mass in the right suprarenal region with fine demarcated outlines, and the result was indicative of an adrenal carcinoma. The patient underwent adrenalectomy. Based on hematoxylin &eosin (H&E) staining and immunohistochemical analysis, the mass was confirmed to be a non-functional ACA with a myelolipomatous metaplasia. The case was uneventful, and the patient was then discharged with recommendation of an annual follow-up. ACA is a rare type of tumor. Myelolipomatous metaplasia found within an adenoma of the adrenocortex is an even more uncommon finding. The correlation between clinical, radiological, and pathological

* Corresponding Author's E-mail: doktermonik@gmail.com.

examination results must be assessed for a more accurate diagnosis. The combination of H&E staining and immunostaining is helpful in facilitating the diagnosis of adrenocortical tumors and metaplasia within the tumor.

Keywords: Adenoma; adrenal; myelolipomatous metaplasia

INTRODUCTION

The adrenal gland is a 4-g organ that lies in the suprarenal region. It can be divided into two regions (cortex and medulla). Each zone secretes different hormones and has its own functions. Adrenal neoplasm is defined as a neoplasm arising from the adrenal cells. A tumor arising from the cortical area of the adrenal gland is basically classified as follows: benign adrenocortical adenoma (ACA) and malignant adrenocortical carcinoma (ACC) if invasion is observed [1].

Nodules that are suspected as neoplasms are commonly identified in autopsies. Some are discovered incidentally during annual check-up or imaging screening for other causes. These nodules are referred to as adrenal incidentaloma. Approximately 80% of adrenal incidentaloma is benign and does not secrete hormones (non-functional). Symptoms may be observed depending on tumor location and whether they are functional or not [1, 2].

The actual incidence of ACA is unknown. Data obtained from 2011 to 2015 in Cipto Mangunkusumo Hospital have reported that only 14 patients presented with adrenal neoplasm; of these patients, 11 were diagnosed with ACA, which is typically a unilateral, solitary, and benign neoplasm. With the widespread use of computed tomography (CT) scan of the abdomen, the diagnosis of such condition is increasing. Some studies have reported that the incidence of non-functional adrenal tumors varies between 1.4% and 8.7% based on autopsy studies. The prevalence of adrenal incidentaloma increases with age, and no differences were observed in terms of prevalence based on race and sex [2, 3].

Different types of metaplasia can develop within the adrenal gland. Occasionally, lipomatous foci or bone cell metaplasia can be found. Myelolipomatous metaplasia within an ACA is an extremely rare cause of adrenal incidentaloma. In 2008, only 17 cases of such condition were reported in the English and Japanese literature. The present study aimed to present a rare case of myelolipomatous metaplasia within an ACA and to establish an effective diagnostic approach from the view point of a pathologist if such condition will be encountered in the future [4].

CASE REPORT

A 40-year-old Indonesian male patient was referred by his office physician to the internal medicine department of a hospital in Jakarta in October 2014. The patient was required to undergo an annual check-up resulting in the incidental finding of a large mass in his abdomen. The patient's family and past medical history was not significant. He was free of symptoms, such as palpitation, weight loss, and hypertension. His electrocardiograph and chest radiograph results showed no abnormalities. The general internist performed ultrasonographic examination and found a mass in the abdomen (Figure 1). A hyperechoic lesion was observed in the right lobus of his liver. The patient was suspected to have a hepatic cellular carcinoma, and the differential diagnosis were hemangioma or a focal fatty infiltration. The internist then recommended whole abdominal contrast-enhanced CT scan and laboratory work up.

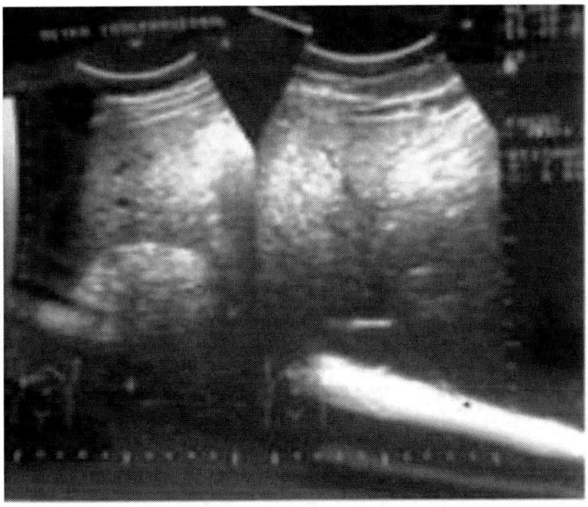

(a)

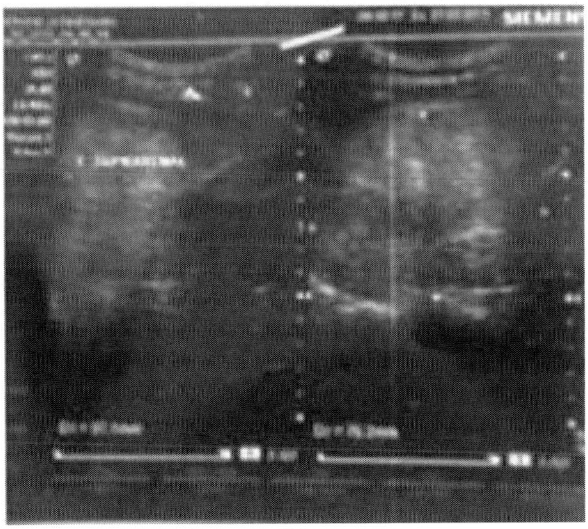

(b)

Figure 1. (a) Result from the first ultrasonography showed a 7×6 cm^2 mass that was suspected to originate from the liver in October 2014. (b) Image from the second ultrasonography in February 2015 showed that the size of the mass increased (9×7 cm^2). After the examination, the tumor was suspected to originate from the suprarenal region.

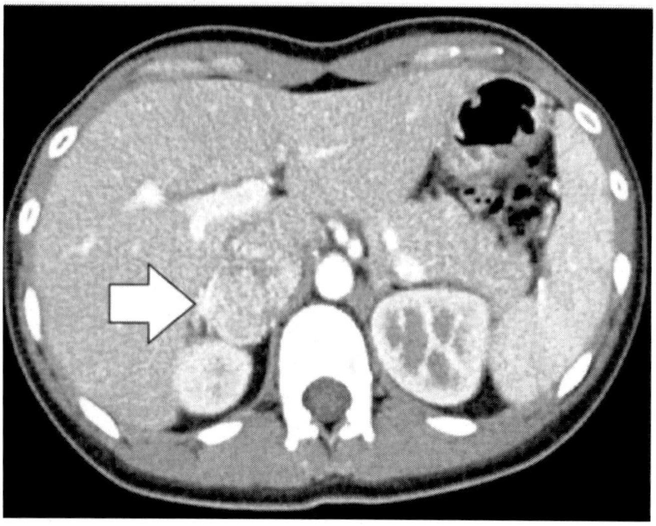

Figure 2. Result of the computed tomography scan revealed a hypervascular mass in the right adrenal gland with early washout enhancing pattern.

The patient had a follow-up consultation a week later with the CT scan and laboratory test results. He was non-reactive for hepatitis C and had normal blood glucose level (fasting glucose level of 85 mg/dL and 2-hour post prandial level of 109 mg/dL), and the following tumor markers were assessed: alpha-fetoprotein (AFP), Ca 19.9, and carcinoembryonic antigen (CEA). The CEA and AFP levels of the patient were within normal limits (CEA: 2.71 [normal value: ≤ 3 ng/mL] and AFP: 2.13 [range: 0–40] ng/mL). The Ca 19.9 level was elevated, which was twice than the normal limit (83.79 U/mL [normal value: < 37 U/mL]). The CT scan result showed a heterogenous mass in the right suprarenal region with fine demarcated outlines, and such result indicated an adrenal carcinoma. The differential diagnosis were changed to adrenal adenoma or adrenal hemorrhage (Figure 2). The patient was then referred to an endocrinologist.

The patient sought consultation from an endocrinologist 4 months after, and the size of the mass increased based on ultrasonographic examination (Figure 1). In February 2015, his body mass index was above the normal limit (26 kg/m^2). His blood pressure was slightly elevated (138/91mmHg). However, the patient's heart rate, respiratory rate, and temperature were normal (99 beats/minute, 17 cycles/minute, and 36.5°C, respectively). The endocrinologist requested for routine blood test, liver function test, uric acid, glucose, bleeding time and electrolyte. All of his laboratory test came back with normal results.

Based on this finding, the endocrinologist referred the patient to a urologist. Three days after, the urologist performed adrenalectomy. The right adrenal gland was resected and was sent to the Department of Anatomycal Pathology at the same hospital. The specimen measured 11.0×10.0×7.0 cm^3, and was a round capsulated mass with fine demarcated outlines, most of which appeared yellow with hemorrhagic areas on the cut surface. Small brown-black lesions that vary in size (0.4–3.0×2.0×2.0 cm^3) were observed (Figure 3).

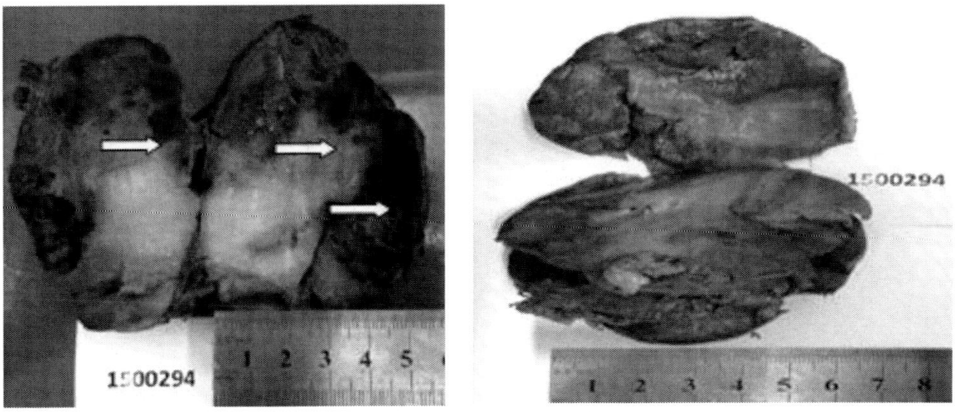

(a) (b)

Figure 3. Macroscopic view of the resected right adrenal gland. (a) View from the longitudinal section showing yellow with brown-black lesions on the cut surface (white arrow showing the brown-black lesion). (b) Posterior view of the image showing yellow-to-brown surface with an intact capsule.

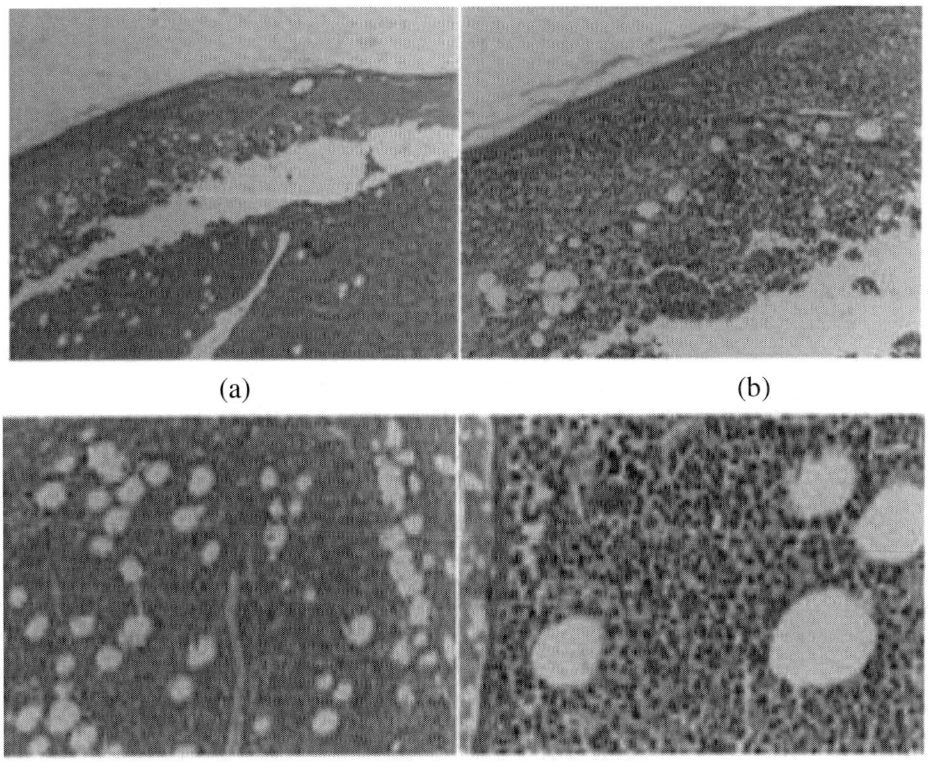

(a) (b)

(c) (d)

Figure 4. Photomicrograph. (a) Finely demarcated mass with well-developed fibrous capsule indicative of an adrenocortical adenoma (Hematoxylin & Eosin staining, 40x). (b). Higher magnification of the adrenocortical adenoma (Hematoxylin & Eosin staining, 100x). (c) Area from the brown-black lesion showing fat tissues and hematopoietic cells (Hematoxylin & Eosin staining, 100×). (d) Higher magnification of foci of the myelolipoma (Hematoxylin & Eosin staining, 400×).

Histologically, the suprarenal tumor showed a mass that was demarcated with a well-developed fibrous capsule. On the peripheral side, there were ACA and brown-black lesions with fat tissues and widely hemorrhagic areas, hematopoietic cells, fibrotic areas, and brownish pigmentations. No signs of malignancies were observed (Figure 4). Immunohistochemistry staining was conducted at the Ciptomangunkusumo Hospital, and results showed positivity for inhibin, Wilms tumor 1 (WT1), neuron-specific enolase (NSE), vimentin, synaptophysin, Melan-A, calretinin, AE 1/3, and chromogranin as well as low positivity for Ki-67 in the area with suspected ACA. The brown-black lesions tested positive for myeloperoxidase (MPO), cluster of differentiation (CD) 117, CD 3, CD 20, CD 15, multiple myeloma (MUM) 1, CD 68, and CD 138 and negative for CD 34 (Figure 5). Hence, the final diagnosis was ACA with myelolipomatous metaplasia.

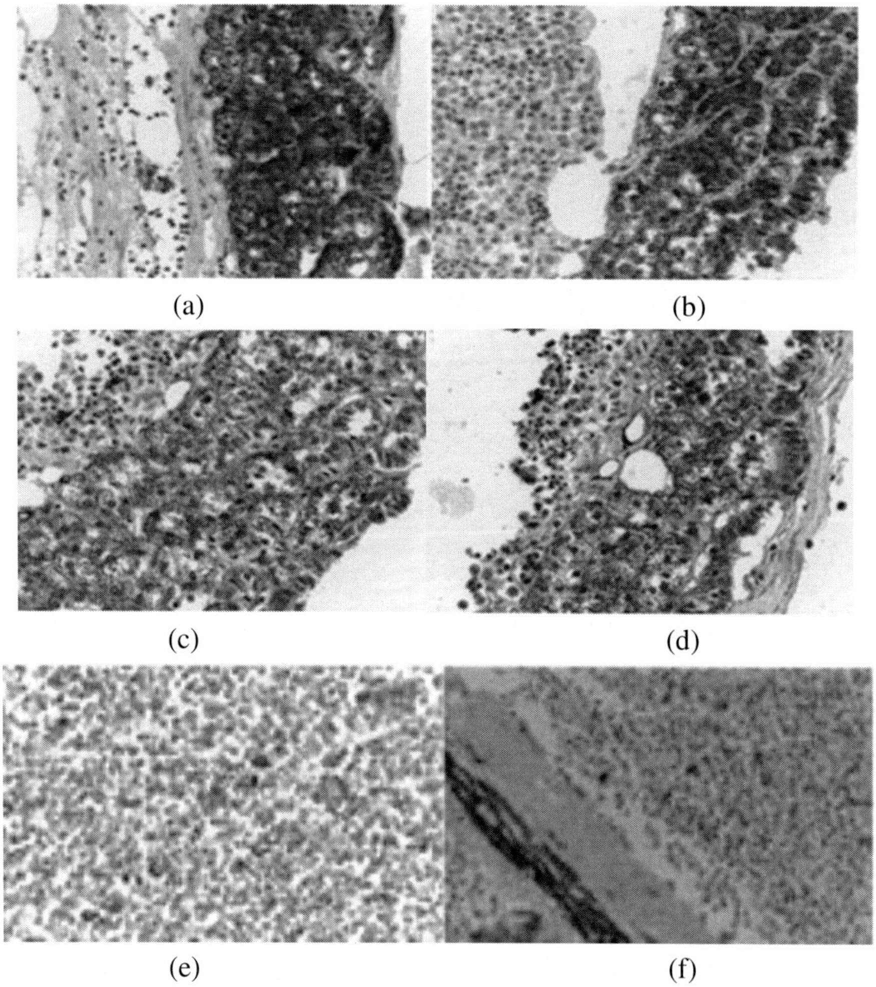

(a) (b) (c) (d) (e) (f)

Figure 5. Immunohistochemistry staining results showing cytoplasmic and cell membrane positivity. (a) Inhibin (400×), (b) NSE (400×), (c) WT1 (400×) and (d) S100 (400×). The brown-black lesions showed (e) cytoplasmic positivity for MPO (400×) and (f) negativity for CD 34 (400×).

DISCUSSION

ACA is a rare type of tumor. Myelolipoma within an ACA is even an extremely rare condition. In 2008, only 17 cases of such condition were reported globally. Thirteen of the patients were women with a mean age of 45 years, and the youngest patient was aged 16 years. In general, ACAs have a predilection for woman, and it can occur in any age groups. Moreover, its incidence is equally distributed in both glands. In this case, a 40-year-old male patient presented with right adrenal lesion. No clinical findings, such as hypertension, hypokalemia, or hormonal imbalance, were observed. Hence, it was suspected as benign and non-functional adrenal lesion [4-9].

The widespread use of imaging has resulted in the increasing diagnosis of adrenal incidentaloma, which is an incidental mass. The World Health Organization defined this lesion as an adrenal mass that is identified serendipitously via radiologic examination in the absence of symptoms and clinical findings indicative of adrenal diseases. Imaging procedures can help in the localization of adrenal cortical adenoma. ACAs account for most adrenal masses incidentally found on CT scan in patients with indications other than suspected adrenal pathology and are typically characterized by a well-defined, round homogenous mass. The primary goal of imaging is to distinguish adrenal adenoma, adrenal carcinoma, pheochromocytoma, and metastatic lesions. The lesion in the abdomen of the patient incidentally found. First, the tumor was suspected as a hepatic carcinoma. However, based on CT scan, which showed a heterogeneous with fine demarcated mass located in the suprarenal region, the physician then suspected the lesion as ACA [1, 5, 6, 10-14].

In the present study, the initial size of the mass was 7x6 cm. After 4 months, the size increased to 9 × 7 cm. The urologist then performed adrenalectomy. According to the American Association of Clinical Endocrinologists and American Association of Endocrine Surgeons (AACE/AAES) medical guidelines for the management of adrenal incidentalomas published in 2009, adrenalectomy after hormonal evaluation is the treatment option for a suspected malignant or indeterminate mass that is ≥ 4 cm on CT scan (Figure 6). Hormonal evaluation was not indicated in this patient due to the lack of obvious clinical signs [13, 15-17].

From the view of a pathologist, a differential diagnosis of a solid adrenal lesion include commonly diagnosed lesions (such as adenoma and pheochromocytoma) and uncommon lesions (including oncocytoma, ganglioneuroma, adrenal/peri-adrenal schwannoma, lipoma, and mature teratoma). We should also accurately differentiate benign lesions from adrenocortical carcinomas due to the fact that the prognosis, follow-up, and therapeutic strategy for ACC are different from those of a benign tumor [2, 14, 18].

The Weiss system is a method widely used to distinguish ACC from benign cortical tumor, including adenoma. The system was established in 1984 and included the following nine-point histopathological criteria: high nuclear grade, more than 5 mitoses per 50 high-power fields, atypical mitotic figures, with < 25% of tumor cells are clear cells, diffuse architecture (more than 33% of tumors), necrosis, venous invasion (smooth muscle in the wall), sinusoidal invasion (no smooth muscle in the wall), and capsular invasion. The presence of three or more criteria highly correlates with subsequent malignant behavior. In this case, only two criteria were observed, and < 25% of tumor cells were clear cells. Moreover, there were 10 mitoses per 50 high-power fields. Thus, based on the Weiss criteria, the adrenal lesion may be a benign lesion [1, 2, 6, 12].

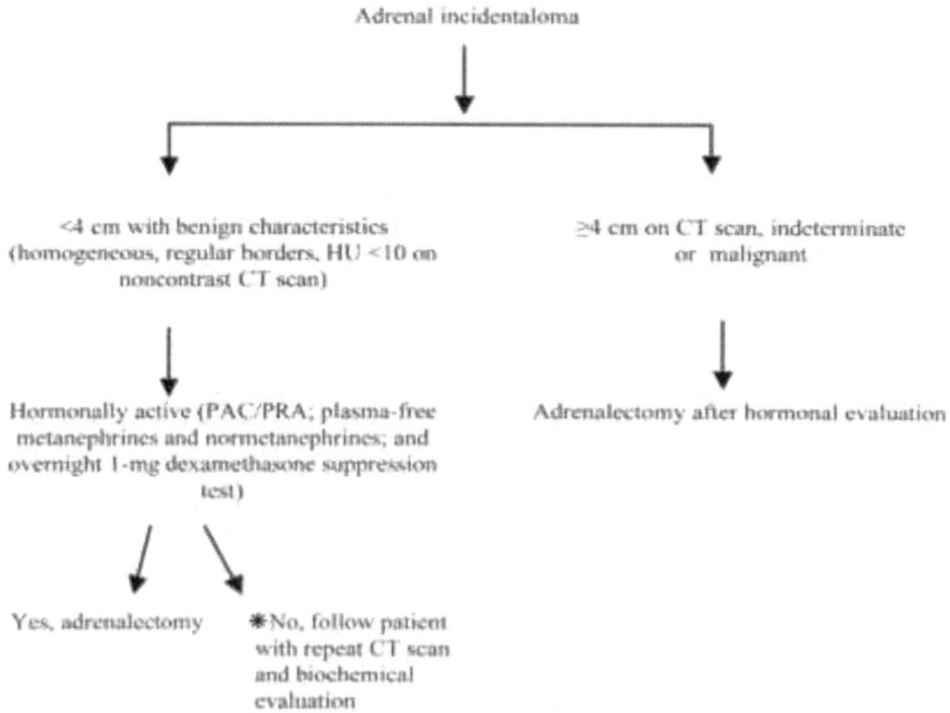

Figure 6. Algorithm for the evaluation and management of an adrenal incidentaloma according to the guidelines of the American Association of Clinical Endocrinologists and American Association of Endocrine Surgeons [13].

Most ACAs are well-circumscribed intra-adrenal tumors, and some are encapsulated. Hemorrhage and necrosis are rarely observed. They can be tan-to -brown or bright yellow in appearance. Gross specimens obtained from oncocytoma are well-circumscribed adrenocortical lesions with dark tan-to-mahogany brown appearance (which is similar to other oncocytic lesions). They are large in size from 3 to 17 cm. Ganglioneuroma is an encapsulated mass with a solid, homogenous gray-white cut surface. Their size can reach up to 18 cm, and their consistency may range from gelatinous to solid. An adrenal/peri-adrenal schwannoma often appears as a solitary, well-circumscribed tumor enveloped in a fibrous capsule with a solid firm white-tan and homogenous cut surface that may contain cystic changes or hemorrhagic regions. Lipoma appears as a well-circumscribed tumor with a homogenous yellowish cut surface indicative of fat tissues. A mature teratoma showed a neoplasm indicating a mature tissue from the endoderm, mesoderm, and/or ectoderm. Lesions may be malignant if they had a coarsely lobulated appearance, with soft, bulging nodules ranging from yellow- orange to tan in color. A high number of areas with necrosis and hemorrhage are commonly observed. Examination of the gross specimen in this case revealed a rounded capsulated mass with fine demarcated outline, most of which appeared yellow with some of hemorrhagic areas and black-to-brown lesions on the cut surface. However, no necrosis was found. These findings were indicative of benign lesions, most probably an adrenal adenoma [1,6,19].

The definitive diagnosis of ganglioneuroma and schwannoma can be obtained via microscopic examination. Ganglioneuroma showed an area of Schwann cells with wavy dark nuclei and inconspicuous nucleoli with scant spindled cytoplasm, admixed with mature ganglion cells and eosinophilic cytoplasm, large vesicular nuclei, and prominent nucleoli. Oncocytomas have mitochondriac-rich cells with abundant compact eosinophilic cytoplasm that is finely granular. Adrenal/peri-adrenal schwannomas are microscopically identical to schwannomas found at any other anatomical sites. Spindle cells with alternating areas of compact hypercellularity with irregular streams and elongated spindle cells (Antoni type A) and of loosely-textured hypocellularity with cystic spaces (Antoni type B). In addition, Verocay bodies between the regions of nuclear palisades and thick walled hyalinized blood vessels may be observed. Mature teratomas are also microscopically identical with teratoma found elsewhere. The diagnosis of mature teratoma can be made if there is a minimum of two mature components observed from the endoderm (respiratory or digestive tract), mesoderm (fat tissue), or ectodermal (skin, bones, and chondrous tissue) without any immature component. ACAs consist of clear cells with abundant intracytoplasmic lipid droplets and compact cells with lipid sparse eosinophilic cytoplasm. These cells form cords and/or nests with relatively abundant vasculature or sinusoidal structures. The microscopic findings from this case were a fine demarcated lesion with mixture of clear and compact cells with eosinophilic cytoplasm indicative of adrenal adenoma and focal areas with myeloid and lipid component indicative of a myelolipoma metaplasia [1, 6, 7, 16, 19].

For further confirmation of the diagnosis of solid adrenal lesions, immune-histochemistry examination was conducted. According to Dabbs et al., stainings for markers, such as inhibin A, WT1, and AE 1/3, can be used to confirm of the lesion originated from the adrenal tissues. To distinguish a benign from a malignant lesion, Jia *et al.* have recommended NSE staining as it shows positivity in the cell membrane and cytoplasm. Staining was also performed to confirm that the brown-black lesions observed in the macroscopic examination were myeloid component. The stainings were positive for MPO, focal positive for CD 117, CD 3, CD 20, CD 15, multiple myeloma (MUM) 1, CD 68, and CD 138, and negative for CD 34. The results are depicted in Table 1 [7, 8, 17].

Table 1. Summary of the immunohistochemical staining confirming the adrenal tissues in this case and comparing them with the reference (+: positive, −: negative, n/a: not available) [7, 9-13]

Immunohistochemistry	ACA	Schwannoma	Ganglio-neuroma	ACC	Present case
S-100	+	+	+	+	+
Synaptophysin	+	−	+	+	+
CD-56	+	−	+	+	+
NSE	+	−	+	−	+
Laminin	−	+	−	−	n/a
Collagen IV	−	+	−	−	n/a
Desmin	−	−	−	−	n/a
CD-34	−	−	−	−	−
Keratin	+	−	−	+	+
Actin	+	−	−	+	n/a
Calretinin	+	−	−	+	+
Inhibin	+	−	−	+	+
Bcl-2	+	−	−	−	n/a
Melan-A	+	−	−	+	+

The adrenal gland may present with different metaplasias that can be observed during microscopic examination. Occasionally, we can find lipomatous foci or bone cell metaplasia and even ovarian thecal metaplasia inside the glands. In this case, we found foci of myelolipomatous metaplasia within ACA. The causes of such metaplasia are not fully elucidated. Currently, the most accepted theories were embolization of the bone marrow, embryonic primitive mesenchymal cells, dysregulation of hematopoietic cell apoptosis, and adrenal response to stimuli, such as necrosis, infections, andstress [4, 20, 21].

The overall prognosis of surgically resected ACAs is good. Jia et al., have reported no recurrences and metastases in any of the benign cases. The incidence rate of a benign adenoma developing into an ACC is not well known. However, such phenomenon is extremely rare [2, 11, 13].

Conclusion

A 40-year-old male patient presented with an incidental mass in the abdomen. The size of the mass increased within 4 months of diagnosis. The patient was then diagnosed with ACA with myelolipomatous metaplasia by Hematoxylin & Eosin staining combined with immunohistochemistry staining. ACA is a rare type of tumor. Myelolipomatous metaplasia within an adenoma of the adrenocortex is an extremely rare finding. The correlation between clinical, radiological, and pathological examination results must be assessed to obtain a more accurate diagnosis. The pathogenesis of myelolipomatous metaplasia is still not fully elucidated.

ACKNOWLEDGMENTS

We would like to thank Evelina Kodrat, MD as pathologist who discovered the case and permitted the case to be reported. Nonetheless, thank you for my seniors and beloved fellow residents for the abundant support and encouragement.

REFERENCES

[1] Lack, E.E.(2007). *Tumors of the adrenal glands and extraadrenal paraganglia*. 3rd series. Washington DC: Armed Forces Institute of Pathology. 1-27.

[2] Lloyd, R.V., Tischer, A.S., Kimura, N., McNicol, A.M.&Young Jr, W.F. Tumours of adrenal gland. In: DeLellis RA, Lloyd RV, Heitz PU, Eng C, editors. *Pathology and Genetics of Tumoursof Endocrine Organs*. Lyon: IARC Press; 2004; 136-146.

[3] Ridho, F. E., Adam, F. M.&Adam, J. M. (2009). Adrenal incidentaloma. *Acta Med. Indones.*, 41 (2): 87-97.

[4] Ong, K., Tan, K.B.&Putti, T.C. (2007). Myelolipoma within a non-functional adrenal cortical adenoma. *Singapore Med. J.*, 48 (7):e200-e202.

[5] Hironobu, S., Yasuhiro, N., Takuya, M., &Takashi, S. Adrenal cortex. In: Lloyd RV, editor. *Endocrine Pathology Differential Diagnosis and Molecular Advances.* Rochester: Springer; 2010; 261-279.

[6] Kanthan, R., Senger, J. L.&Kanthan, S. (2012). Three uncommon adrenal incidentalomas: a 13 year surgical pathology review. *World J. Surg. Oncol.*, 10 (1):1-11.

[7] Wang, C., Sun, Y., Wu, H., Zhao, D., Chen, J. (2014). Distinguishing adrenal cortical carcinomas and adenomas: a study of clinicopathological features and biomarkers. *Histopathology*, 64 (4): 567-576.

[8] Zhang, P. J., Genega, E. M., Tomaszewski, J. E., Pasha, T. L.&LiVolsi, V. A. (2003). The role of calretinin, inhibin, melan-A, BCL-2, and C-kit in differentiating adrenal cortical and medullary tumors: an immunohistochemistry study. *Mod. Pathol.*,16 (6): 591-597.

[9] Delellis, R. A., Shin, S. J.&Treaba, D. O.Immunohistology of endocrine tumors. In: Dabbs DJ. Editor. *Diagnostic Immunohistochemistry Theranosticand Genomic Applications*. 3rd edition. Philadelphia, PA: Saunders-Elsevier; 2011; 291-329.

[10] Lack, E. E. Tumors of the adrenal glands and extraadrenal paraganglia AFIP Atlas of tumor pathology. 4th series. Washington DC : *Amer. Registry of Pathology*: 2007; 91-106.

[11] Jia, A. H., Du, H. Q., Fan, M. H., Li, Y. H., Xu, J. L., Niu, G. F., Niu, G.F., Bai, J., Zhang, G.Z. &Ren, Y.B. (2015).Clinical and pathological analysis of 116 cases of adult adrenal cortical adenoma and literature review. *Onco Targets and Ther*, 8:1251-1257.

[12] Lu, H. S., Gan, M. F., Chen, H. S.,& Huang, S. Q. (2008). Adrenal myelolipoma within myxoid cortical adenoma associated with Conn's syndrome. *J. Zheijang University Sci.* B,9 (6):500-505.

[13] Zeiger, M. A., Thompson, G. B., Duh, Q. Y., Hamrahian, A. H., Angelos, P., Elaraj, D, Fishman, E.&Kharlip, J.(2009).American association of clinical endocrinologists and American association of endocrine surgeons medical guidelines for the management of adrenal incidentalomas. *Endocr. Pract.*, 15 (Suppl 1):S1-S20.

[14] Ctvrlik, F., Koranda, P.&Tichy, T. (2014). Adrenal disease: a clinical update and overview of imaging. A review. *Biomed. Pap. Med. Fac. Univ. Palacky Olomouc Czech Repub.*, 158 (1):23-34.

[15] Willatt, J., Chong, S., Ruma, J. A. & Kuriakose, J. (2015). Incidental adrenal nodules and masses: the imaging approach. *Int. J. Endocrinol.*, 2015:1-6.

[16] Moreira, S. G. & Pow-sang, J. M. (2002). Evaluation and management of adrenal masses. *Cancer Control*,9 (4):326-334.

[17] Anagnostis, P., Karagiannis, A., Tziomalos, K., Kakafika, A. I., Athyros, V. G. &Mikhailidis, D. P. (2009) Adrenal incidentaloma: a diagnostic challenge. *Hormones*, 8 (3):163-184.

[18] Bialas, M., Okon, K.&Stachura, J. (2008). Primary adrenal tumor- a 16 year experience in a single institution. *Pol. J. Pathol.*, 59:101-106.

[19] Lloyd, R. V. (2011). Adrenal cortical tumors, pheochromocytomas and paragangliomas. *Mod. Pathol.*, 24 (Suppl 2): S58-S65.

[20] Bishop, E., Eble, J. N., Cheng, L., Wang, M., Chase, D. R., Orazi, A.&O'malley, D. P. (2006). Adrenal myelolipomas show non random X-chromosome inactivation in hematopoietic elements and fat: support for a clonal origin of myelolipomas. *Am. J. Surg. Pathol.*, 30 (7):838-843.

[21] Seyle, H. & Stone, H. (1950).Hormonally induced transformation of the adrenal into myeloid tissue. *Am. J. Pathol.*, 23 (2):211-233.

In: Case Reports in Surgery
Editors: Ahmad Jabir Rahyussalim et al.
ISBN: 978-1-53616-582-1

Chapter 28

CHRONIC MYELOID LEUKEMIA IN A BCR-ABL1-POSITIVE PATIENT WITH PANCYTOPENIA AND EXCESSIVE FIBROSIS

Dian Sari Oethia Vathonati[1]
and Agnes Stephanie Harahap[2,*]
[1]Anatomical Pathology Residency Program, Faculty of Medicine,
Universitas Indonesia, Jakarta, Indonesia
[2]Department of Anatomical Pathology, Faculty of Medicine,
Universitas Indonesia, Jakarta, Indonesia

ABSTRACT

Chronic myeloid leukemia (CML) is a myeloproliferative neoplasm of the hematopoietic stem cells, in which granulocytes are the major proliferative component. It is characterized by the chromosomal translocation between chromosomes 9 and 22, resulting in the *BCR-ABL1* fusion gene. *The clinical manifestation*, bone marrow features, and laboratory test results *at the time of diagnosis vary among reported patients and depend on* the phase of CML. Approximately 50% of newly diagnosed cases are asymptomatic and discovered when an abnormal white blood cell count is detected. In some cases, the bone marrow shows variable stages of fibrosis, whereas severe reticulin fibrosis is rarely observed. In this article, we present a patient with uncommon initial features of CML (i.e., pancytopenia, severe bone marrow fibrosis, and the absence of splenomegaly). Histopathological examination of the bone marrow revealed a hypercellular bone marrow with a normal myeloid to erythroid ratio showing myeloid maturation into segmented neutrophils. The number of megakaryocytes with atypical nuclei was increased, forming a cluster. Reticulin staining showed that fibers were

* Corresponding Author's E-mail: agnharahap@gmail.com.

increased diffusely and densely with extensive intersections. This increasing number of megakaryocytes and excessive fibrosis resembles primary myelofibrosis. The presence of the *BCR-ABL1* fusion gene confirmed the *diagnosis* of CML. The aim of this report is to share the experience of diagnosing a case of CML with a rare initial clinical course and excessive fibrosis of the bone marrow.

Keywords: *BCR-ABL1*-positive, chronic myeloid leukemia, pancytopenia

INTRODUCTION

Chronic myeloid leukemia (CML) is an acquired myeloproliferative neoplasm, in which granulocytes are the major proliferative component. It arises in hematopoietic stem cells and is associated with chromosomal translocation between the ABL1 gene of chromosome 9 and the BCR gene of chromosome 22. This results in the formation of the Philadelphia (Ph) chromosome [1]. The translocation leads to the production of an abnormal tyrosine kinase enzyme, which causes excessive proliferation and reduced apoptosis in myeloid cells [2, 3]. Notably, the etiology of CML is unknown in most cases. There is an assumption that high-dose ionizing radiation may be linked to an increased incidence of CML. However, most CML cases reported thus far were not exposed to radiation [4].

The incidence of CML varies among countries, ranging from 0.4/100,000 individuals in non-Western countries to 1.75/100,000 individuals in the USA [4]. It can occur in all age groups; however, it is predominantly reported in middle and old age, accounting for 20% of adult leukemia cases [5]. The median age at the time of diagnosis is 57-60 years CML is very rare in children. The male to female ratio is 1.2-1.7:1 [4]. From 2013 to 2016, a total of 41 cases of CML were diagnosed in the Anatomical Pathology Department of the Faculty of Medicine of Cipto Mangunkusumo Hospital, Jakarta, Indonesia. All patients were adults, with most cases reported in fifth decade of life.

CML is characterized by the increased and unregulated proliferation of myeloid cells without loss of their capacity to differentiate [6]. Cells in the myeloid cell line are those arising from myeloid progenitor cells, eventually becoming mature blood cells. These mature blood cells include basophils, neutrophils, eosinophil, monocytes, erythrocytes, and platelets. Although *BCR-ABL1* is found in all myeloid lineages, the initial major finding suggestive of CML is neutrophilic leukocytosis. The BCR-AB1 translocation may also be found in *some lymphoid* and *endothelial cells. Of note,* this *translocation* is *found* in 10% of patients with acute lymphoblastic leukemia [1, 7].

In the USA, CML is diagnosed asymptomatically or incidentally in 40-50% of patients. The condition is often diagnosed following a routine physical examination or blood test. White blood cell counts are increased, and the cells are differentiated and mature [8]. Common signs and symptoms of the chronic phase (CP), usually resulting from anemia and splenomegaly [2], include fatigue, weight loss, malaise, and left upper quadrant fullness or pain [1].

Based on the number of immature white blood cells (blasts cells) observed in the blood or bone marrow as well as other characteristic criteria, CML can be classified into three phases. These phases are important for prognosis and treatment [1]. The phases are CP, the accelerated phase (AP), and the blast phase (BP). The vast majority (90-95%) of patients are diagnosed during the CP, which is the earliest *phase of CML* [2]. The median duration of the CP is 5-6 years and, if left untreated, the disease usually progresses to the AP or BP. The duration of the AP and BP is 6-9 months and 3-6 months, respectively. The BP is the terminal phase of CML [9].

Approximately 30% of patients with CML present with marrow fibrosis, commonly mild or moderate. Notably, advanced bone marrow fibrosis occurs in <5% of patients [10]. In general, almost all myeloid neoplasms have the potential to induce fiber deposition. Although the highest fibrotic risk is related to an underlying *BCR-ABL1*-negative primary myelofibrosis, it may also be found in *BCR-ABL1*-positive CML [11]. Rarely, CML may present with an unusual profile, rendering the diagnosis challenging [12]. CML may present with excessive bone marrow fibrosis and atypical presence of megakaryocytes, potentially resembling primary myelofibrosis [13, 14].

The aim of this report was to share the experience of diagnosing CML with unusual features, such as pancytopenia and atypical megakaryocytes with excessive fibrosis of the bone marrow. Targeted therapy against CML leads to life-saving remission. Therefore, it is very important to recognize CML at the time of initial diagnosis. In this case, the patient was diagnosed by the presence of the BCR-ABL fusion gene along with results obtained through clinical, laboratory, and histopathological examinations.

CASE REPORT

A 50-year-old male visited Siloam Hospital (Jakarta, Indonesia) in July 2017 with complaints of generalized body weakness, which worsened in the previous 5 days. Dizziness and blurred vision were noted. The patient had a history of two blood transfusions performed in May 2017 in Manado, Indonesia. His vital signs were normal and there was no palpable organomegaly in his abdomen. Laboratory tests, including a complete blood count, were conducted and the results revealed anemia and leukopenia. Therefore, the patient was advised to undergo *bone marrow aspiration and biopsy*.

In August 2017, the patient returned to the same hospital with similar complaints. The laboratory results showed pancytopenia with differential cell count, low blast cell count, and normal segmented neutrophils count (Table 1).

Table 1. Results of the laboratory blood test

Tests	Result, July 2017	Result, August 2017	Unit	Reference interval
Hemoglobin	6.5	3.7	g/dL	13.0-18.0
Hematocrit	18.5	10.4	%	40.0-54.0
Erythrocytes	2.25	1.36	$10^6/\mu L$	4.50-6.20
MCV	82.2	76.5	fL	81.00-96.00
MCH	28.9	26.5	pg	27.0-36.0
MCHC	35.1	14.6	g/L	31.0-37.0
White blood cells (WBC)	2.6	1.0	$10^3/\mu L$	4.00-10.00
Differential count				
Basophils	0		%	0-1
Eosinophils	0		%	0-4
Band neutrophils	2		%	2-6
Segmented neutrophils	62		%	50-70
Lymphocytes	27		%	20-40
Monocytes	7		%	2-8
Platelets	268	77	$10^3/\mu L$	150-400

His pancytopenia was managed mainly through the transfusion of red blood cells and platelets. The level of lactate dehydrogenase in the serum was increased. The liver function test, and the levels of creatinine, bilirubin, and electrolytes were within the normal range. C*hest* radiography showed pneumonic infiltration. Ultrasonography of the abdomen and pelvis revealed a slightly enlarged liver with homogeneous parenchyma. The spleen, bladder, and prostate were normal.

The results of the bone marrow aspiration showed a myeloid to erythroid ratio within the normal range (Table 2). Maturation in the myeloid series presented into segmented neutrophils and the number of blasts was not elevated.

A review of the bone marrow biopsy was also performed at Cipto Mangunkusumo hospital. A histopathological examination revealed a hypercellular bone marrow (Figure 1 a, 1 b) with a normal myeloid to erythroid ratio, showing myeloid maturation into segmented neutrophils (Figure 2 a, 2 b). In addition, the number of megakaryocytes with atypical nuclei was increased, forming a cluster (Figure 3 a, 3 b).

Table 2. Bone marrow aspiration performed in July, 2017

Tests	Result	Unit	Reference interval
Thrombopoiesis			
Megakaryocytes count	-		
Myeloid series			
Myeloblasts	0.0	%	0-1
Promyelocytes	1.0	%	1-5
Myelocytes	*0.0*	%	2-10
Metamyelocytes	*2.0*	%	5-15
Bands	*2.0*	%	10-40
Segmented neutrophils	29.0	%	10-30
Basophil	0.0	%	0-1
Eosinophil	0.0	%	0-3
Myeloid total	34	%	
Erythroid series			
Pro-erythroblasts	0.0	%	0-1
Erythroblasts basophils	*0.0*	%	1-4
Polychromatic erythroblasts	6.0	%	10-20
Orthochromatic erythroblasts	7.0	%	5-10
Erythroid total	13.0	%	
Male to female ratio	2.6:1	%	(2-4):1
Other series			
Lymphocytes	40	%	0-15
Monocytes	7	%	0-2
Plasmocytes	6	%	0-1

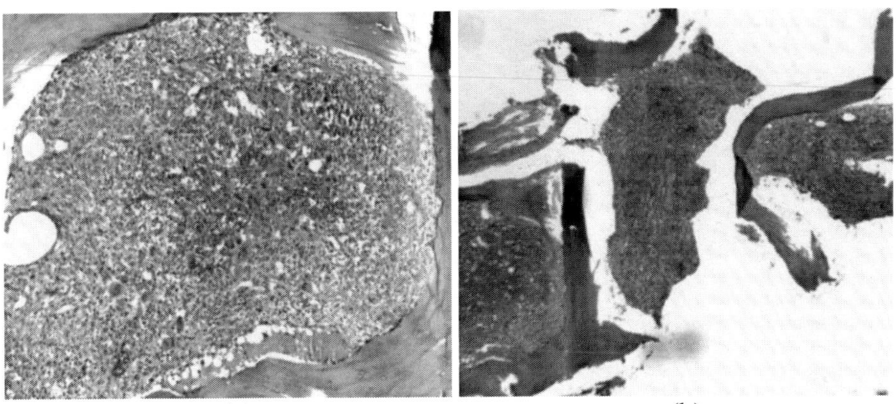

(a) (b)

Figure 1. (a, b) Bone marrow biopsy showed a hypercellular bone marrow (H&E, 40×, 100×).

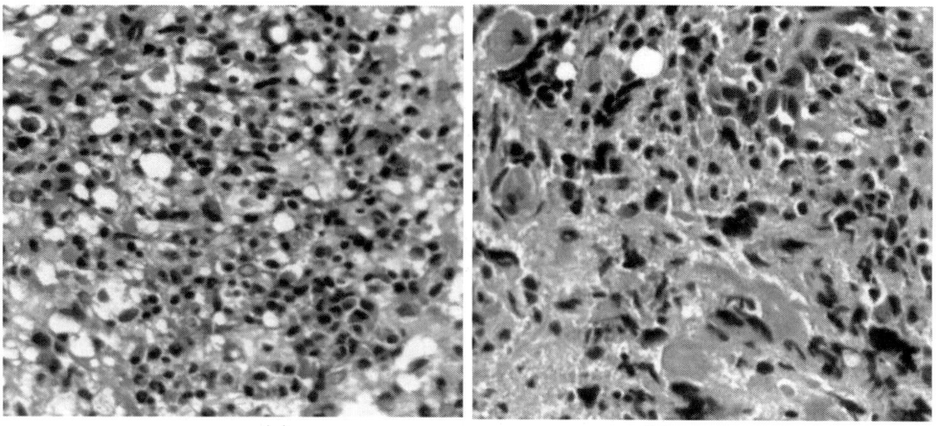

(a) (b)

Figure 2. (a, b) Higher magnification revealed a normal myeloid to erythroid ratio, showing myeloid maturation into segmented neutrophils. The number of blasts was not increased (H&E, 400×).

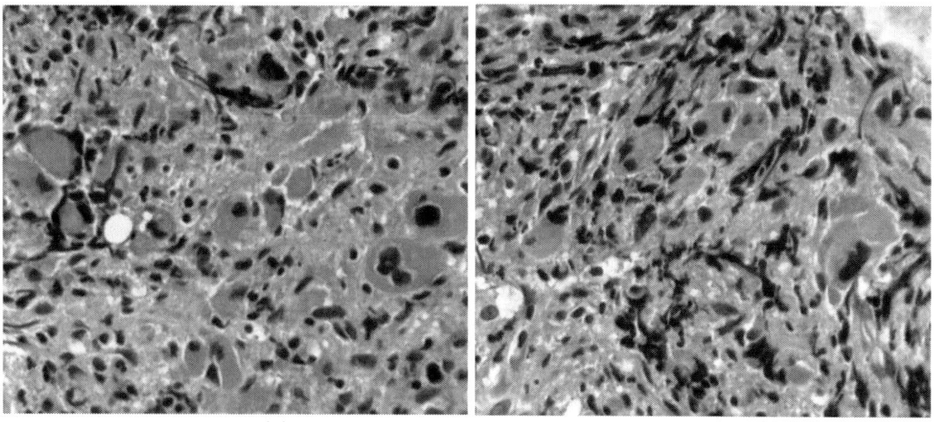

(a) (b)

Figure 3. (a, b) The number of megakaryocytes with atypical nuclei was increased, forming a cluster (H&E 400×).

Staining with Periodic Acid Schiff (PAS) showed that the number of megakaryocytes was increased. Some megakaryocytes were scattered with small, hypolobated nuclei (Figure 4 a, 4 b). Reticulin staining showed that the fibers were increased diffusely and densely with extensive intersections (Figure 5 a, 5 b). Trichrome staining showed the presence of focal bundles of collagen fibers (Figure 6 a, 6 b). According to the definition established by the World Health Organization, the grade of marrow fibrosis was marrow fibrosis 3. Hence, this patient was diagnosed with a myeloproliferative neoplasm, suggestive of primary myelofibrosis.

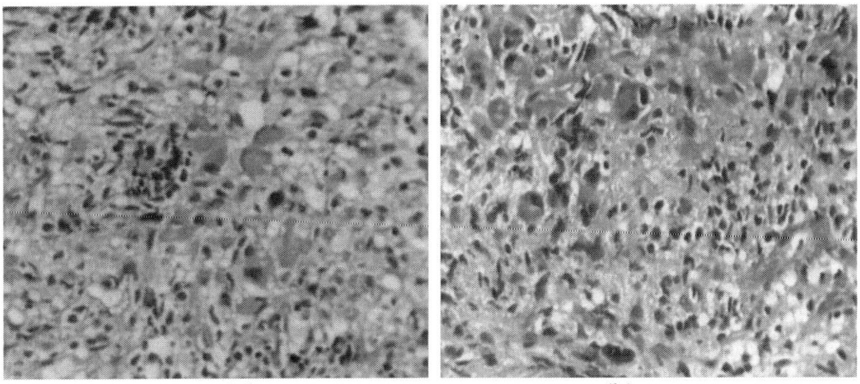

(a) (b)

Figure 4. (a, b) Increased megakaryocytes. Some scattered megakaryocytes were small with hypolobated nuclei (PAS, 40×).

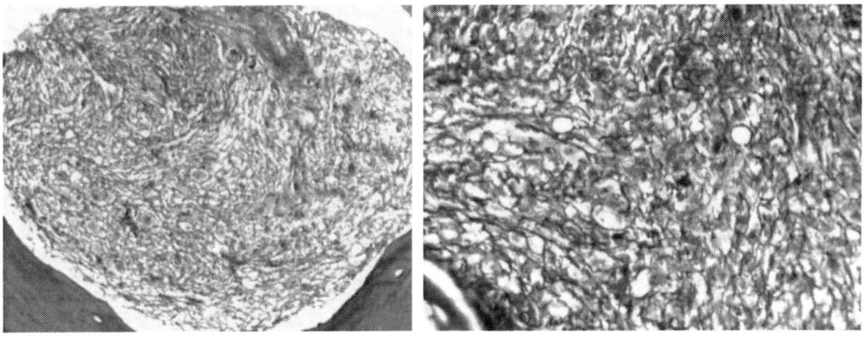

(a) (b)

Figure 5. (a) Reticulin fibers were increased diffusely and densely (Reticulin, 4×). (b) Extensive intersections of reticulin fibers (Reticulin, 40×).

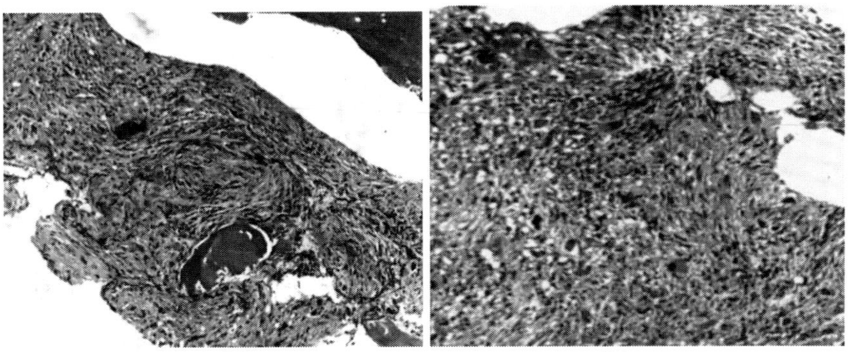

(a) (b)

Figure 6. (A-B) The bone marrow exhibited focal bundles of collagen fibers (Trichrome, 10×).

Subsequently, an evaluation of mutations in the JAK2 gene and the presence of the BCR-ABL1 fusion gene was performed using blood samples to reach a definitive diagnosis.

The presence of the BCR-ABL1 fusion gene was determined through real-time quantitative polymerase chain reaction. The analysis for mutations in the JAK2 gene yielded negative results. The presence of the BCR-ABL1 abnormality confirmed the diagnosis of CML in this patient. Based on the presence of excessive bone marrow fibrosis and thrombocytopenia (unrelated to therapy), CML at that time was considered to be at the AP.

This patient exhibited uncommon clinical, laboratory, and morphologic bone marrow features to meet the criteria for the diagnosis of CML. In this, case the condition included pancytopenia, absence of splenomegaly, and excessive bone marrow fibrosis, with some megakaryocytes showing atypical nuclei. Owing to the uncommon clinical features, this patient also consulted a pathologist in Germany. He preferred to diagnose this case as CML because of the presence of the *BCR-ABL1* fusion gene. The treating physician had previously encountered a number of similar CML cases with excessive fibrosis and the absence of an increase in size of the spleen. In this case, the majority of megakaryocytes exhibited atypical nuclei. However, a number of megakaryocytes exhibited the "dwarf form," which is typical in CML.

Discussion

The clinical hallmark of CML is leukocytosis, i.e., the uncontrolled production of maturing granulocytes including neutrophils, basophils, and eosinophils in the peripheral blood [15]. Of note, the number of platelets is normal or slightly increased and mild to moderate anemia is usually noted. In our case, the initial peripheral blood findings revealed pancytopenia. The patient had abnormally low levels of red blood cells, white blood cells, and platelets. This condition may be the result of myelofibrosis, which accompanies CML [14]. Myelofibrosis is the presence of reticulin and deposition of collagen, replacing bone marrow hematopoietic cells with fibrous material. The exact pathogenesis of myelofibrosis is not fully understood. However, evidence has demonstrated the role of activating mutation involving CALR, the deregulated expression of pro-inflammatory cytokines, and the impaired bone marrow microenvironment [6].

The bone marrow microenvironment is composed of cells, structural fibrils, and the extracellular matrix. The cellular components include macrophages, fibroblastic cells, adipocytes, and endothelial cells. The most common structural fibrils in the bone marrow are collagen and reticulin. The ground substance includes water, salts, glycosaminoglycans, and glycoproteins. These elements provide a connective tissue structure for the bone marrow and physical support for the hematopoietic progenitor cells. Consequently, the bone marrow microenvironment plays an important role in hematopoiesis [12].

The elevation of pro-inflammatory cytokines is a major biological hallmark of bone marrow fibrosis. This effect is thought to be a consequence of the malignant clone as a modifier of the bone marrow microenvironment. One neoplastic cell type thought to be a major contributor to fibrosis is the megakaryocyte, which exhibits aberrant proliferation [11]. Megakaryocytes produce the transforming growth factor β. This cytokine potently stimulates fibroblasts to produce the extracellular matrix. Moreover, it increases the expression of proteases that inhibit enzymes involved in the degradation of the extracellular matrix [6]. Hence, megakaryocytes are important mediators in the development of bone marrow fibrosis [12].

In our case, the predominance of fibrosis and atypical megakaryocytes at presentation confounded the initial diagnosis. This raised the possibility of a differential diagnosis, such as primary myelofibrosis. Mohamed et al. reported a CML case with advanced myelofibrosis resembling primary myelofibrosis. That case also presented with anemia, thrombocytopenia, and an absence of splenomegaly; however, the white blood count was within the normal range. Therefore, it is recommended that a molecular analysis is performed in patients with myelofibrosis [10].

In patients with CML, various grades of megakaryocytic proliferation can be observed in bone marrow biopsies or cytological smears at the time of diagnosis [15]. CML with marrow fibrosis is more commonly developed in patients with a marked megakaryocytic proliferation [10]. In our case, the histopathological examination of the bone marrow through reticulin staining showed that fibers were increased diffusely and densely with extensive intersections. This finding was consistent with the observed increase in the number of megakaryocytes. This case presented with advanced (grade 3) fibrosis.

CML is classified into three phases that assist in predicting the prognosis. The phases are determined mainly according to the number of immature white blood cells (blasts cells) observed in the blood or bone marrow (Table 3) [1].

The recognition of disease progression, during which the CP develops into the AP and BP, is important for treatment and prognostic purposes. Unfortunately, the clinical and morphological differences between the CP, AP, and BP are not always clear. Large clusters or sheets of small, abnormal megakaryocytes with marked reticulin or collagen fibrosis are suggestive of AP, especially if accompanied by any of the hematological parameters [1]. In our case, the number of megakaryocytes with atypical nuclei was increased, forming a cluster. In addition, thrombocytopenia (unrelated to therapy) was noted. These findings are indicative of the AP.

In the CP, splenomegaly is observed in approximately 70% of CML patients, caused by the infiltration of the red pulp cords by mature and immature granulocytes [1]. In the AP and BP, splenomegaly is due to extra-medullary hematopoiesis. This patient did not exhibit splenomegaly.

The diagnosis of CML is based on the detection of the *BCR-ABL1* fusion gene, which is the underlying abnormality of this disease [12]. This mutation leads to persistently enhanced tyrosine kinase activity. This activity is responsible for maintaining proliferation and inhibiting differentiation and apoptosis. This leads to an excessive number of neoplastic clones in the bone marrow, Furthermore, neoplastic cells replace non-neoplastic hematopoietic and mesenchymal cells (adipocytes) [14]. The real-time quantitative polymerase chain reaction is used to detect the presence of the *BCR-ABL1* mutation. It can detect a single CML cell in 100,000 normal cells isolated from blood or bone marrow samples [16]. The results of this test are reported using the international scale. This analysis was performed in the present patient, showing positivity for *BCR-ABL1*, with 6% on the international scale.

Table 3. Phases of Chronic myeloid leukaemia according to WHO

CML phase	WHO definition
Chronic phase (CP)	- Peripheral blood (PB) shows leukocytosis (12-1000x10^9/L) - Blasts less than 2% of the white blood cells (WBC) - Basophilia is invariably present, eosinophilia is common - Monocytosis may be present, but usually <3% - Platelet ranges from normal to greater than 1000x10^9/L, thrombocytopenia is uncommon. - Bone marrow cellularity is increased - Blasts account < 5% of the marrow cells - Erythroid islands are usually reduced - Megakaryocytes may be normal or slightly decreased in number, 40-50% exhibit moderate to marked proliferation. - Megakaryocytes are smaller than normal and have hyposegmented nuclei (dwarf megakaryocytes) - Moderate to marked reticulin fibrosis correlates with increased numbers of megakaryocytes and associated with an enlarged spleen was found in 30-40% of biopsies
Accelerated phase (AP)	Presence of ≥1 of the following hematological/cytogenetic criteria or provisional criteria concerning the response to therapy with tyrosine kinase inhibitors (TKIs). Hematological/cytogenetic criteria: – Persistent or increasing WBC (>10 × 10^9/L), unresponsive to therapy – Persistent or increasing splenomegaly, unresponsive to therapy – Persistent thrombocytosis (>1,000 × 10^9/L), uncontrolled by therapy – Persistent thrombocytopenia (unrelated to therapy) – Basophil ≥20% in the PB – 10-19% blasts in the PB or bone marrow

CML phase	WHO definition
Accelerated phase (AP)	– Additional clonal chromosomal abnormalities in the Philadelphia (Ph) chromosome, including major route abnormalities (a second Ph chromosome, trisomy 8, isochromosome 17q, and trisomy 19), a complex karyotype, and abnormalities of 3q26.2 – Any new clonal chromosomal abnormality in Ph+ cells that occurs during therapy – Criteria for the provisional response to TKIs – Hematological resistance (or failure to achieve complete hematological response) to the first TKI – Any hematological, cytogenetic, or molecular indication of resistance to sequential treatment with two TKIs – Occurrence of at least two mutations in the *BCR-ABL1* fusion gene during TKI therapy. Large clusters or sheets of small, abnormal megakaryocytes with marked reticulin or collagen fibrosis
Blast phase	– Blasts ≥20% of the PB WBC, or of the nucleated cells of the bone marrow – Extramedullary blast proliferation

CONCLUSION

CML is an acquired myeloproliferative neoplasm, in which granulocytes are the major proliferative component. It develops in hematopoietic stem cells and is characterized by a chromosomal translocation, resulting in the *BCR-ABL1* fusion gene and the formation of the Ph chromosome. The majority of CML cases are diagnosed on the basis of findings in the peripheral blood and bone marrow biopsy, combined with the detection of the Ph chromosome. Rarely, a number of CML cases exhibit atypical peripheral blood test results and uncommon histopathological features in the bone marrow biopsy, resembling primary myelofibrosis in the overt fibrotic stage. Therefore, the diagnosis of CML should not be immediately excluded prior to confirming the presence of the Ph chromosome or *BCR/ABL1* rearrangement.

The diagnosis of CML with atypical features (i.e., pancytopenia and excessive fibrosis of the bone marrow) requires the combination of clinical, laboratory, and histopathological examinations, accompanied by the presence of an acquired genetic abnormality, the *BCR/ABL1* fusion gene. An increased awareness of this disease, especially at the CP, may prevent progression to the AP or BP.

REFERENCES

[1] Vardiman, JW; Melo, JV; Baccarani, M; Radich, JP; Kvasnicka, HM. WHO Classification of Tumours of Haematopoietic and Lymphoid Tissues. 5th ed. Lyon: *International Agency for Research on Cancer*; 2017.

[2] Jabbour, EJ. Chronic myeloid leukemia: 2016 update on diagonis, therapy and monitoring. *Am J Hematol*. 2016; 91: 252-65.

[3] Cardama, AQ; Cortes, J. Molecular biology of bcr-abl1 positive chronic myeloid leukemia. *Blood*, 2009; 113: 1619-30.

[4] Hoglund, M; Sandin, F; Simonsson, B. Epidemiology of chronic myeloid leukaemia: An update. *Ann Hematol*. 2015; 94: 241-7.

[5] Frazer, R; Irvine, AE; McMullin, MF. Chronic myeloid leukaemia in the 21st century. *Ulster Med J*. 2007; 76: 8-17.

[6] Zahr, AA; Salama, ME; Carreau, N; Tremblay, D; Verstovek, S; Mesa, R; et al. Bone marrow fibrosis in myelofibrosis: Pathogenesis, prognosis and targeted strategies. *Haematologica*. 2016; 101: 660-71.

[7] Ismail. S; Naffa, R; Yousef, AF. Incidence of BCR-ABL fusion transcripts in healthy individuals. *Mol Med Rep*. 2014; 9:1271-6.

[8] Al-Achkar, W; Wafa, AS; Moassass, F; Klein, E; Liehr, T. Multiple copies of BCR-ABL fusion gene on two isodicentric Philadelphia chromosomes in an imatinib mesylate-resistant chronic myeloid leukemia patient. *Oncol Lett*.2013; 5: 1579-82.

[9] Schiffer, CA; Hehlman, R; Larson, R. Perspective on the treatment of chronic phase and advanced phase CML and Philadelphia chromosome positive ALL. *Leukemia*. 2003; 17: 691-99.

[10] Mohamed, M; Beamish, M; Grabek, J. Chronic myeloid leukemia masquerading as primary myelofibrosis. *J Clin Pathol. Suppl*. 2014; 46: 75-7.

[11] Hussein, K; Stucki-Koch, A; Gohring, G; Kreipe, H; Suttorp, M. Increased megakaryocytic proliferation, pro-platelet deposition and expression of fibrosis-associated factors in children with chronic myeloid leukemia with bone marrow fibrosis. *Leukemia*. 2017; 31: 1540-6.

[12] Kuter, DJ; Bain, B; Mufti, G; Bagg, A; Haserjian, RP. Bone marrow fibrosis: Pathophysiology and clinical significance of increased bone marrow stromal fibres. *Br J Haemtol*. 2007; 139: 351-62.

[13] Dunphy, CH; Hasserjian, RP; George, TI. *Neoplastic Hematopathology: An Atlas and Concise Guide*. New York: Demos Medical; 2013.

[14] Koshy, J; Alperin, J; Jana, B; Markowitz, A; Qian, YW. A case of Philadelphia chromosome positive myeloproliferative neoplasm in a pregnant woman with unusual primary myelofibrosis features. *Case Rep Hematol* 2013;2013: 702831.

[15] Busche, G; Kreipe, HH. *Chronic Blood and Bone Marrow Pathology*. 2nd ed. Churchill Livingstone: Elsevier; 2011.

[16] Bauer, S; Romvari, E. Interpreting molecular monitoring results and international standardization in chronic myeloid leukemia. *J Adv Pract Oncol*. 2012; 3: 151-60.

In: Case Reports in Surgery
Editors: Ahmad Jabir Rahyussalim et al.
ISBN: 978-1-53616-582-1

Chapter 29

CLEAR CELL CHONDROSARCOMA: A CASE REPORT

Ros Nirmawati[1], Evelina Kodrat[1,*] and Errol Untung Hutagalung[2]
[1]Department of Anatomical Pathology, Faculty of Medicine, Universitas Indonesia, Cipto Mangunkusumo Hospital, Jakarta, Indonesia
[2]Department of Orthopaedics and Traumatology, Faculty of Medicine, Universitas Indonesia, Cipto Mangunkusumo Hospital, Jakarta, Indonesia

ABSTRACT

Clear cell chondrosarcoma is a rare variant of low-grade malignant cartilaginous tumor, representing approximately 2% of all chondrosarcomas. In this article, we report a rare case of clear cell chondrosarcoma in a 21-year-old male. Histopathological findings showed abundant clear cytoplasm or a faintly acidophilic cytoplasm with distinct cytoplasmic borders. The nuclei were round, vesicular, and centrally located, with prominent nucleoli. Mitotic figures are uncommon. Follow-up immunohistochemical staining showed positivity for S-100 protein and negativity for other epithelial markers, supporting the diagnosis of clear cell chondrosarcoma. Clear cell chondrosarcoma mostly involves the epiphyseal of long bones, especially in the femur or humerus. Complete surgical excision is the treatment of choice.

Keywords: chondrosarcoma, clear cell chondrosarcoma

INTRODUCTION

Clear cell chondrosarcoma is a rare variant of low-grade malignant cartilaginous tumor, representing approximately 2% of all chondrosarcomas [1]. Unni et al. first

* Corresponding Author's E-mail: elina_1610@yahoo.com.

described it in 1976, the clear cell chondrosarcoma entity was formerly known as "Clear-cell Variant of Chondrosarcoma" [2,3]. The cytoplasm appears clear due to the abundance of glycogen in tumor cells [1,4]. This condition tends to arise in the epiphyseal area of long bones [1,4-6]. The peak incidence is observed during the third and fourth decades of life [4].

We report this case to avoid the risk of inaccurate diagnosis and recognize the differential diagnosis.

Case Report

A 21-year-old male had a chief complaint of pain ranging from knee up to left hip for almost 2 years and 4 months. The patient then underwent pelvic X-ray and lumbosacral *magnetic resonance imaging* (MRI) examination. The Pelvic X-ray showed an expansile lytic lesion with a wide transition zone on the left proximal femoral. There was no cortical destruction, presence of a soft-tissue mass, or periosteal reaction (Figure 1). MRI results showed lesions that destructed the left femoral head and also appeared a signal with the same intensity as lesions in the surrounding soft tissue and left hip joint (Figure 2.). These findings indicated the presence of an aggressive primary bone tumor.

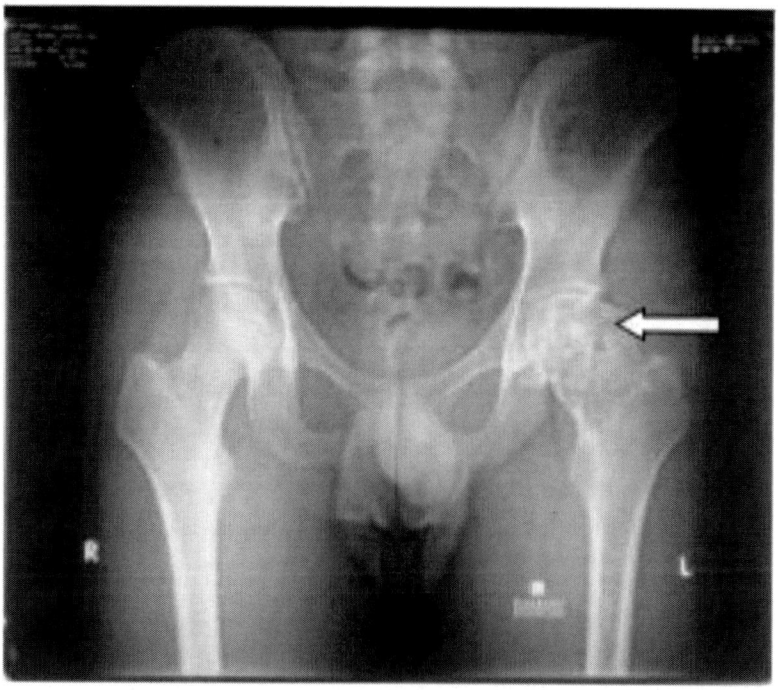

Figure 1. Pelvic X-ray examination showed the presence of an expansile lytic lesion with a wide transition zone. There was no cortical destruction, presence of a soft-tissue mass, or periosteal reaction (arrow).

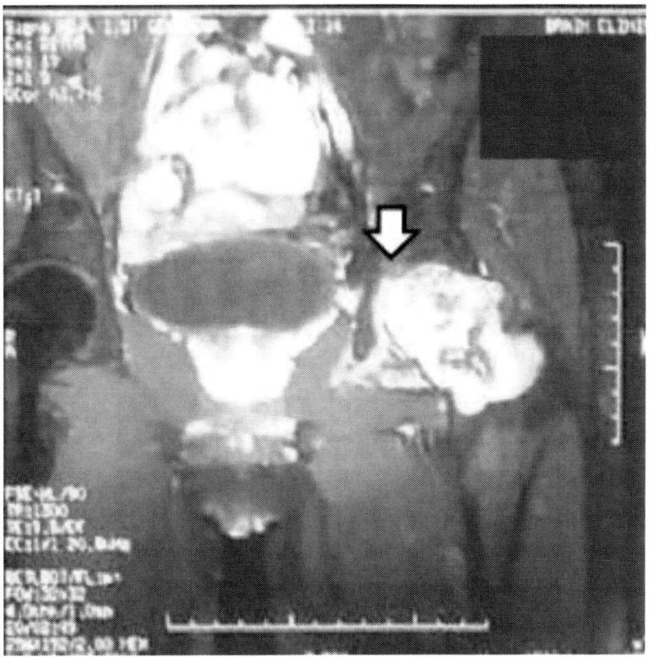

(a)

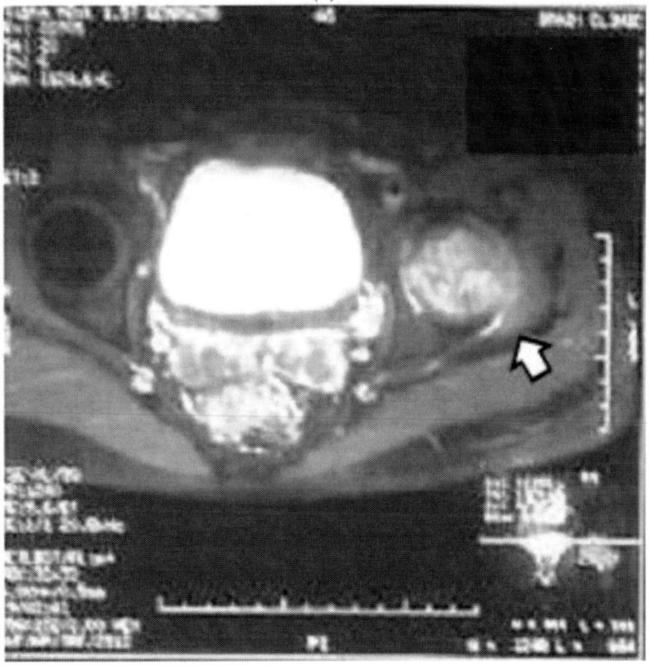

(b)

Figure 2. Coronal (a) and axial (b) lumbosacral MRI. The MRI results showed lesions that destructed the left femoral head and also appeared a signal with the same intensity as lesions in the surrounding soft tissue and left hip joint. These findings indicated the presence of an aggressive primary bone tumor.

Later, the patient underwent an open biopsy of his left femoral head at a hospital. Histological report revealed fragments of lesional tissue, comprising cellular nests of polygonal cells with central nuclei, conspicuous nucleoli, and pale eosinophilic to clear cytoplasm, admixed with small trabeculae of new reactive bone. Scattered multinucleated giant cells were present. In other area of the tumor, small foci resembling conventional chondrosarcoma were present. The tumor cells were immunoreactive for S-100 but negative for MNF116. These results were consistent with clear cell chondrosarcoma.

After one month, the patient underwent a wide excision procedure in another private hospital. The specimen from wide excision was sent to the laboratory of anatomic pathology. By report, the histopathological features showed a solid tumor mass with formation of a malignant osteoid. The tumor cells consisted of chondroblastic and epitheloid cells with pleomorphic and hyperchromatic nucleoli. Mitotic activity was easily observed. Osteoclast-like giant cell, necrotic area, hemorrhage, and bone marrow were visible in the tumor mass. Based on these findings, this patient was diagnosed as conventional osteosarcoma rather than chondrosarcoma.

Due to the differences in histological results, this case was discussed at our weekly Clinicopathological Conference (CPC) and suggested to repeat immunohistochemical staining on resection specimen as we were not able to have the slides and paraffin block from the first open biopsy.

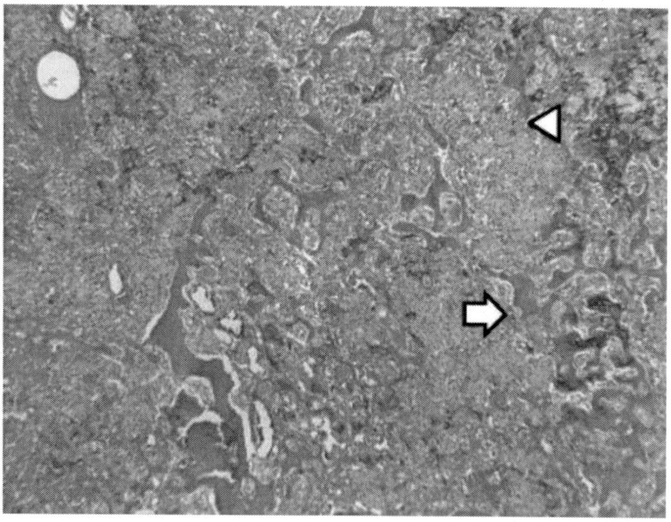

Figure 3. The solid mass consisted of bony trabeculae, with osteoblastic rimming among the tumor cells (arrow). Production of cartilage matrix was also found (arrow head)(H&E, ×40).

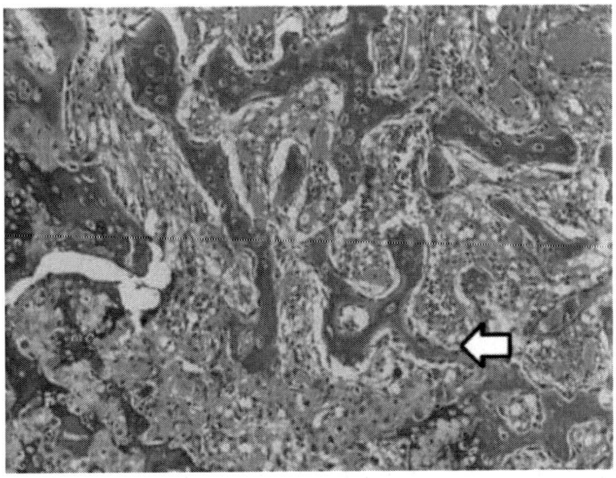

Figure 4. Irregular bony trabeculae with osteoblastic rimming (arrow) (H&E, ×100).

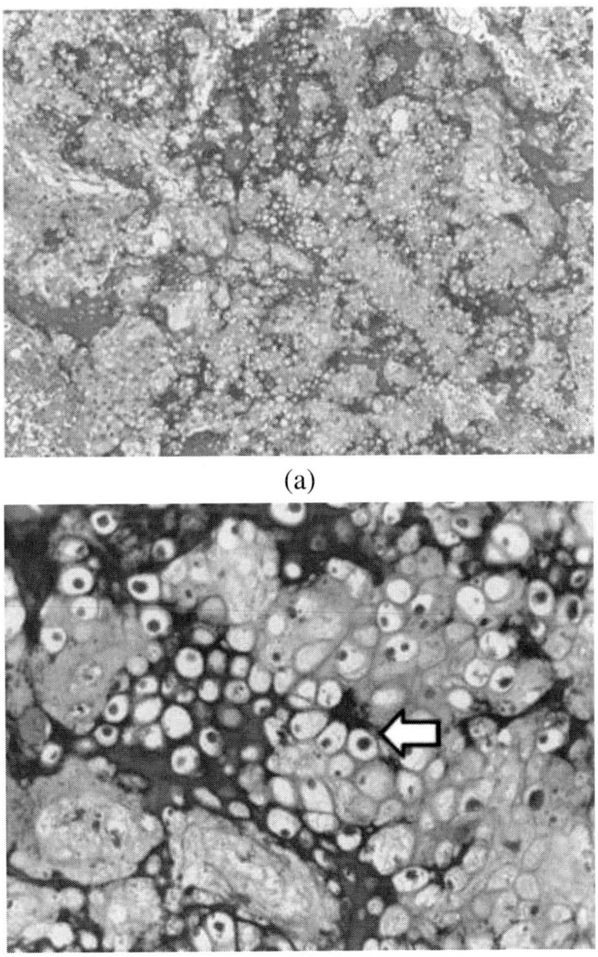

(a)

(b)

Figure 5. (a) An area of clear cell chondrosarcoma with production of chondro-osseous matrix (H&E, ×100). (b) The clear cell chondrosarcoma consisted of large round cells with centrally located nuclei, distinct cytoplasmic borders (arrow), and abundant clear and pale eosinophiliccytoplasms (H&E, ×400).

Based on the slides provided, the histological appearance under low magnification showed that the solid mass consisted of bony trabeculae, with osteoblastic rimming among the tumor cells. The tumor cells were round, with slightly-moderately pleomorphic nuclei; there were large cells with distinct cytoplasmic borders in several areas, prominent nucleoli, and abundant clear or pale eosinophilic cytoplasm. Mitotic activity was infrequent. Multinucleated giant cells and production of cartilage matrix were also visible (Figure 3-6). The repeated immunohistochemical staining results showed that the neoplastic cells were positive for S-100 (Figure 7) and negative for AE1/3, CK8, CK18, CK7, and CK20. These morphological and immunohistochemical staining features were consistent with clear cell chondrosarcoma.

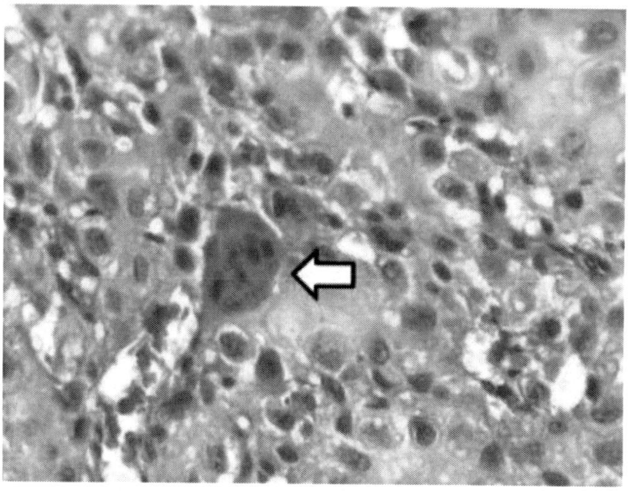

Figure 6. A scattered multinucleated giant cell (arrow) in the tumor (H&E, ×400).

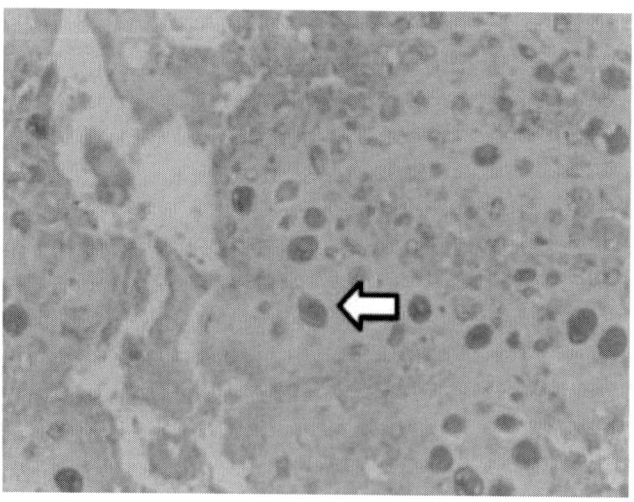

Figure 7. The nuclei of neoplastic cells were positive for the S-100 protein (H&E, ×400).

DISCUSSION

Clear cell chondrosarcoma is a rare variant of chondrosarcoma [1]. It mostly occurs in adults (third to fifth decades of life) with a 2.4:1 male-to-female ratio [1, 4]. The initial symptom is local pain in the affected area, developing in the longterm due to the slow growth of the tumor [1, 2, 4, 6]. Our patient was a 21-year-old male, who had been suffering from pain on his left knee for 2 years prior to his admission to the hospital.

Clear cell chondrosarcoma usually involves the epiphysis of long bones, especially the femur or humerus [1, 4]. Chondroblastoma and GCT of the bone exhibit similar localization with clear cell chondrosarcoma, whereas conventional chondrosarcoma is usually found in the metaphysis or diaphysis of long bones [5].

Clear cell chondrosarcoma is characterized by a distinctive histologic feature i.e., the presence of "clear cells" (abundant clear to faintly acidophilic cytoplasm with distinct borders), whose nuclei are large, vesicular, and centrally located. The nucleoli are usually prominent and mitotic figures are uncommon [1-6]. Histologically, it may resemble chondroblastoma, GCT of the bone, osteoblastoma, or even conventional osteosarcoma [5].

The most common radiological of clear cell chondrosarcoma findings are well-marginated radiolucent areas with distinct reactive borders, an absence of cortical destruction or periosteal reaction, and unusual soft-tissue extension [3,5,7]. The radiological findings of clear cell chondrosarcoma must be differentiated from those of other benign epiphyseal lesions, such as chondroblastoma and GCT of the bone [7-9]. In this report, the pelvic X-ray examination was an expansile lytic lesion with a wide transition zone. There was no cortical destruction, presence of a soft-tissue mass, or periosteal reaction.

Chondroblastoma arises in the epiphysis or epimetaphysis of long bones, more commonly in male and younger patients [10,11]. Radiologically, chondroblastoma is typically a small (3-6 cm), well-demarcated lytic lesion and generally with no bone expansion. Periosteal reaction is frequent and occasionally distant from the primary lesion [10]. Microscopically, the tumor cells are usually surrounded by fine lines of calcification, which are typical in both clear cell chondrosarcomas and chondroblastomas. However, chondroblastoma does not show a clear cytoplasm, which is typical for clear cell chondrosarcoma. Instead, it shows an oval nucleus with a nuclear groove and a faintly acidophilic cytoplasm [2]. In general, the distinction between chondroblastoma and clear cell osteosarcoma do not necessarily require immunohistochemistry staining. However, in several difficult cases, SOX9 and cytokeratins are useful to distinguish both entities. The expression of SOX9 and cytokeratins is found in chondroblastoma, while it is negative in clear cell chondrosarcoma [10].

Moreover, GCT of the bone affects the same site as clear cell chondrosarcoma [5]. Notably, the radiological and histopathological features are evidently different from those observed for clear cell chondrosarcoma. GCT of the bone is usually found in patients aged 20-40 years, with a slight predominance observed in female patients [12,13]. Plain radiography of GCT showed a large expansile lytic-sclerotic lesion with cortical thinning (the “soap-bubble appearance”). The presence of numerous osteoclast-like giant cells, which contain >20 nuclei, is the hallmark of GCT [4,13,14]. In contrast, scattered multinucleated giant cells in clear cell chondrosarcoma are not associated with the neoplastic process, and they usually contain only 6-8 nuclei [5].

In addition, clear cell chondrosarcoma has a scattered osteoid matrix and a bony trabeculae appearance among the tumor cells resembling conventional osteosarcoma. Osteoid matrix with lace-like appearance and accompanied with an increase level of alkaline phosphatase in the serum prior to surgery should be considered as osteosarcomas, especially in young patients [5,9]. Radiographically, conventional osteosarcoma exhibits a permeative pattern with periosteal reaction, cortical destruction, and the extension of soft-tissue mass [4,15,16]. Meanwhile, clear cell chondrosarcoma exhibits a well-marginated radiolucent area with distinct reactive borders and an absence of cortical destruction [1,3,4]. Conventional osteosarcoma features high-grade nuclei, such as severe nuclear anaplasia and pleomorphism with occasional mineralization [15]. The absence of a clear cell population among the intertrabecular spaces and its location may distinguish osteosarcoma from clear cell chondrosarcoma [4,15].

The presence of an interanastomosing osteoid with osteoblastic rimming may also be considered as osteoblastoma. Osteoblastoma is composed of osteoblasts that are rich in vascularity. The absence of the clear cell feature distinguishes this tumor from clear cell chondrosarcoma [2,4,5,17].

The patient was initially diagnosed with clear cell chondrosarcoma based on histological report from the open biopsy specimen. He underwent wide excision at another private hospital with result showing conventional osteosarcoma. Due to the differences in histological results, the case was presented at CPC and was suggested to repeat the immunohistochemical staining to confirm the diagnosis. The immunohistochemical staining showed positivity for the S-100 protein and negativity for other epithelial markers (i.e., AE1/3, CK8, CK18, CK7, and CK20). The final diagnosis was clear cell chondrosarcoma.

Ancillary staining, such as histochemistry and immunohistochemistry, may assist in confirming the diagnosis of clear cell chondrosarcoma. The content of glycogen in the cytoplasm explains the clear cytoplasm feature and yields positive staining for periodic acid-Schiff [1,4,7]. The nuclei in clear cell chondrosarcomas are strongly positive for the S-100 protein [1,3,4,7,18,19]. Matsuura S et al. investigated the immunohistochemical expression profiles of cytokeratins (i.e., CAM5.2, AE1/AE3, CK7, CK8, CK18, and CK20), epithelial membrane antigen, sex-determining region Y-box 9 (SOX9), type II collagen, runt-related transcription factor 2 (RUNX2), and osteocalcin in clear cell chondrosarcoma. The results were compared with those observed in chondroblastoma, conventional chondrosarcoma, and osteosarcoma. Both clear cell chondrosarcoma and chondroblastoma showed epithelial and chondrogenic markers. Clear cell chondrosarcomas stain negative for CAM5.2 and the epithelial membrane antigen. The type II collagen immunohistochemistry showed 100 % positivity in clear cell chondrosarcoma while in chondroblastoma showed positivity for about 54%. The cartilagenous component of clear cell chondrosarcoma and chondroblastoma express SOX9 respectively 20% and 54%. Osteocalcin is not detected in the cytoplasm of clear cells; however, it is expressed in osteoblasts and osteocytes within woven bone. RUNX2 up-regulated the promoter activity of osteocalcinin osteosarcoma cell lines, but not in chondrosarcoma or chondrocyte cell lines [19].

The treatment of choice for clear cell chondrosarcoma is a wide and complete surgical excision. Chondrosarcoma has a relatively low proliferation rate, thus, radiotherapy remains ineffective as it aims at actively dividing cells. Systemic treatments, such as chemotherapy, have also been shown to be ineffective [20].

Inappropriate treatment results in recurrence in 16% of patients. En bloc excision is preferable to marginal excision or curettage. Although clear cell chondrosarcoma is commonly considered an indolent tumor; however, lung, brain, and bone metastases have been reported. The average rate of mortality is approximately 10%, while disease-free survival after incomplete removal is 13 years. The overall survival rate in patients with metastasis after initial therapy is approximately 7 years [4].

CONCLUSION

Clear cell chondrosarcoma is a rare variant of low-grade malignant cartilaginous tumor, representing approximately 2% of all chondrosarcomas. Increased awareness regarding this disease may prevent misdiagnosis. Histologically, it may resemble other tumors, such as chondroblastoma, GCT, osteoblastoma, and conventional osteosarcoma. Immunohistochemical features are able to distinguish between the differential diagnoses. Clear cell chondrosarcomas are strongly positive for the S-100 protein. Sufficient clinical data, including location, radiological finding combined with microscopic features, and appropriate ancillary staining are mandatory to avoid misdiagnosis.

CONFLICTS OF INTEREST

None declared.

REFERENCES

[1] McCarthy, E. F., Hogendoorn, P. C. W. (2013). Clear cell chondrosarcoma. In: Fletcher, C. D. M., Bridge, J. A., Hogendoorn, P. C. W., Mertens, F., editors. *WHO classification of tumours of soft tissue and bone* (4th ed. pp.273-274). Lyon: IARC.

[2] Unni, K. K., Dahlin, D. C., Beabout, J. W., Sim, F. H. (1976). Chondrosarcoma: Clear cell variant. A report of sixteen cases. *J. Bone Joint Surg.*, 58-A, 676-683.

[3] Ayoub, K. S., Grimer, R. J., Carter, S. R., Mangham, D. C., Davies, A. M., Tillman, R. M. (1999). Clear cell chondrosarcoma of bone. *Sarcoma.*, 3, 115-119.

[4] Czerniak, B. (2016). *Dorfman and Czerniak's bone tumor.* (2nd ed). Philadelphia: Elsevier Saunders.

[5] Bjornsson, J., Unni, K. K., Dahlin, D. C., Beabout, J. W., Sim, F. H. Clear cell chondrosarcoma of bone. Observations in 47 cases. *Am. J. Surg. Pathol.*, 8, 223-230.

[6] Itälä, A., Leerapun, T., Inwards, C., Collins, M., Scully, S. P. (2005). An institutional review of clear cell chondrosarcoma. *Clin. Orthop. Relat. Res.*, 440, 209-212.

[7] Present, D., Bacchini, P., Pignatti, G., Picci, P., Bertoni, F., Campanacci, M. (1991). Clear cell chondrosarcoma of bone. A report of 8 cases. *SkeletalRadiol.*, 20, 187-191.

[8] Collins, M. R., Koyama, T., Swee, R. G., Inwards, C. Y. (2003). Clear cell chondrosarcoma: radiographic, computed tomographic, and magnetic resonance findings in 34 patients with pathologic correlation. *Skeletal Radiol.*, 32, 687-694.

[9] Ishida, T., Yamamoto, M., Goto, H., Yamamoto, A., Machinami, R. (1999). Case Report: Clear cell chondrosarcoma of the pelvis in skeletally immature patient. *Skeletal Radiol.*, 28, 290-293.

[10] Kilpatrick, S. E., Romeo, S. (2013). Chondroblastoma. In: Fletcher CDM, Bridge JA, Hogendoorn PCW, Mertens F, editors. *WHO classification of tumours of soft tissue and bone.* (4th ed. pp. 262-263). Lyon: IARC.

[11] Kaim, A. H., Hügli, R., Bonèl, H. M., Jundt, G. (2002). Chondroblastoma and clear cell chondrosarcoma: radiological and MRI characteristics with histopathological correlation. *Skeletal Radiol.*, 31, 88-95.

[12] Sobti, A., Agrawal, P., Agarwala, S., and Agarwal, M. (2016). Giant cell tumor of bone-an overview. *Arch. Bone Jt. Surg.*, 4, 2-9.

[13] Athanasou, N. A., Bansal, M., Forsyth, R., Reid, R. P., Sapi, Z. (2013). Giant cell tumour of bone. In: Fletcher, C. D. M., Bridge, J. A., Hogendoorn, P. C. W., Mertens, F., editors. *WHO classification of tumours of soft tissue and bone.* (4th ed. pp. 321-324). Lyon: IARC.

[14] Wülling, M., Engels, C., Jesse, N., Werner, M., Delling, G., Kaiser, E. (2001). The nature of giant cell tumor of bone. *J Cancer Res Clin Oncol.*, 127, 467-474.

[15] Klein, M. J., Siegal, G. P. (2006). Osteosarcoma, anatomic and histologic variants. *Am J Clin Pathol.*, 125, 555-581.

[16] Rosenberg, A. E., Cleton-Jansen, A. M., de Pinieux, G., Deyrup, A. T., Hauben, E., Squire, J. (2013). Conventional osteosarcoma. In: Fletcher, D. M., Bridge, J. A., Hogendoorn, P. C. W., Mertens, F., editors. *WHO classification of tumours of soft tissue and bone*. (4th ed. pp.282-288). Lyon: IARC.

[17] Lucas, D. R. (2010). Osteoblastoma. *Arch. Pathol. Lab. Med.*, 134, 1460-1466.

[18] Aigner, T., Dertinger, S., Belke, J., Kirchner, T. (1996). Chondrocytic cell differentiation in clear cell chondrosarcoma. *Hum. Pathol.*, 27, 1301-1305.

[19] Matsuura, S., Ishii, T., Endo, M., Takahashi, Y., Setsu, N., Yamamoto, H., et al. (2013). Epithelial and cartilaginous differentiation in clear cell chondrosarcoma. *Hum. Pathol.*, 44, 237-243.

[20] Gelderblom, H., Hogendoorn, P. C. W., Dijkstra, S. D., Rijswijk, C. S., Krol, A. D., Taminiau, A. H. M., et al. (2008). The Clinical approach towards chondrosarcoma. *The Oncologist.*, 13, 320-329.

In: Case Reports in Surgery
Editors: Ahmad Jabir Rahyussalim et al.
ISBN: 978-1-53616-582-1

Chapter 30

Hürthle Cell Carcinoma: A Rare Case with Unique Morphological Features

Familia Bella Rahadiati[1], Agnes Stephanie Harahap[2,*] and Maria Fransiska Ham[2]
[1]Anatomical Pathology Residency Program,
Faculty of Medicine, Universitas Indonesia, Jakarta, Indonesia
[2]Department of Anatomical Pathology, Faculty of Medicine,
Universitas Indonesia, Jakarta, Indonesia

Abstract

Hürthle cell carcinoma (HCC) of the thyroid is an unusual and relatively rare type of thyroid cancer. Small series of HCC patients have been reported in the literature, but because of its relative rarity, its pathological and clinical significance have not been well documented. A 55-year-old woman presented with rapid neck mass enlargement and hoarseness. Thorax X-ray imaging suggested intrathoracic struma. Ultrasonographic examination showed struma nodosa in the right lobe. Fine-needle aspiration biopsy results suggested a follicular neoplasm of Hürthle cell type. Grossly, the right thyroid size was 6 × 5 × 4 cm and was brown, firm, and encapsulated. The cut surfaces were brown and lobulated, with no papillary growth or calcification. A histological examination showed large tumor cells in a trabecular arrangement, rounded nuclei, coarse chromatin, some vesicular with prominent nucleoli, and abundant granular eosinophilic cytoplasm. Another section revealed capsular invasion, and a solid area containing scattered bizarre giant cells with irregular nuclei. The histopatological features and imunohistochemical staining results supported a diagnosis of encapsulated angioinvasive HCC with bizarre nuclei. HCC is a rare type of carcinoma that remains controversial and difficult to diagnose. Careful assessment should be performed to look for bizarre nuclei to prevent overdiagnosis.

[*] Corresponding Author's E-mail: agnharahap@gmail.com.

Keywords: carcinoma, Hürthle cell, morphology, thyroid, unique

INTRODUCTION

Thyroid carcinoma is the most common endocrine malignancy. Most these cancers are derived from the follicular epithelial cells of the thyroid gland. The cancers are further divided into sub-groups, depending on the degree of differentiation, and range from well-differentiated thyroid carcinoma (WDTC) to rare undifferentiated (UTC) or anaplastic thyroid carcinoma (ATC) [1, 2].

Hürthle cell tumor (HCT) is a rare thyroid neoplasm of the follicular cell origin, with >75% being composed of cells with oncocytic features. The ability to classify each tumor with oncocytic features as either benign or malignant has remained controversial [3]. HCT has no specific imaging characteristics. Ultrasound alone is unable to distinguish Hürthle cell carcinoma (HCC) from other histological variants. There are preoperative and intraoperative difficulties in discriminating adenoma from carcinoma [4, 5]. Small series of HCC patients have been reported in the literature, but HCC is an understudied cancer with poor prognosis. Because of its relative rarity, its pathological and clinical significance have not been well documented [3, 6].

HCC of the thyroid gland is unusual. It accounts for only approximately 3%-10% of all differentiated thyroid cancers and has the highest incidence of metastasis among the differentiated thyroid cancers [7]. HCC has a more aggressive natural history than that of follicular carcinoma, with a higher rate of locoregional recurrence, distant metastases, and mortality [8]. In the last five years, we have registered nine cases of HCT in Cipto Mangunkusumo Hospital (CMH), which include one case of Hürthle cell adenoma (HCA), four cases of minimally invasive HCC, and four cases of HCC.

HCC is a malignant thyroid neoplasm composed of oncocytes derived from follicular cells crowded with mitochondria, which are also called Hürthle cells, Askanazy cells, or oxyphylic cells [9]. The behavior of Hürthle cell neoplasms is unpredictable [4]. Differentiation of HCA and HCC is performed based on capsular or vascular invasion and the presence of metastases [8]. The prognosis of the malignant types of these tumors remains debatable because some authors have reported that HCA occasionally behaves like HCC [3]. In many HCC, the amount of cytoplasm is less abundant than that in adenoma, which results in an increased nuclear/cytoplasm ratio. A greater percentage of cells are tall, cuboidal or columnar, and scattered bizarre hyperchromatic forms maybe seen only in the adenoma [9].

According to the literature, both benign and malignant thyroid lesions contain so-called "cells of endocrine atypia" or cells with bizarre nuclei. These manifest as single cells or small groups displaying marked cellular and nuclear enlargement, some degree of pleomorphism, marked cellular hyperchromasia, and occasionally macronucleoli randomly dispersed among otherwise differentiated thyroid follicular cells. The presence of these enormous cells can be extremely worrisome and should be carefully assessed to arrive at the correct diagnosis [10]. We describe a rare case of HCC with unique morphological features that were identified in CMH.

CASE REPORT

A 55-year-old woman came to CMH on July 21, 2014, with a chief complaint of neck mass enlargement for the previous 10 months (Figure 1). Her past medical history revealed that the patient had lived with a small nodule the size of a corn kernel in her right neck for the last 12 years but she did not have any nodule-related complaints. However, she noticed that the neck mass began enlarging and had reached the size of a chicken egg over the previous 10 months. She went to the doctor and began taking levothyroxine once a day. She had been taking the drug for one month but then felt exhaustion and experienced palpitation, so she stopped taking the medicine. She also became hoarse but did not feel any pain, experience dyspnea, or notice exophthalmus. She went to a primary health care facility and was then referred to the CMH Internal Medicine department with a diagnosis of toxic struma nodosa and hypertension. She began taking amlodipin 10 mg once a day. She had no history of diabetes mellitus (DM), asthma, or allergy. Her family medical history showed that the patient's father had a history of tumor, the mother had a carcinoma of the cervix, and a sibling had type II DM. The patient was managed in the CMH Internal Medicine department and was scheduled to undergo a fine-needle aspiration biopsy (FNAB) procedure, ultrasound examination, administration of thyroid-stimulating hormone (TSH), and free thyroxine (fT4) laboratory tests.

Chest X-ray showed a soft tissue mass in the right inferior colli that pushed the trachea to the left and suggested intra-thoracic struma (Figure 2). Ultrasound examination of the right lobe showed an isoechoic, rounded heterogeneous lesion that was well demarcated with a regular edge and fully loaded the thyroid's right lobule. The lesion size was 3.7 × 3.34 × 3.3 cm. Intra-lesion calcification was not seen. Doppler technique showed intra-lesion vascularization. The thyroid's left lobe was normal in size and shape, with no focal pathological lesion or calcification. A lesion with a solid and cystic component was seen in the isthmus. The trachea was located in the midline. Lymph node enlargement was not found. Radiological examination identified a struma nodosa in the right lobe of the thyroid and an isthmus nodule (Figure 3). Laboratory examination showed normal sensitive TSH (sTSH) and fT4. The sTSH level was 1.210 μIU/mL, and the fT4 level was 1.420 ng/dL.

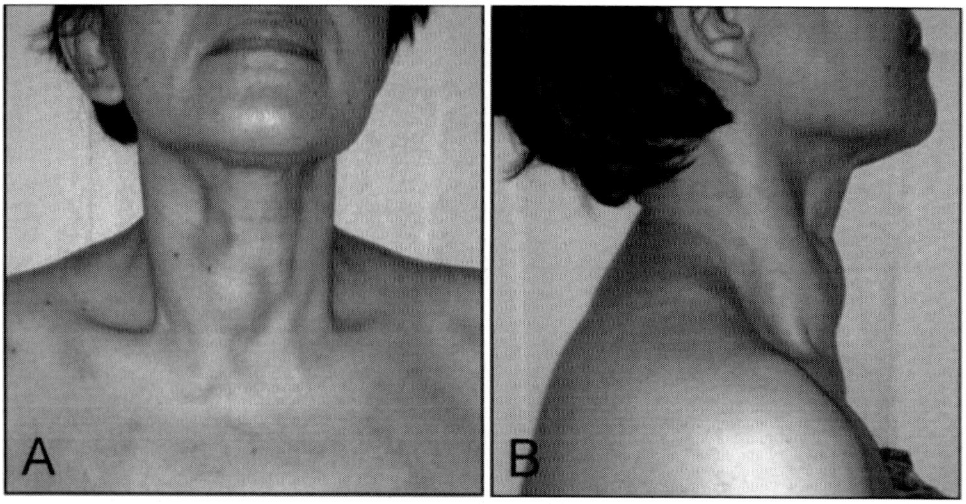

Figure 1. A lump in the right anterior of the neck that moved upward when swallowing. The lump had a diameter of 6 cm and a firm distinct border. The left lateral border was in the midline, the right lateral border was in the medial sternocleidomastoideus muscle, the inferior border was in the sternal notch, and the superior border was in the hyoid bone.

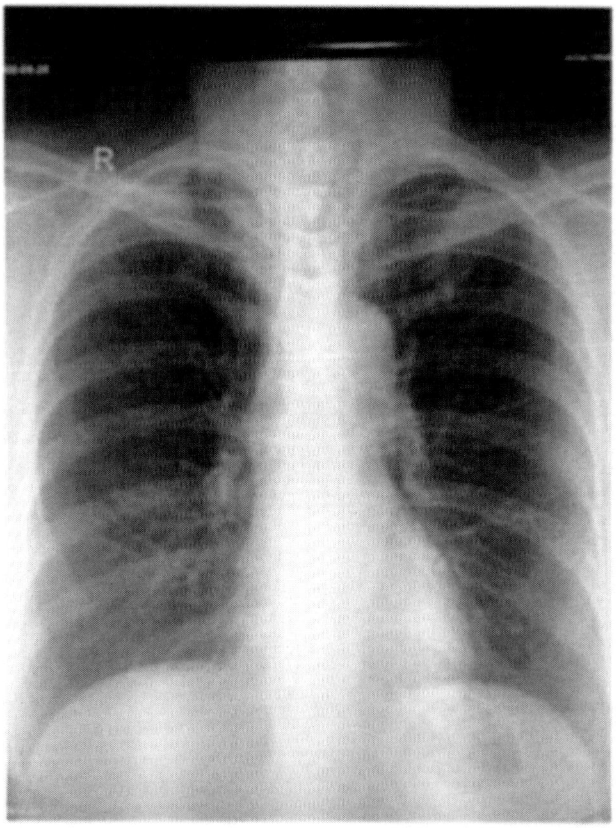

Figure 2. Chest X-ray image showing a soft tissue mass in the right inferior colli, suggesting an intrathoracic struma. The heart and lung were normal.

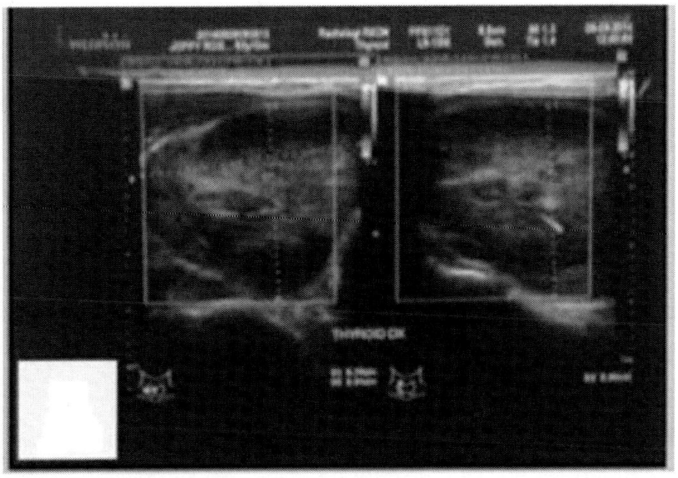

A

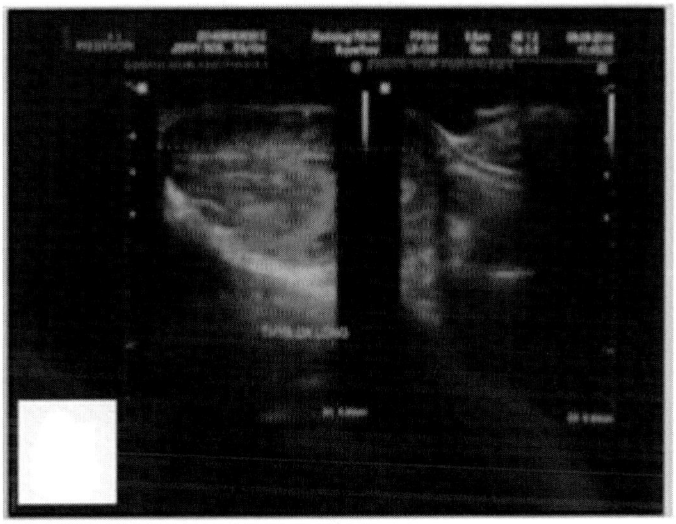

B

Figure 3. Ultrasound examination of the right lobe showing a rounded heterogeneous isoechoic lesion with awell-demarcated regular edge and that fully loaded the right lobule of the thyroid. The lesion size is 3.7 x 3.34 x 3.3 cm. Intralesion calcification is not seen.

FNAB was performed on August 14, 2014, and the results suggested a follicular neoplasm of Hürthle cell type. Then, the patient was sent to the CMH Surgical Oncology Department. The physical examination revealed a nodule in the right anterior of the neck that moved upward when the patient swallowed. The nodule had a size of approximately 5 × 4 × 3 cm and a firm, mobile, smooth surface. The temperature was the same as that of the surrounding tissue. Jugular, submandible, and submental lymph nodes were not palpable (Figure 1).

On February 6, 2015, the patient underwent isthmolobectomy surgery. Her last laboratory tests showed a normal blood count, except for a differential count, and the routine biochemical blood test results were within normal ranges. Euthyroid state was confirmed by the laboratory result. The preoperative clinical diagnosis was struma nodosa non-toxic suspected as a malignant T3N0M0. Intraoperative pathological consultation using frozen sections supported a diagnosis of WDTC transformed to ATC. According to this result, the surgeon decided to perform a total thyroidectomy in this patient. Tissue samples were sent to the CMH Anatomical Pathology Department.

Cytology Findings

FNAB smears contained diffuse clusters of large cells with abundant granular eosinophylic cytoplasm. These cells had pleomorphic nuclei, coarse chromatin, and some showed prominent nucleoli. There were scattered giant cells and multinucleated giant cells. More than 75% of the aspirate was composed of these oncocyte cells. The FNAB findings suggested a diagnosis of folicular neoplasm of the Hürthle cell type.

Macroscopic and Histologic Presentation

Grossly, the resected right thyroid measured 6 × 5 × 4 cm and was brown to red, firm, and encapsulated. The surface was smooth, and the cut surface was brown and lobulated. Calcification and papillar growth were not seen (Figure 4). The left thyroid lobe measured 3 × 1.5 × 0.5 cm and was brown to black and firm. The sentinel lymph nodes were also sent to the Anatomic Pathology Department.

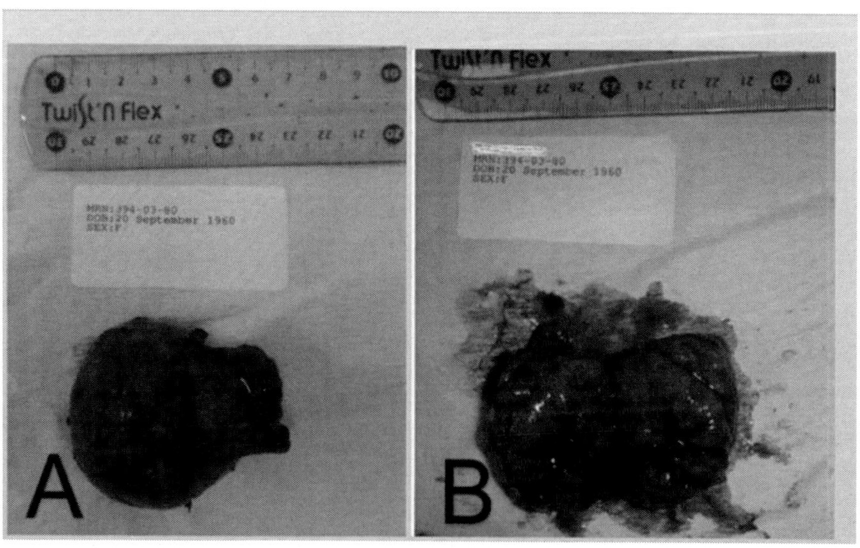

Figure 4. Gross appearance. The thyroid size is approximately 6 x 5 x 4 cm and is brown to red, firm, and encapsulated. The surface is smooth, and the cut surface is brown tinted and lobulated. Calcification and papillary growth are not seen.

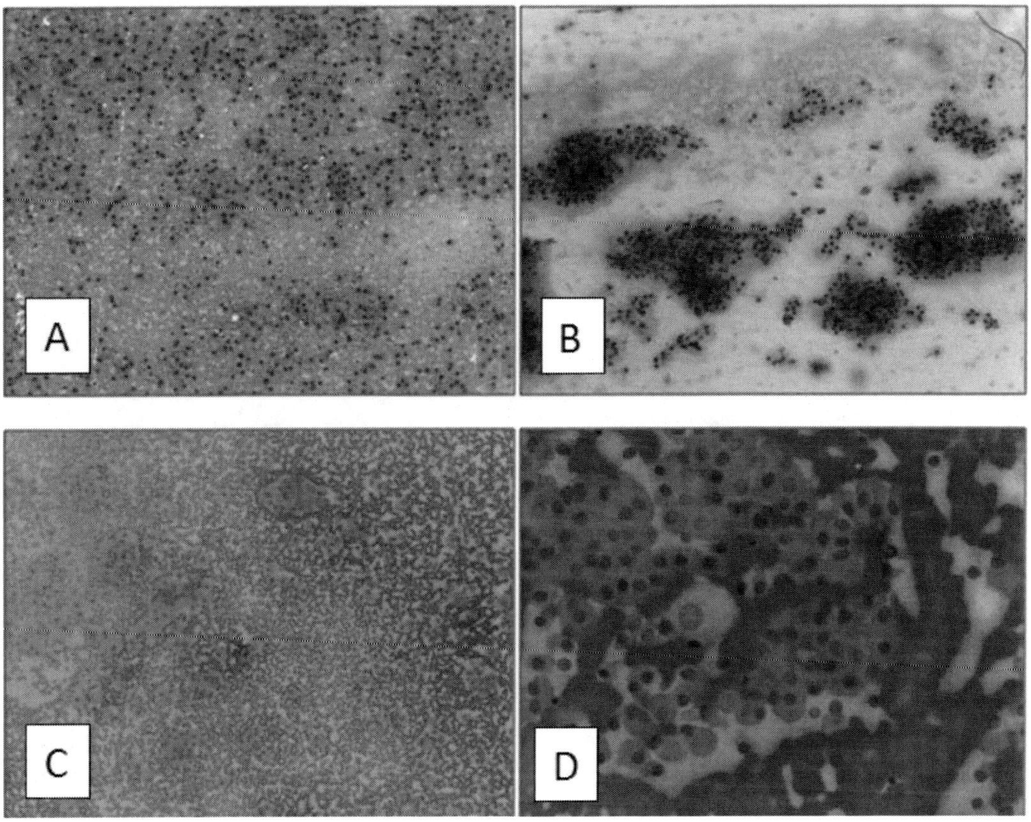

Figure 5. Cytologic features of FNAB. (a, b) Dispersed cluster of epithelial cells with atypical enlarged nuclei and abundant eosinophylic (Giemsastain, 10×). (c, d) The cells have granular eosinophylic cytoplasm (Papanicolaoustain A.100×, B 400×).

Histologic examination showed large tumor cells in a trabecular arrangement, small follicles with scanty colloid, and a solid pattern. The cells were polygonal to square shaped, had distinct cell borders, rounded nuclei, coarse chromatin, some vesicules with prominent nucleoli, and abundant granular eosinophilic cytoplasm (Figure 7). One section shows an area containing bizarre giant cells with irregular hypercromatic nuclei and prominent nucleoli (Figure 8). Another area shows tumor cells with eosinophylic cytoplasm and heights three times their width (Figure 9). The tumor was diagnosed as a mixed tall cell variant of papillary thyroid carcinoma (TCVPTC) and HCC transformed to ATC. Tissue sampling from the left lobe shows adenomatous struma. Non-sentinel nodes were considered to indicate non-specific chronic lymphadenitis. Second opinions and further investigation proved that the correct diagnosis was HCC with bizarre nuclei. ATC is difficult to manage, its management often need combination of surgery, radiotherapy and chemotherapy [2]. HCC is radio-iodine resistant and the best theraphy approach has emerge controversy between expert. Some expert recommend conservative management while others suggest aggressive treatment [3].

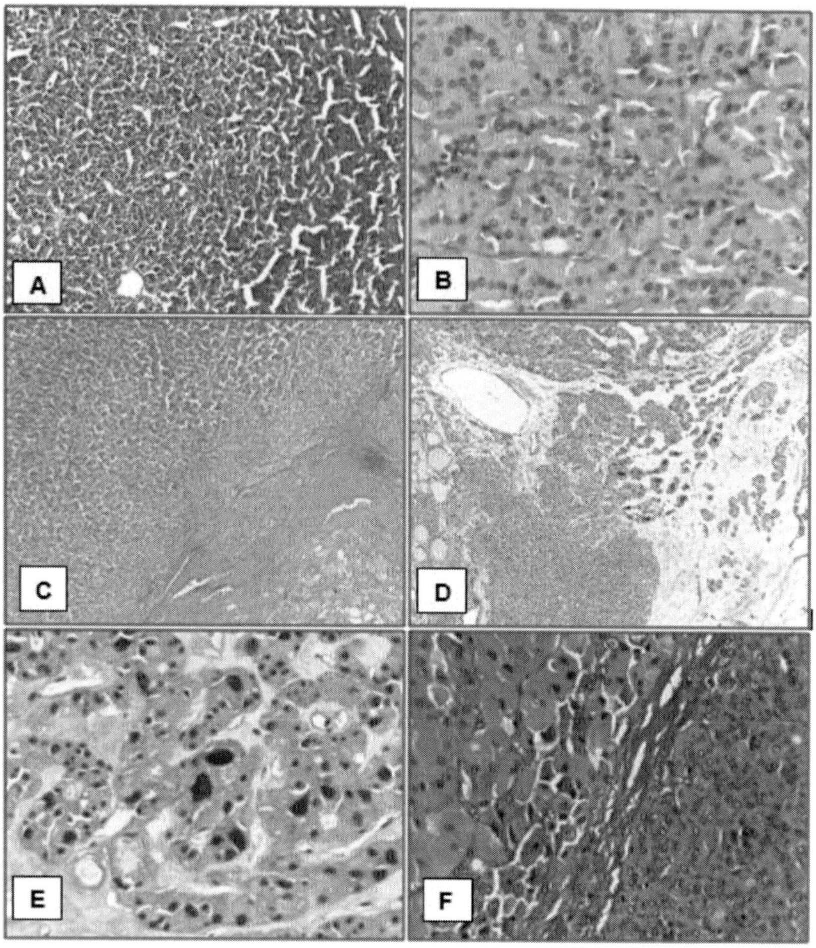

Figure 6. Variable appearance of HCC. (a) The cells are arranged in a trabecular pattern and have columnar to square shapes [hematoxylin and eosin (HE) 10×]. (b) HCC has abundant granular cytoplasm with vesicular nuclei and prominent nucleoli (HE, 4000×). (c) Area of capsular invasion (HE, 40×). (d) Area containing bizarre giant cells with hyperchromatic irregular nuclei (HE, 40×). (e) The tumor shows a follicular pattern with scanty colloid and bizarre cells dispersed among the other cells (HE, 400×). (f) Solid area composed of polygonal large cells with abundant cytoplasm and pleomorphic nuclei (HE, 400×).

DISCUSSION

FNAB is regarded worldwide as the first approach to thyroid nodule evaluation. It is a simple, safe, and cost-effective method for correctly characterizing the nature of a lesion in >70% cases [11, 12]. In our case, the smears showed dispersed and clustered monotonous proliferation of Hürthle cells and scanty colloid without nuclear features of papillary thyroid carcinoma. The observed features matched the diagnostic criteria for a follicular neoplasm of Hürthle cell type. In general, it is recommended that all patients with cytologically suspicious HCT undergo surgical resection [13-15].

Our patient initially underwent isthmolobectomy. Frozen section examination revealed WDTC transformed to ATC, so the surgeon decided to perform a total thyroidectomy on this patient. The mainstay of treatment for all differentiated thyroid cancers is surgical resection, and HCC is no exception. Once an HCC is histologically confirmed following diagnostic thyroid lobectomy, a complete thyroidectomy should be considered. Histopathological analysis remains the gold standard for diagnosis, although it may be apparent preoperatively if there is evidence of metastasis. Malignant HCT requires aggressive surgery because it is poorly responsive to chemotherapy, does not concentrate iodine, and is generally not radiosensitive.

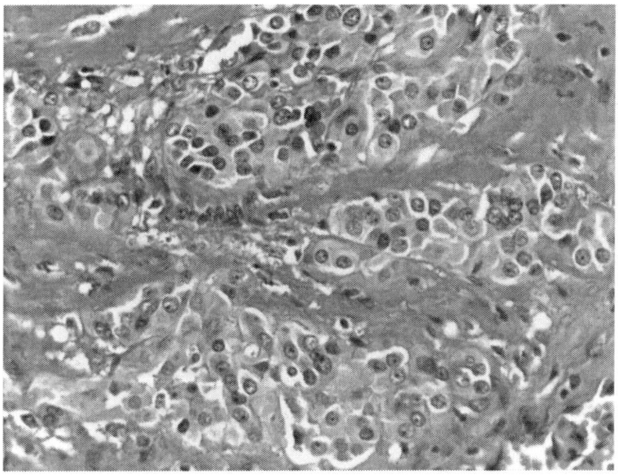

Figure 7. Hürthle cells showing polygonal to square shapes with distinct cell borders, rounded nuclei, coarse chromatin, vesicules with prominent nucleoli, and abundant granular eosinophilic cytoplasm (HE, 400×).

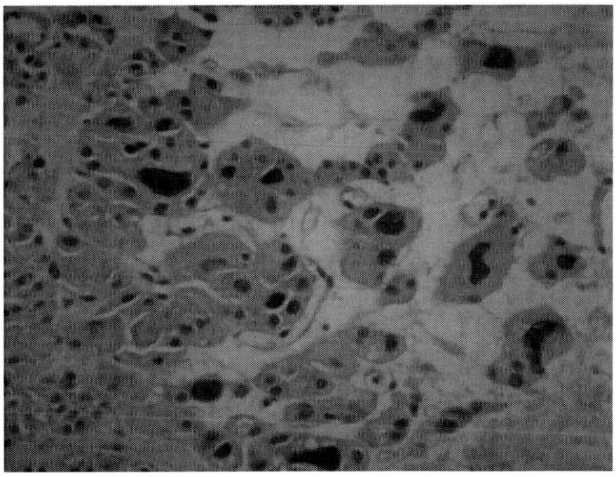

Figure 8. HCT may contain bizarre giant nuclei. This is not an indicator of malignancy, however (HE, 400×).

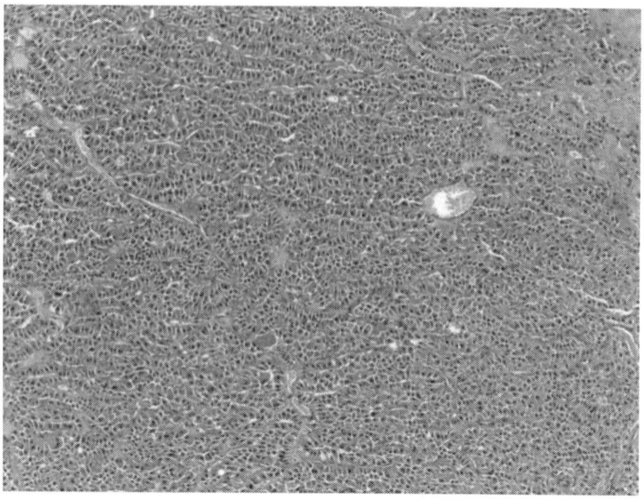

Figure 9. HCT arranged in a trabecular pattern. The cells are tall or columnar. Note the hyperchromatic nuclei. There are no nuclear features of papillary thyroid carcinoma (HE, 100×).

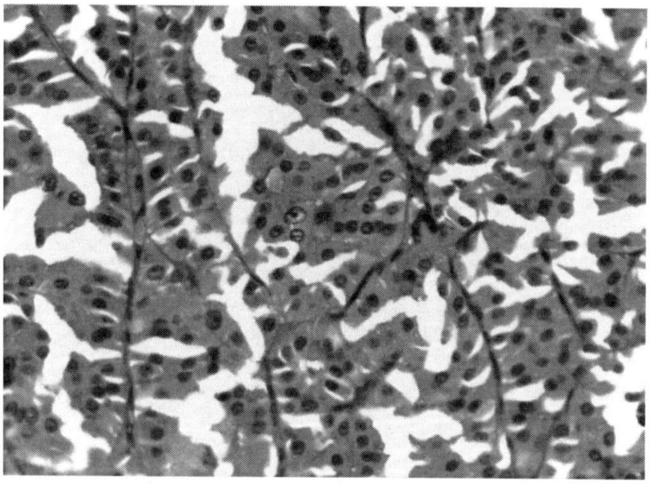

Figure 10. Discohesive growth of neoplastic cells can simulate papillary structure. This is not true papillary growth (HE, 400×).

Indeed, because of the relatively reduced avidity of HCC for radioactive iodine, and the resultant compromised efficacy of treatment, complete surgical resection is important [5, 12]. ATC is uncommonly identified as a small incidental finding after surgical resection of a predominantly non-anaplastic tumor. The role for total thyroidectomy when an initial lobectomy has been performed is based more on the characteristics of non-anaplastic malignancy than on the incidental finding of ATC [16].

A paraffin block histopathology examination led to a diagnosis of mixed HCC and TCVPTC transformed to ATC. Further examination of the resected thyroid mass showed thyroid tissue containing a malignant tumor mass in a small follicular with scanty colloid trabecular arrangement and some solid areas. The neoplastic cells were mostly polygonal to square in shape, with distinct borders and abundant eosinophilic granular cytoplasm.

Some cells were columnar with hyperchromatic nuclei. Nuclear grooves, nuclear clearing, nuclear crowding, and pseudoinclusion were not present. This finding excluded a diagnosis of TCVPTC.

Hürthle cells are large polygonal cells with distinct borders derived from thyroid follicular epithelium. They contain abundant granular cytoplasm, because of excess mitochondria, and have a large nucleus with a prominent nucleolus. Hürthle cells can be observed in both benign and malignant conditions. The mechanism behind mitochondrial abundance in these conditions is not completely understood, but it is probably a reflection of excessive mitochondrial proliferation and/or decreased mitochondrial degradation [5, 17]. This is a phenomenon of metaplasia that occurs in inflammatory disorders, such as thyroiditis, or other situations that result in cellular stress. Oncocytes proliferation gives rise to hyperplastic and neoplastic nodules [7].

The genetic abnormalities identified in HCT include aneuploidy, H-RAS mutations, allelic alterations, and alterations in mitochondrial DNA [14]. HCT have lower prevalences of RAS gene mutation and PAX8/PPARG rearrangement than those of their counterparts lacking oncocytic change. The TP53 mutation has been identified in 10%-20% of oncocytic follicular carcinomas lacking high-grade or poorly differentiated features, sometimes in association with PTEN mutations [17, 18].

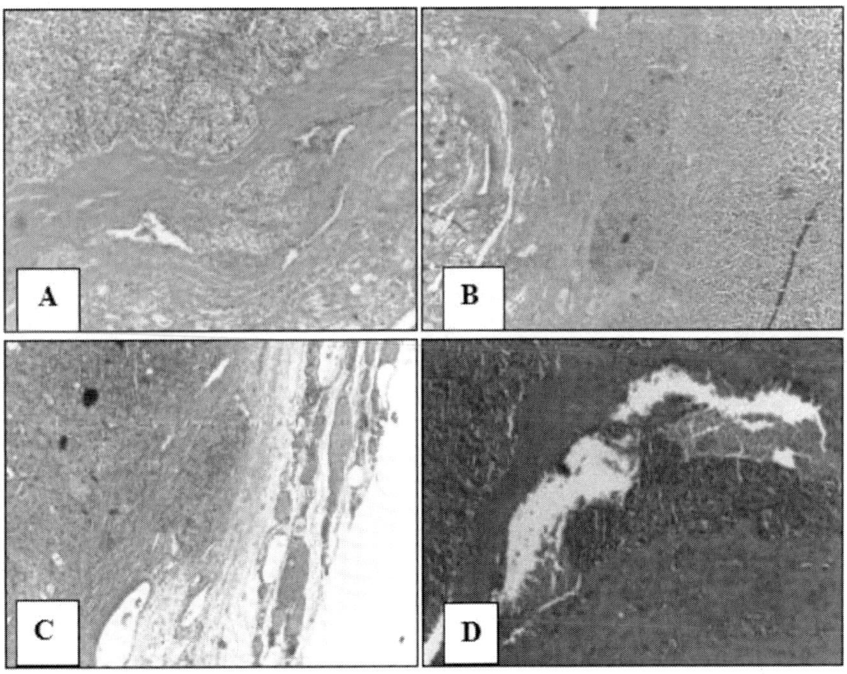

Figure 11. (a-c) Capsular invasion of the tumor. (d) Vascular invasion (a-d, HE, 100×).

HCC is currently classified as a variant of follicular carcinoma and is also known as oncocytic or oxyphilic carcinoma, which is defined as a thyroid malignancy consisting of ≥75% Hürthle cells. HCC differs from its benign counterpart by the presence of capsular and/or vascular invasion or the presence of metastatic disease [3, 8, 17]. The histologic distinction between HCA and HCC is determined by the presence or absence of capsular and/or vascular invasion [5-19]. HCA can be distinguished from HCC with criteria similar to those for non-Hürthle follicular tumors. HCA is an encapsulated tumor, and no invasion is seen. HCT with capsular invasion is classified as minimally invasive HCC. HCT with limited vascular invasion (<4 vessels) and extensive vascular invasion (≥4 vessels) is classified as an encapsulated angioinvasion HCC. Widely invasive HCC shows extensive invasion of the thyroid and extra-thyroidal soft tissue [20]. In our case, we found several foci of capsular invasion and one focal of vascular invasion. Therefore, we categorized our case as an encapsulated, angioinvasive HCC.

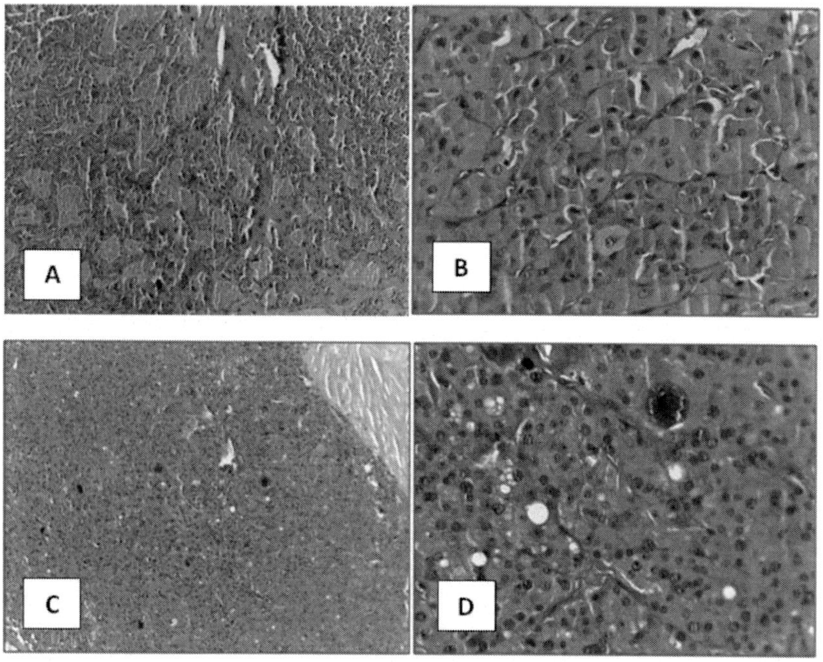

Figure 12. Another feature of HCC. (a) HCC can show hemorrhagic areas. These areas can develop spontaneously or be an effect of previous FNAB (HE, 100×). (b) Solid area with voluminous eosinophilic cytoplasm, vesicular nuclei with prominent nucleoli (HE, 400×). (c, d) Predominantly solid with scattered bizarre nuclei (HE, 10×, HE, 40×).

HCC prognosis is related to the extent of vascular invasion. The more veins are invaded by tumors, the less favorable the prognosis. Factors other than vascular invasion are associated with overall survival in HCC patients. Goffredo et al. [17] determined that older age, larger tumor size, extrathyroidal tumor extension, and not undergoing surgery were associated with reduced overall survival of HCC. Tumor size is an important feature of biological behavior. A Hürthle cell tumor that is ≥3.5 cm has a 67% risk of malignancy [20].

There are some additional morphological and architectural features that can reliably differentiate benign from malignant HCT. The more accurate parameters for a carcinoma diagnosis include the concept of small-cell dysplasia, large-cell dysplasia, syncytia, crowding, and a dispersive cellular pattern [20]. The presence of mitosis, a solid or trabecular growth pattern, extrathyroidal extension, and presence of lymph node metastases are among the histologic features that predict recurrence [17].

In some neoplasm areas, bizarre giant cells are seen. The cells show large, irregular, bizarre, markedly atypical, hyperchromatic nuclei, and some vesicular with prominent nucleoli. The number of cytoplasms ranged from high to abundant, with eosinophilic and granular characteristics. These findings were previously interpreted as characteristic of the giant cell type of ATC. A second opinion pointed out that giant cells are seen in HCC. According to the literature, both benign and malignant thyroid lesions contain so-called "cells of endocrine atypia" or cells with "bizarre nuclei", these manifest as single cells or small groups displaying marked cellular and nuclear enlargement, some degree of pleomorphism, marked cellular hyperchromasia, and occasionally macronucleoli randomly dispersed among otherwise differentiated thyroid follicular cells. Their occurrence can be extremely worrisome. When these enormous cells are observed in HCT, it is probably better not to definitively diagnose such a case as ATC [10].

We performed some immunohistochemical analyses to support our diagnosis as HCC rather than ATC. HCC will show reactivity to TTF-1 and thyroglobulin, whereas ATC will not react to either marker [10, 21]. In our case, the TTF-1 and thyroglobulin were positive in all areas, including the solid area and the area containing bizarre giant cells.

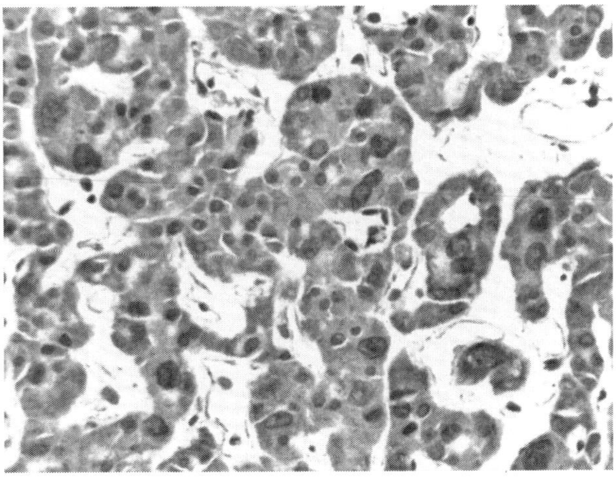

Figure 13. The tumor showed reactivity to thyroglobulin marker (IHC 400×).

A small portion of HCC undergoes transformation to ATC [20]. HCC have a greater propensity for malignant transformation to anaplastic carcinomas than do other WDTC [7]. In our case, the immunohistochemical analyses failed to show the ATC transformation since a thyroglobulin marker showed reactivity in all tumor areas. Overdiagnosis of HCC to ATC can cause unnecessary alarm because ATC has short-term survival, with a mortality rate >90% and a mean survival time of six months after diagnosis, whereas HCC has higher survival rates ranging from 85% for minimally invasive lesions to near 10% for widely invasive cases [20].

Conclusion

Hürthle cell proliferation can lead to hyperplastic or neoplastic nodules. HCT is a rare thyroid neoplasm of follicular cell origin, and >75% of these neoplasms are composed of cells with oncocytic features. The diagnoses of HCA and HCC are differentiated based on capsular or vascular invasion and the presence of metastases. HCC's histologic appearance is highly variable. An accurate HCC diagnosis, accompanied by identification of prognostic factors, enables evidence-based management decisions. Bizarre nuclei can occur in benign and malignant HCTs and should be assessed carefully to prevent overdiagnosis.

References

[1] Eloy, C; Ferreira, L; Saldago, C; Soares, P; Sobrinho-Simoes M. Poorly differentiated and undifferentiated thyroid carcinomas. *Turk Patoloji Derg* 201531, 48-59.

[2] Li M; Milas M; Nasr C; Brainard JA; Khan MJ; Burkey BB; et al. Anaplastic thyroid cancer in young patient: A contemporary review. *Am. J. Otolaryngol.* 201334, 636-40.

[3] Barnabei, A; Ferretti, E; Baldelli Procaccini, A; Spriano, G; Appetecchia, M. Hürthle cell tumors of the thyroid. Personal experience and review of the literature. *Acta Otorhinolaryngol. Ital.* 200929, 305-11.

[4] Okere, PCN; Olusina, DB; Enyinnah, MO. Hurthe cell tumor of the thyroid gland: Report of a rare case and review of literature. *Niger J. Clin. Pract.* 201417, 375-7.

[5] Ahmadi, S; Stang, M; Jiang, XS; Sosa, JA. Hürthle cell carcinoma: current persepectives. *Onco Targets Ther.* 20169, 6873-84.

[6] Ganly, I; Filho, JR; Eng, S; Ghossein, R; Morris, LGT; Liang, Y; et al. Genomic dissection of Hürthle cell carcinoma reveals a unique class of thyroid malignancy. *J. Clin. Endocrinol. Metab.* 201498, 962-72.

[7] Aytug S. *Hürthle cell carcinoma.* [Internet]. 2015. [cited 2015 April 13] Available from: http://emedicine.medscape.com/article/279462-overview.

[8] Mills, SC; Haq, M; Smellie, WJB; Harmer, C. Hürthle cell carcinoma of thyroid: Retrospective review of 62 patients treated at Royal Marsden Hospital between 1946 and 2003. EJSO200935, 230-4.

[9] Rosai, J; De Lellis, RA; Carcangiu Frable, WJ; Tallini, G. Thyroid tumors with oncocytic (Hürthle cell) features. In: Caton MQ; Thomas DS; Silve MC; Black AN; editors. Atlas of tumor pathology tumors of thyroid and parathyroid glands. 4th series. Washington; DC. Armed Forces Institute of Pathology. 2014.

[10] Talbot, I; DO; Wakely PE. Undiffentiated (anaplastic) thyroid carcinoma: Practical immunohistochemistry and cytologic look-alikes. *Seminars in Diagnostic Pathology*. 201532, 305-10.

[11] Faquin, WC; Michael, CW; Renshaw, AA; Vielh, P. Folicular neoplasm; Hürthle cell type/suspicious for a follicular neoplasam; Hürthle cell type. In: Ali SZ; Cibas ES; editors. *The Bethesda system for reporting cytopathology*. 2010. London: Springer; 2010. p. 51-73.

[12] Ristevka, N; Satojanoski, S; Gjorceva, DP. Appearance of Hürthle cell carcinoma soon after surgical extirpation of Hürthle cell adenoma and follicular adenoma of the thyroid gland. *Radiol. Oncol*. 201549, 26-31.

[13] Lee, KH; Shin, JH; Ko, ES; Hahn, SY; Kim, JS; Kim, JH; et al. Predictive factors of malignancy with cytologically suspicious for Hürthle cell neoplasm of thyroid nodules. *Int. J. Surg. Res*. 201311, 898-902.

[14] Cannon, J. The significance of Hürthle cells in thyroid disease. *Oncologist* 201116, 1380-7.

[15] Tai, P; Korzeniowski, M; Sadikov, E; Joseph, K; Kirbi, A; Tonita, J; et al. Issues in managing Hürthle cell carcinoma of thyroid: A case report. *Cureus* 20179, 1-6.

[16] Smallridge, RC; Ain, KB; Asa, Sl; Bible, KC; Brierley, JD; Burman, KD; et al. American thyroid association guidelines for management of patients with anaplastic thyroid cancer. *Thyroid* 201222, 1104-37.

[17] Goffredo, P; Roman, SA; Sosa, JA. Hürthle cell carcinoma: A population-level analysis of 3311 patients. *Cancer* 20132, 505-11.

[18] Máximo, V; Lima, J; Prazeres, H; Soares, P; Sobrinho-Simoes, M. The biology and the genetics of Hürthle cell tumors of the thyroid. *Endocr. Relat. Cancer* 201219, 131-47.

[19] Sandoval, MA; Paz-Pacheco, E. Hürthle cell carcinoma of the thyroid. *Case Reports* 20112011, bcr1120103536.

[20] LiVolsi, V; Baloch, ZW; Simoes, SM; Tallini, G. Hürthle (oncocytic) tumors. In: DeLellis, RA; Lloyd, RV; Heinz, PU; Eng, C; editors. *World Health Organization classification of tumors of endocrine organ*. Lyon: IARC; 2017. p. 96-9.

[21] Liu, H; Lin, F. Application of immunohistochemistry in thyroid pathology. *Arch. Pathol. Lab. Med*. 2015139, 71-82.

In: Case Reports in Surgery
Editors: Ahmad Jabir Rahyussalim et al.

ISBN: 978-1-53616-582-1

Chapter 31

INVASIVE BREAST CARCINOMA MIMICKING SECRETORY CARCINOMA: A CASE REPORT

Patricia Fransisca Julianty, Primariadewi Rustamadji** *and Hartono Tjahjadi

Department of Anatomical Pathology, Faculty of Medicine,
Universitas Indonesia, Jakarta, Indonesia

ABSTRACT

Secretory carcinoma is an exceptionally rare typeof invasive breast cancer in the special subtype classification of World Health Organization 2012. It occurs in <0.15% of all breast cancers and has a distinct histomorphology, which is characterized by the presence of intracellular and extracellular eosinophilic secretory materials. It generally shows triple negativity for estrogen receptor, progesterone receptor, and human epidermal growth factor 2and shows strong reactivity for S-100 protein. We report the case of a 54-year-old woman with invasive breast carcinoma. The histomorphology mimicked that of secretory carcinoma, with unusual immunohistochemical findings typical of secretory carcinoma. However, secretory carcinoma is associated with a characteristic translocation that creates *ETV6–NTRK3* gene fusion, which was not observed in this case. Despite the considerable resemblance with secretory carcinoma, this case was ultimately diagnosed as invasive breast carcinoma of no special type.

Keywords: Invasive breast carcinoma, no special type, secretory carcinoma

* Corresponding Author's E-mail: primariadewi@yahoo.com.

INTRODUCTION

Invasive breast carcinoma is the most common carcinoma occurring in women and accounts for 23% of all cancers in women globally and 27% in affluent countries. The World Health Organization (WHO) Classification of Tumours of the Breast,Fourth Edition[1], categorizesbreast cancers that do not havesufficient characteristics as a specific histological typeknown as "carcinoma of no special type" (NST). Invasive NST carcinoma is the most common type of invasive carcinoma of the breast, accounting for 40%–75% of cases in published series [1].

Secretory carcinoma (SC) is anexceptionally rare type of breast cancer in the special subtype classification of WHO. It occurs in < 0.15% of all breast cancers [2]. Itwas first observedin young children and was therefore initially calledjuvenile breast; later, it was observed to occur in all ages and soTavassoli and Norris recommended the term SC as abetter description of its clinical spectrum and behavior [3]. SCoccurs in both females and malesof ages 9–69 (median, 25) years. Moreover, it can occur in any part of the breast, with the central region being the most frequentlocation[4]. SC has a distinct histomorphology, which is characterized by the presence of intracellular and extracellular eosinophilic secretory materials with papillary, solid, microcystic, and tubular architecture. A consistent findingis thepresence of intracellular and extracellular secretory materials that is positive for periodic acid–Schiff (PAS) staining, resistant to PAS-diastase, and positive for Alcian blue (AB) staining [2, 3]. Moreover, the cells are oflow to moderate nuclear grade and exhibit low mitotic activity [2-4]. SC generally shows triple negativity for estrogen receptor (ER), progesterone receptor (PR), and human epidermal growth factor 2 (HER2), and strong reactivity for S-100 protein [4, 5]. It is associated with a characteristic translocation, t (12;15), whichcreates the *ETV6–NTRK3* gene fusion [2].

Invasive carcinoma NST has prognostic characteristic and management are similar or slightly worse compared to breast cancer as a whole.The prognosisis greatly influenced byclassical variables such as histological grade, tumor size, lymphnode status, vascular invasion, and the predictors of therapeutic response [1]. The prognosis forSC is better thaninvasive carcinoma NST:recurrence and distant metastasis are extremely rare [4], and even lymph node metastasis is associated with excellent prognosis if only a few lymph node are involved [6]. Themanagement of invasive NST carcinoma depends on the prognostic and predictive characteristics [1].There areno consensus guidelines for the treatment of SC because of its rarity, but modified radical mastectomy can be an option for tumors larger than 2 cm in diameterwith poor gross circumscription [6, 7].

Here, we report a case of a 54-year-old woman withinvasive breast carcinoma that mimickedSC; however,it was ultimately found not to have the fusion gene specific to SC. The histomorphology features were deceptive, and little is known about SCand its mimicking; it is therefore useful to report such cases as maximum information can be made available for precise diagnosis.

CASE REPORT

A54-year-old woman presented with a painless lump in herright breast, which she had first noticedtwo yearspreviously. It had gradually increased in size during the previous year and, 7 months previously, the patient also noticed a mass in the axillary region. There was no history of breast carcinoma in herfamily. She attended our hospital on September 19th 2016.

A physical examination revealed amobile, hard, firm, painless nodule with a well-defined border, locatedin the upper medial quadrant of herright breast inthe areolar region. There was noskin ulceration or nipple discharge. Ultrasonography showed a heterogenous hypoechoic mass with calcification in the upper inner quadrant of the right breast; itmeasured 2×2×2.4cm, with an ill-defined margin. In addition, there was enlargement of the right axillary lymph node without a central hilum, measuring 1.5×0.8cm. Abdominal ultrasonography and thoracic X-ray imaging showed no signs of metastatic lesions.

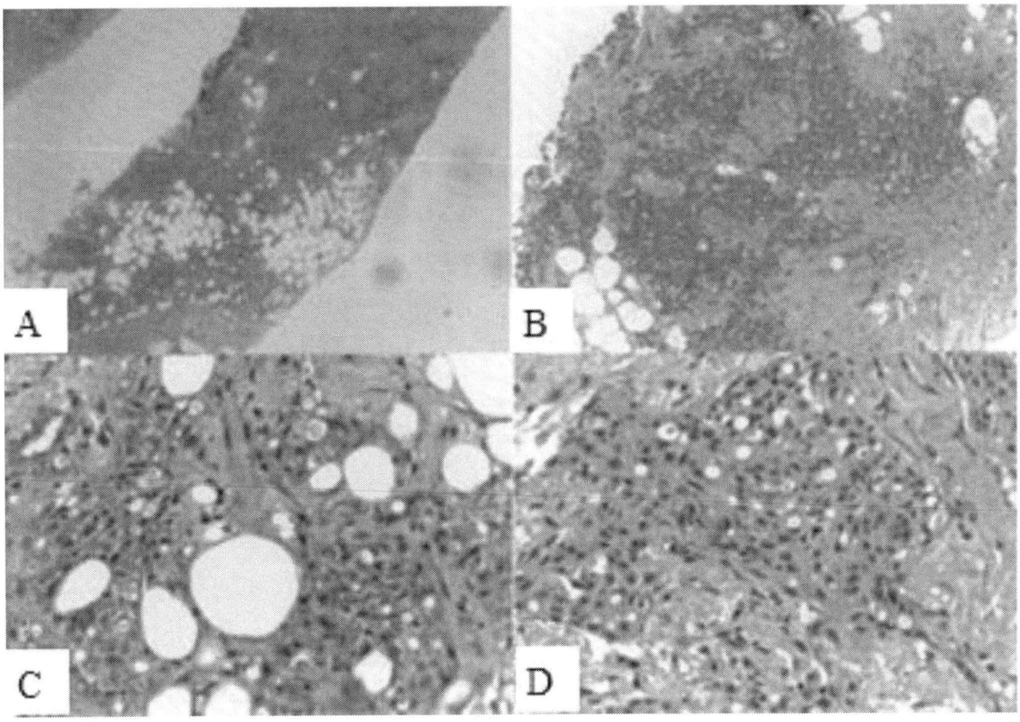

Figure 1. Core biopsy. (a, b) The tumor cells were arranged in a trabecular infiltrative nest. (a) H&E stain,40×. (b) H&E stain,100×. (c, d) The nuclei were moderate in size and hyperchromatic with eosinophilic cytoplasm. Both H&E stain,400×. H&E, hematoxylin and eosin.

A coreneedle biopsy was performed on September 29th. The specimen showed epithelial neoplastic cells arranged in a trabecular infiltrative nest with no tubule formation. The nuclei were moderate in size andhyperchromatic, with eosinophilic cytoplasm (Figure 1). The mitotic count was fewer than 5 per 10 high-power fields. No vascular invasion wasobserved. The tumorwas diagnosed as invasive NSTcarcinoma, grade 2 (tubule score = 3; nuclear score = 2; mitotic score = 1; total score = 6).

A fineneedle aspiration biopsy was performed on November 21st as part of aspecial educational and experimental study. Thisrevealed the tumor cells to be clustered and dispersed, withpleomorphic nuclei, coarse chromatin, and irregular membranes, with eosinophilic cytoplasm and intracytoplasmic vacuolization (Figure 2). The diagnosis was breastcarcinoma.

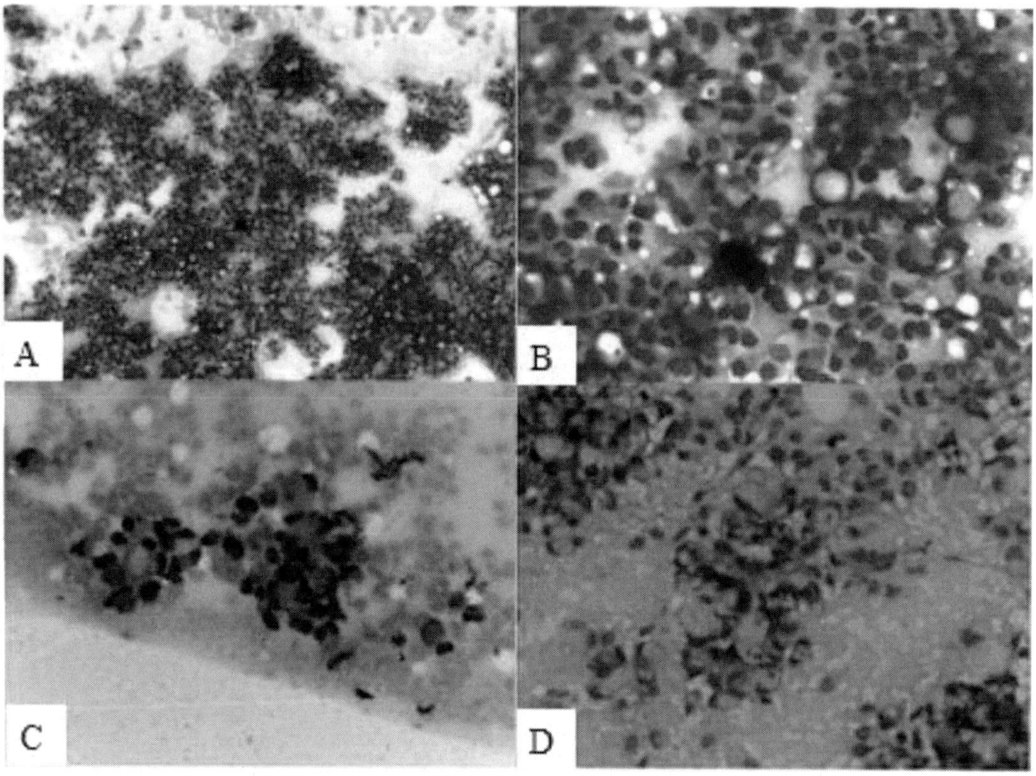

Figure 2. Fine needle aspiration biopsy smears. (a) The tumorcells were clustered. Giemsa stain,100×. (b, c) The tumor cells hadpleomorphic nucleiwith eosinophilic cytoplasm and intracytoplasmic vacuolization. Giemsa stain, 400×. (d) Clusters of tumorcells. Papanicolaou stain, 400×.

A modifiedradical mastectomy was performed on December 7th and the specimen was sent for pathological examination. On gross examination, the tumor was 3×2.5×2.5cm in size, ill-defined, firm, and white to tan (Figure 3). It waslocated 2 cm from the areola in the upper inner quadrant.

Microscopic examination showed the tumor mass had asolid pattern with infiltrative nests. Tubule formation was observedin less than 10% of the tumor area. The tumorcells hadround or oval nucleithatvaried in size from moderate to large. They were vesicular, with scattered nucleoli andeosinophilic to pale cytoplasm.The cytoplasm was vacuolated,with abundant eosinophilic material in the lumina (Figure 4). The mitotic count was 6per10high-power fields.

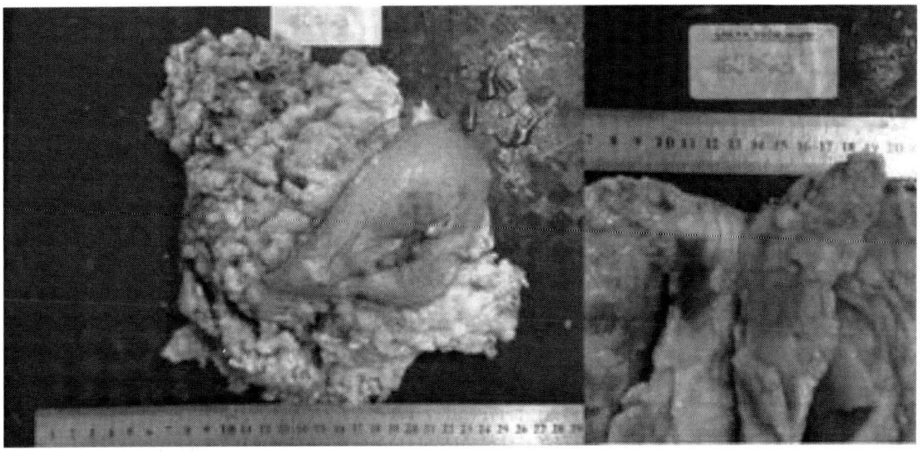

Figure 3. Gross specimen. The tumorwas firm andill-defined.

There was notumor infiltration into the areola, skin, orsurgical margins. When the secretory material was stained with PAS and AB, the PAS staining persisted after diastase digestion (Figure 5). Specimens from dissection of theaxillary lymph nodes at levels I and II revealedmetastasis in one ofthethree lymph node. On the basis of these findings, the tumorwas diagnosed as SC, grade 2 (tubule score = 3; nuclear score = 3; mitotic score = 1; total score = 7), with a recommendation for immunostaining.

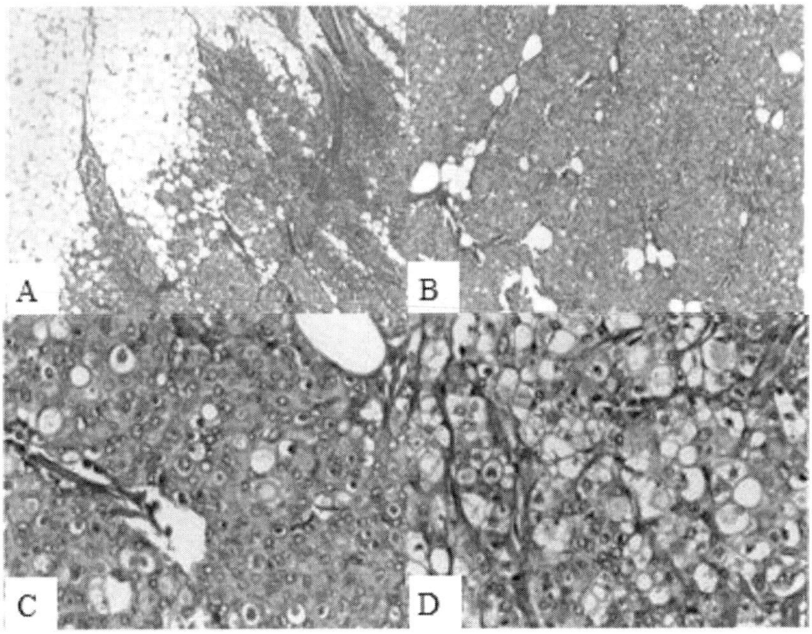

Figure 4. (a, b) Tumor cells showing the solidpattern and infiltrative nest. (a) H&E stain,40×. (b) H&E stain, 100×. (c, d) The tumorcells hadround or oval, moderate to large nuclei, which were vesicular, with scattered nucleoli andeosinophilic to pale cytoplasm. The cytoplasm was vacuolated with eosinophilic material. H&Estain, 400×. H&E, hematoxylin and eosin.

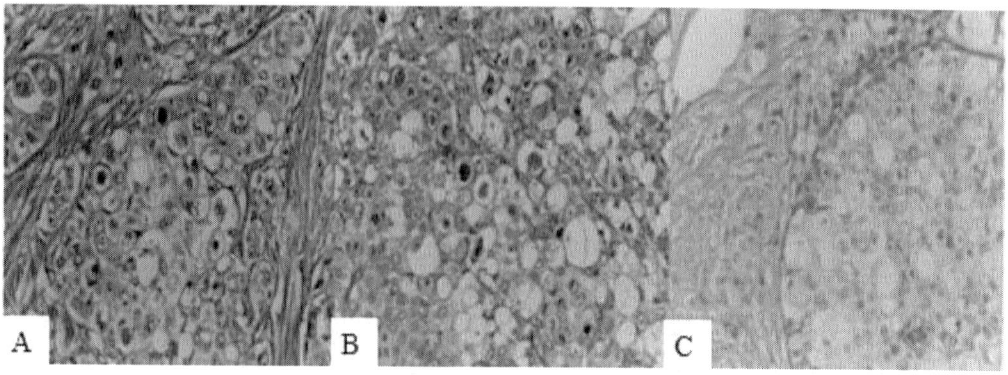

Figure 5. The eosinophilicmaterial. The specimen was (A)positive forperiodic acid–Schiff (PAS) staining, (B)resistant to PAS-diastase, (C)and positive for Alcian bluestaining. All 400×.

Immunohistochemically, the neoplastic cells were positive for ER (80%), negative for PR, and expressed HER2 with a score of 2+ (weak membranous staining). Subsequent chromogenic in situ hybridization showed no amplification of HER2. In addition, 15% of the tumor cells were positive for Ki67, and the cells were negative for S-100 protein, positive for carcinoembryonic antigen, positive forE-cadherin, and negative for CD117 (Figure 6).

A paraffin-embedded cell block was tested for the *ETV6–NTRK3* fusion gene, which characterizes SC, at the Prince of Wales Hospital, Hong Kong, using a fluorescence in situ hybridization break-apart probe kit. This demonstrated the absence of the *ETV6–NTRK3* fusion gene (Figure 7).

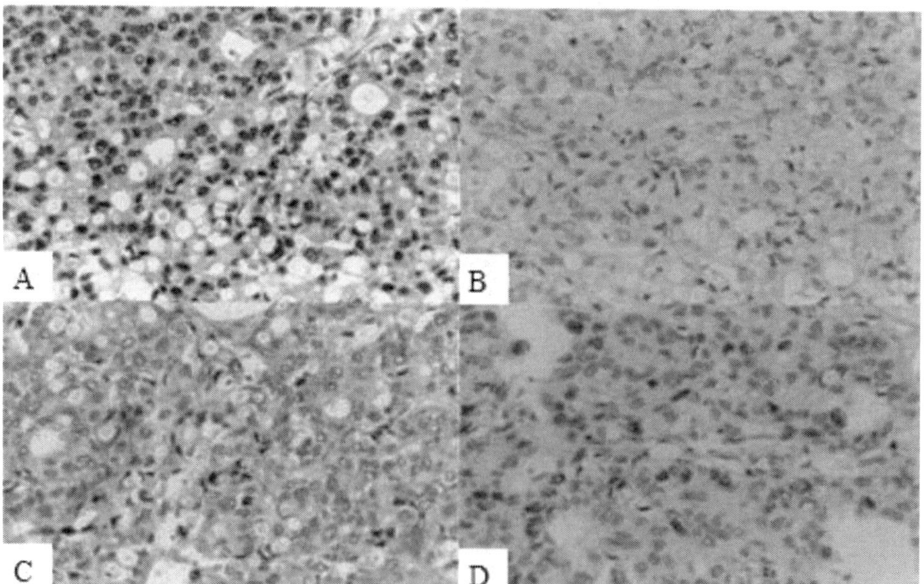

Figure 6. (Continued).

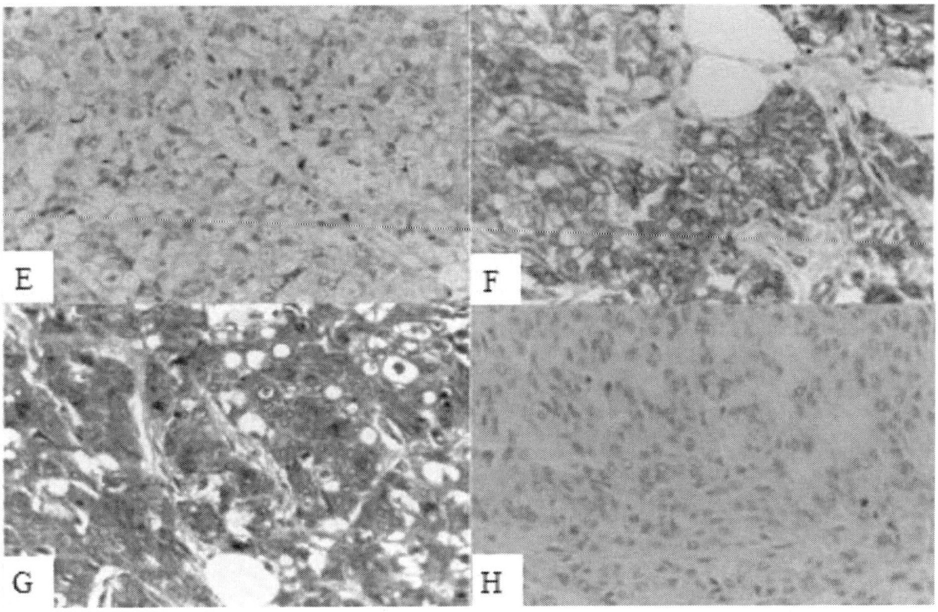

Figure 6. Immunohistochemical staining showed that the cells were (a) estrogen receptor-positive, (b) progesterone receptor-negative, (c) did not overexpress HER2, (d) positive for Ki67 (15%of the cells), (e) negative for S-100 protein, (f) positive for E-cadherin, (g) positive for carcinoembryonic antigen, (h) andnegative for CD117. All 400×.

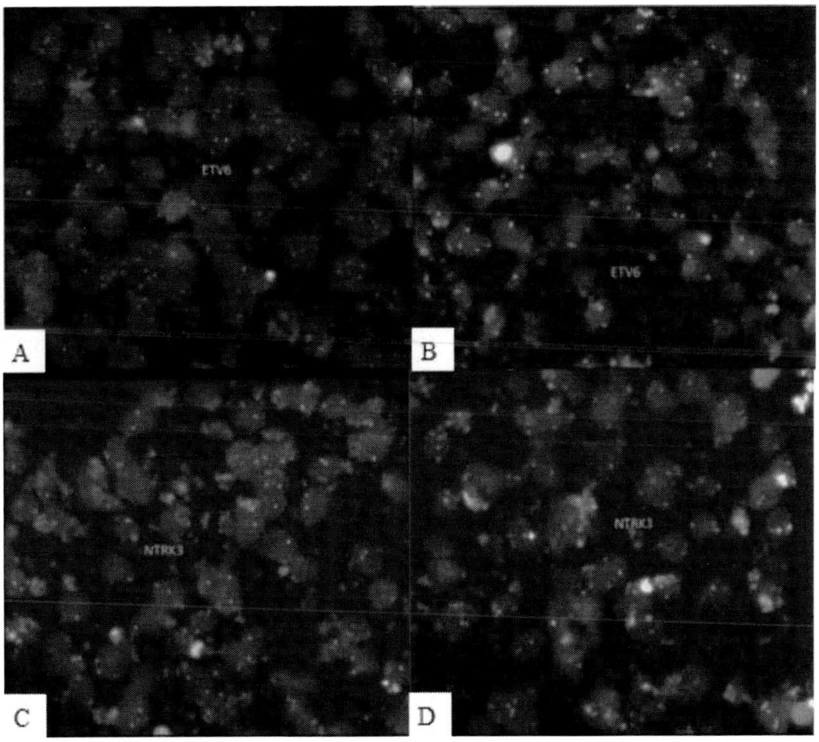

Figure 7. Results of the *ETV6–NTRK3* fusion gene test using a fluorescence in situ hybridization break-apart probe. (a, b) The cells were negative for the *ETV6* translocation. (c, d) The cells were negative for the *NTRK3* translocation.

The patient was administered aromatase inhibitor hormonal therapy, anastrozole, without chemotherapy or radiotherapy. At 10 months after the surgery, she remains well, without local recurrence or distant metastases.

Discussion

SC is a rare subtype of breast malignancy that accounts for less than 0.15% of all breast cancer [2]. During a six-year period, from January 2011 until December 2016, our hospital experienced only three cases, although none of these were tested for the fusion gene.

The signs and symptoms of our patient initially appeared to be consistent with SC. She was aged 54years; SC has been stages from 9 to 69 [3], with about one-half of cases older than 20 years, and a substantial number aged between 50 and 69 years [8]. The nodule in her right breast was painless and was first noticed two years two years previously, gradually increasing in size over the previous year. SC is a slow-growing, painless, well-circumscribed, mobile, palpable mass [2,6]. In our patient, the single mass was 3×2.5×2.5 cm in size, ill-defined, firm, and white to tan in color, and it was located 2 cm from the areola in the upper inner quadrant. SC can occur in any part of the breast, with the central region of the breast the most prevalent location. It usually grows as a single mass and ranges in size from 0.5 to 12 cm (mean, 3 cm) [2, 8]. The cut surface varies from grayish-white or yellow to tan in color [2, 3].

Fine needle aspiration smears of SC are characterized by the presence of a globular structure comprising small, centrally located, mucoid material, usually covered by two or three, or occasionally more, epithelial cells. The presence of grape-like clusters of vacuolated cells can be another helpful cytologic feature. Other findings of SC include prominent intracytoplasmic vacuolization and occasional signet ring cells. Some cells contain granular cytoplasm. The nuclei are crescent-shaped or ovoid, with moderate to low nuclear-to-cytoplasmic ratios. Most of the cells have a bland appearance, although some can appear malignant [8-12]. In our case, the fine needle aspiration smears revealed tumor cells that were clustered and dispersed. It showed a frankly malignant appearance, with pleomorphic nuclei, coarse chromatin, and irregular cell membranes, with eosinophilic cytoplasm and prominent intracytoplasmic vacuolization. Some parts of the smears contained structures that mimicked the globular structures and grape-like clusters that are the most characteristic features of SC [8]. However, although we observed globular structures and prominent intracytoplasmic vacuolization, the tumor cells showed a frankly malignant appearance, which is unusual for SC.

The core biopsy specimen showed the same histological features as the mastectomy specimen. Microscopically, SC is usually circumscribed, although itsometimes exhibits overtly infiltrative growth. It is arranged in papillary, microcystic, ductal, and solid patterns [2, 8]. Our case showed aninfiltrative tumor arranged inasolid nest.

SC tumor cells can have secretory orapocrine features. The cytoplasm of the SC cells of a secretory nature ispale to clear, pink or amphophilic, and containsabundant secretions. The nuclei appear to be low-grade and aresmall to moderate in size, and those withpale chromatin usually contain small uniform nucleoli. The chromatin ranges from dark and finely dispersed topale and granular. Cells with apocrine features contain granular eosinophilic cytoplasm and the nuclei are characteristic of those of apocrine cells. It is usual to observe both secretory and apocrine types of cell in a carcinoma, although one type can predominate [8]. In our case, the tumor cells had round or oval nuclei that weremoderate to large in size, vesicular and with scattered nucleoli. InSC, the tumor cells typically have a blander appearance, with nuclei that are small to moderate in size and less pleomorphic, but SC with intermediate or high nuclear atypiahasbeen reported [13]. SC is usually associated with low mitotic activity [2, 4, 6]. The mitoticactivity of our case was as low as that found in SC.

The presence of intracellular and extracellular secretory material that is PAS-positive, PAS-diastase resistant, and AB-positiveis aconsistent finding in SC [2]. The secretionaccumulates within the tumor cells, in glands formed by the tumor cells, and in the microcystic spaces associated with the tumor cells. With hematoxylin and eosin staining, thesecretory material appears pale pink or amphophilic, and it often contains lacunarthat give the appearance of bubbles [8]. In our case, thevacuolated cytoplasm with abundant eosinophilic material that wasPAS-positive, PAS-diastase resistant, and AB-positiveledus to diagnose it as a special type of breast carcinoma.

On immunostaining, SC generally shows astriple negative for ER, PR, and HER2, with strong reactivity for S-100 [5]. Ourcase was ER-positive, butPR-negative and HER2-negative. Although there have beensome reported cases of SC that were positive for ER, this is unusual [14-16]. Ourcase was negative for S-100 protein. We were unable to find any previous reports ofS-100 protein-negative SC, so thisfinding didnot support the SC diagnosis.

In SC, Ki67 levels varyfrom less than 1% to 34%, and E-cadherin is positive [8]. In our case, Ki67 was positive in 15% of the nuclear tumor cells and E-cadherin was positive. Positivity or negativity for the carcinoembryonic antigen varies in SC, whereas CD117 is positive in 70% of cases [4, 8]. Ourcase was positive forthe carcinoembryonic antigen and negative for CD117.

The differential diagnosis includedacinic cell carcinoma, cystic hypersecretory carcinoma, carcinoma with apocrine differentiation, cribriform carcinoma, glycogen-rich carcinoma, and lipid-rich carcinoma, as well asinvasive NSTcarcinoma [4, 6, 17]. Acinic cell carcinomas, which are even less common than SC, present with cells containing basophilic granules. They can closely resemble SC; as with SC, they are triple negative for ER,PR, and HER2 and usually positive forS-100 protein [4]. Osako *et al.* proposed four markers for distinguishing between SC, acinic cell carcinoma, cystic hyper secretory carcinoma, and common invasive breast carcinoma: *ETV6* rearrangement, amylase, αlactalbumin, and adipophilin [17]. Cystic hyper secretory carcinomas comprise grossly evident cystic spaces filled with densely eosinophilic secretory material, with scant cytoplasm [4]. Carcinomas with apocrine differentiation are invasive, with all or nearly all of the tumor cells exhibiting apocrine cytologic features, and nointracellular vacuoles. They are usually negative for ER and PR and positive for androgen receptors [6]. Cribriform carcinomas typically have less cytoplasm and lack the foamy eosinophilic quality. There is often secretion, but this is not darkly eosinophilic, and they are usually positive for ER and PR and negative for HER2 [4]. Glycogen-rich carcinomas show PAS-positivity andare sensitive to diastase digestion, whereas lipid-rich carcinomas show abundant microvacuolated, foamy, or clear cytoplasm due to lipids that are not stained by PAS or AB [6].

Fusion of the *ETV6* and *NTRK3*genes results in a chimeric tyrokinase protein that displays potent transforming activity for fibroblast and mammary ductal epithelial cells. It is characteristic of SC, detected using fluorescence in situ hybridization [2, 8, 18-20]. The absence ofthe*ETV6–NTRK3* fusion gene in our case confirmed that the diagnosis was not SC, despite all its morphological resemblance with SC. Because there were insufficient characteristics to achieve a specific histological type classification, the case was ultimately classified as invasive NST carcinoma.

The prognosis for invasive NST carcinoma is influenced profoundly by the classical variables of histological grade, tumor size, lymphnode status, and vascular invasion and by predictors of the therapeutic response. Invasive NST carcinoma and other invasive breast carcinomas are routinely graded based on an assessment of tubule/gland formation, nuclear pleomorphism, and mitotic count. Grade is a powerful prognostic factor [1]. According to the Elston–Ellis system, our case was grade 2 (moderately differentiated). Invasive carcinomas are divided into four subtypes based on protein expression patterns: luminal A, luminal B, HER2-enriched, and basal [1]. The subtype of our case was luminal A, which has a favorable prognosis.

It is important to differentiate between SC and invasive NST carcinoma because they differ in their prognosis [8, 17]. The prognosis is more favorable for SC: even patients with lymph node metastasis have an excellent prognosis if only a few lymph nodes are involved [6, 21], andrecurrenceand distant metastases are extremely rare [4].

Invasive NST carcinoma should be managed according to its prognostic and predictive characteristics. Most casesbenefit from hormonal treatment, but thebenefit of chemotherapy less clear [1]. Because of its rarity, there are no consensus guidelines for the treatment of SC. A recentreport describes the successful treatment of a patient with SC with targeted therapy, the tyrokinase inhibitor larotrectinib [22]. In our case, after the modified radical mastectomy and axillary lymph node dissection, the patient was given anastrozole, anaromatase inhibitor, and hormonal therapy.

SUMMARY

SCis a rare breast malignancy, which consistently showsthepresence of intracellular and extracellular secretory material that is PAS-positive, PAS-diastase resistant, and AB-positive, and is usually triple negative for ER, PR, and HER2, with strong reactivity for S-100 protein. It is associated with a characteristic translocation that creates *ETV6–NTRK3* gene fusion. The presentcase showed histomorphologythat mimicked SC, with prominent eosinophilic secretory material that stained positive for PAS, PAS-diastase, and AB; however, the nuclear features were more pleomorphic than is typical of SC, andimmunostaining showedfeatures unusual for SC (ER-positive and S-100 negative). Cases with histomorphology features of SC but has unusual immunohistochemical findings typical ofSC must be tested for the *ETV6–NTRK3* fusion geneprior diagnosed as SC. Despite the resemblance to SC in this case, the absence of the *ETV6–NTRK3* fusion gene excludedSC as a diagnosis and this case was ultimately diagnosed as invasive NSTcarcinoma.

ACKNOWLEDGMENTS

I would like to thank Gary Tse for helping us with fusion gene examination and his guide, Dr. DiahriniSpPA(K), for support during the process of writing this report. I also would like to thank fellow residents and my beloved friends for theirassistance and support.

REFERENCES

[1] Colditz, G; Chia, KS. Invasive breast carcinoma: introduction and general features. In: Lakhani SR, Ellis IO, Schnitt SJ, Tan PH, Vijver MJ, editors. *WHO classification of tumours of the breast*. 4th ed. Lyon: IARC; 2012. 14-31.

[2] Eusebi, V; Ichihara, S; Salomon, AV; Sneige, N; Sapino, A. Special subtypes. In: Lakhani SR, Ellis IO, Schnitt SJ, Tan PH, Vijver MJ, editors. *WHO classification of tumours of the breast*. 4th ed. Lyon: IARC; 2012. 39-76.

[3] Tavassoli, FA; Norris, HJ; Secretory carcinoma of the breast. *Cancer*, 1979;45:2404-13.

[4] Hicks, DG; Lester, SC. Secretory carcinoma. In: Bennet NI, Cannon TL, Ferrel TW, Gervais LA, Concannon KE, Fassett EC, editors. *Diagnostic pathology breast.* 2nd ed. Philadelphia: Elsevier; 2016. 357-64.

[5] Li, Dali; Xiao, X; Yang, W;Shui, R;Tu, X; Lu, H; et al. Secretory breast carcinoma: a clinicopathological and immunophenotypic study of 15 cases with a review of the literature. *Mod. Pathol.*, 2011;25:567-75.

[6] Vasudev, P; Onuma, K. Secretory breast carcinoma, unique, triple-negative carcinoma with a favorable prognosis and characteristic molecular expression. *Arch. Pathol. Lab. Med.*, 2011;135:1606-11.

[7] Matos, E. Secretory breast carcinoma-case report and review of the medical literature. *Breast*, 2004;13:353-5.

[8] Koerner FC. Secretory carcinoma. In: Hoda SA, Brogi E, Koerner FC, Rosen PP, editors. *Rosen's breast pathology*. 4th ed. Philadelphia: Wolters Kluwer; 2015. p. 689-701.

[9] Tse, G; Tan, PH; Schmitt, F. *Fine needle aspiration cytology of the breast.* 1sted. Philadelphia: Springer; 2013.

[10] Field, AS. Fine needle aspiration biopsy cytology of breast : a diagnostic approach based on pattern recognition. In: Field AS, Zarka MA, editors. *Practical cytopathology*. Philadelphia: Elsevier; 2017. 147 -231.

[11] Kocjan, G. Diagnostic dilemmas in FNAC cytology-difficult breast lesion. In: *Fine needle aspiration cytology*. Philadelphia: Springer; 2006. 186-211.

[12] Shanthi V, Krishna BA, Rao NM, Sujatha C. Cytodiagnosis of secretory carcinoma of the breast. *J. Cytol.,* 2012;29:63-5.

[13] Han, Y; Zhang, Q; Li, B; Jiang, N;Qiao, Z; Yu, X; et al. Secretory breast carcinoma: a clinicopathological and immunohistochemical study of 7 cases. *Int. J. Clin. Exp. Pathol.* 2016;9:1893-900.

[14] Gabal, S;Talaat, S. Secretory carcinoma of male breast: case report and review of the literature. *Int. J. Breast Cancer*, 2011;2011:1-5.

[15] Yorozuya, K; Takahashi, E;Kousaka, J;Mouri, Y; Yoshida, M;Fujii, K; et al. A case of estrogen receptor positive secretory carcinoma in a 9-year-old girl with ETV6-NTRK3 fusion gene. *Jpn. J. Clin. Oncol.*, 2011;42:208-11.

[16] Diallo, R; Schaefer, K;Bankfalvi, A; Decker, T;Ruhnke, M;Wulfing, P; et al. Secretory carcinoma of the breast: a distinct variant of invasive ductal carcinoma assessed by comparative genomic hybridization and immunohistochemistry. *Hum. Pathol.,* 2003; 34:1299-305.

[17] Osako, T; Takeuchi, K; Horii, R; Iwase, T; Akiyama, F. Secretory carcinoma of the breast and its histopathological mimics: value of markers for differential diagnosis. *Histopathology*, 2013;63:509-19.

[18] Euhus, DM; Timmons, CF; Tomlinson, GE. ETV6-NTRK3—Trk-ing the primary event in human secretory breast cancer. *Cancer Cell*, 2002;2:347-8.

[19] Makretsov, N; He, M; Hayes, M; Chia, S;Horsman, DE; Sorensen, PH; et al. A fluorescence in situ hybridization study of ETV6-NTRK3 fusion gene in secretory breast carcinoma. *Gene Chromosome Canc*, 2004;40:152-7.

[20] Tagnon, C;Knezevich, SR; Huntsman, D;Roskelley, CD;Melnyk, N;Mathers, JA; et al. Expression of the ETV6-NTRK3 gene fusion as a primary event in human secretory breast carcinoma. *Cancer Cell*, 2002;2:367-76.

[21] Vieni, S;Cabibi, D;Cipolla, C;Fricano, S;Graceffa, G;Latteri, MA. Secretory breast carcinoma with metastatic sentinel lymph node.*World J Surg Oncol.* 2006;4:88-94.

[22] Shukla, N; Roberts, SS;Baki, MO;Mushtaq, Q; Goss, PE; Park, BH; et al. Successful targeted therapy of refractory pediatric ETV6-NTRK3 fusion-positive secretory breast carcinoma. *JCO Precis Oncol*, 2017;1-8.

In: Case Reports in Surgery
Editors: Ahmad Jabir Rahyussalim et al.
ISBN: 978-1-53616-582-1

Chapter 32

LANGERHANS CELL HISTIOCYTOSIS WITH UNUSUAL NODULAR PATTERN

Imelda Setiana Silitonga[1] and Endang Sri Roostini Hardjolukito[2,*]
[1]Anatomical Pathology Residency Program, Faculty of Medicine,
Universitas Indonesia, Jakarta, Indonesia
[2]Department of Anatomical Pathology, Faculty of Medicine,
Universitas Indonesia, Jakarta, Indonesia

ABSTRACT

Langerhans cell histiocytosis (LCH) is a rare clonal proliferative disorder of Langerhans cells with unknown etiology, which occurs predominantly in male children. Histopathology features show polymorphous cells arranged in diffuse sheets. This case study involved the case of a patient who exhibited a nodular pattern that was unusual for LCH. The aim of this case report is to share experience about the unusual histology of LCH. An eleven-month-old boy presented with enlarged neck and inguinal lymph nodes. Ultrasound showed multiple enlargements of the lymph nodes with hypervascularization and a regular and distinct border. The patient underwent open surgical biopsy and the specimen was sent for histopathology analysis. The histopathology showed a nodular pattern with the characteristics of Langerhans cells that have abundant eosinophilic cytoplasm and the presence of nuclear grooves, nuclear folding, and inflammatory cells. The immunostaining was positive for CD1a, Langerin, S100, and CD68. In most cases of LCH, the morphology features showed polymorphous cells arranged in diffuse sheets. There are to our knowledge no published reports to date that show LCH in the nodular pattern. Whether or not there is different pathogenesis or biological behavior in nodular LCH remains unclear.

Keywords: histopathology, immunostaining, langerhans cell histiocytosis

---

* Corresponding Author's E-mail: ensrhardjo@gmail.com.

INTRODUCTION

Langerhans cell histiocytosis (LCH) is a rare disease that involves the clonal proliferation of cells with dendritic cell features that can affect many organs. The lesion consists of LCH cells that resemble epidermal antigen-presenting dendritic Langerhans cells [1,2]. LCH was named after the founder Paul Langerhans in 1868, and the Langerhans cell is mononuclear cell, approximately 10 to 15 μm in diameter and contains the Birbeck granules [3].

Patients with LCH can be of any age, but it occurs most commonly in children, with a greater occurrence in males (ratio ranging from 1.2:1 to over 2:1) [3,4,5].

Many names have been used previously to refer to LCH, including histiocytosis X, eosinophilic granuloma, Letterer Siwe disease, and Hand Schüller Christian disease. To date the etiology of LCH is unknown, and there is a lack of understanding regarding the pathogenesis of LCH. The clinical presentation of LCH also varies from isolated single system disease to a life-threatening multisystem condition. Patients may have systemic symptoms like fever, pancytopenia, skin manifestations, widespread bone lesions, lymphadenopathy, and hepatosplenomegaly [1,4-7].

LCH is classified as either a single system or multi system disease whereby the single system disease is when the disease affects only one organ, and the multi system affects two or more organs [7]. Lymph node involvement can be part of a widespread disease that also involves other organ systems. However, LCH can also be localized to one region.

Histology and immunostaining are used to diagnose LCH. Histopathology reveals polymorphous cells arranged in diffuse sheets. There are no reports that show cells arranged in a nodular pattern. The nuclear characteristics are irregular with prominent folds, grooves, fine chromatin, inconspicuous nucleoli, and having moderately abundant eosinophilic cytoplasm. Patients with LCH typically present with a background of inflammatory cells like eosinophils, neutrophils, macrophages, and lymphocytes and the mitotic activity varies in number. LCH is characterized by the expression of CD1a, S100, and Langerin [3,4,8,9]. In 1987, the Histiocyte Society Writing group defined the criteria for the diagnosis of LCH by the presence of Birbeck granules visible via electron microscopy or by positive CD1a immunostaining. Presence of positive CD1a and Birbeck granules in the lesion is the current gold standard for the diagnosis of LCH [5,6,10].

Treatment decisions depend on whether there is a low or high risk of organ involvement and the extent of the disease at the time of diagnosis. Treatment options may include surgery, chemotherapy, radiation, and corticosteroid therapies. Patient prognosis depends on age, the extent of organ involvement, and response to initial treatment [4]. In this research study, we report the clinical and pathologic features of an eleven-month-old boy with LCH and nodular morphologic features.

CASE REPORT

An 11-month-old boy with multiple lumps on his neck for 10–12 days came to a private hospital on 5th December 2014. He underwent a neck ultrasound and chest X-ray on 6th December 2014, and the ultrasound examination showed multiple enlargements of the lymph nodes with hypervascularization and a regular and distinct border. The size of the largest lymph node was 1.42× 1.35 cm on the right side of the neck and 1.62 × 0.97 cm on the left side of the neck. The thyroid was normal. Lymphadenopathy was concluded from the ultrasound.

The chest X-ray showed the widening of the superior mediastinum with normal heart and hilum, and therefore interstitial pneumonia was concluded.

On the 19th of December 2014, the patient came to the Cipto Mangunkusumo Hospital complaining of a high fever that had persisted for one month. The other complaints were productive cough for one week and multiple lumps on the left and right side of his neck which initially looked like a bean and became bigger within the final two weeks. There was no weight loss, no history of going pale, bleeding, or of abdominal enlargement. There was also no family history of these symptoms. On physical examination, the patient was conscious, had no fever, was 76 cm tall, and weighed 9.1 kg. There were enlarged lymph nodes on the neck and submandible, with the largest size being 1.5 × 2 cm. The nodules were not tender but rather were firm in consistency and fixed to the surrounding tissue. These nodules were also accompanied by an enlarged inguinal lymph node approximately 0.5 cm in diameter.

On pulmonary examination, there were no rales or wheezing. The patient was then diagnosed with bilateral neck lymphadenopathy, and a biopsy was ordered.

On the 20th December 2014, the patient was referred to the pediatric hematology division, and it was suspected that he had a malignancy because there was no response to the antibiotic. Therefore, the next plan for this patient was to wait for the results of the biopsy. The blood test results from the 20th of December 2014 showed a hemoglobin concentration of 9.2 g/dl, 29.7% hematocrit, leukocyte 8920/uL, thrombocyte 614.000/uL, ureum 22 mg/dl, and creatinin 0.20 mg/dl. On the 22nd of December 2014, the laboratory test for LDH was 573 U/L, and on the 24th of December the patient underwent abdominal and neck ultrasound. The result of the abdominal ultrasound was normal while the neck ultrasound showed lymphadenopathy colli with suspected malignancy.

The biopsy was done on the 23rd December 2014, and the histopathology features showed some lymph nodes with the capsule consisting of a tumor mass that had a diffuse pattern and some tumor masses with a nodular pattern that was separated by connective tissue. The tumor cells had round/oval nuclei, some with a nuclear groove, and fine chromatin with abundant eosinophilic cytoplasm.

There were also multinucleated histiocytes. Mitosis was <10/10 HPF. Eosinophils, lymphocytes, and neutrophils were also present. Based on these features we concluded that the patient had Langerhans cell histiocytosis and therefore recommended immunostaining analysis (Figure 1-4).

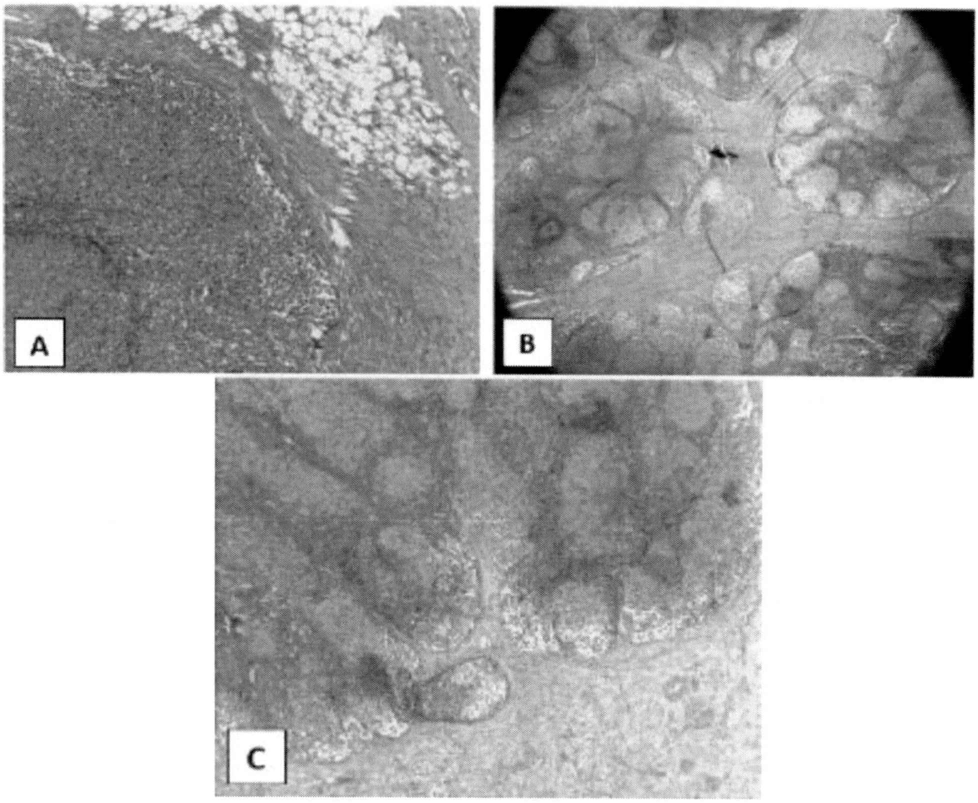

Figure 1. Histopathology features. (a) Diffuse (HE 100x). (b) Nodular (HE 25x). (c) Nodular (HE 40x).

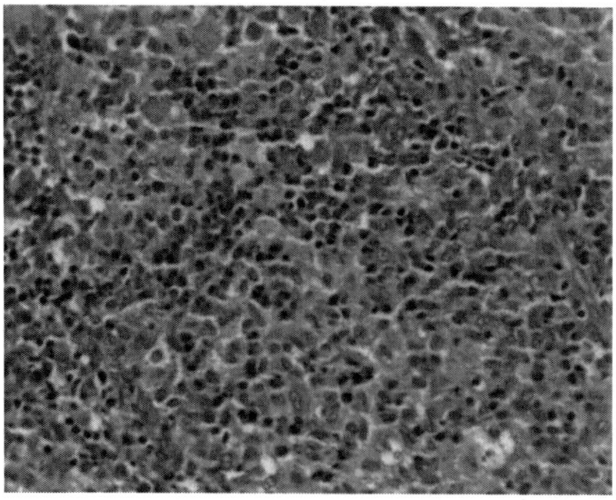

Figure 2. Many eosinophils as background (HE 400x).

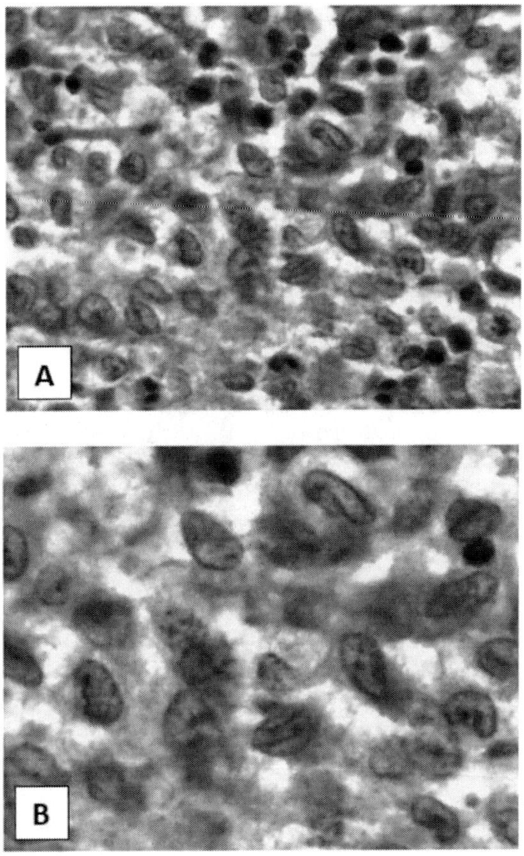

Figure 3. Nuclei characteristics showing nuclear folding and nuclear grooves (a) HE 100x,(b) HE 400x.

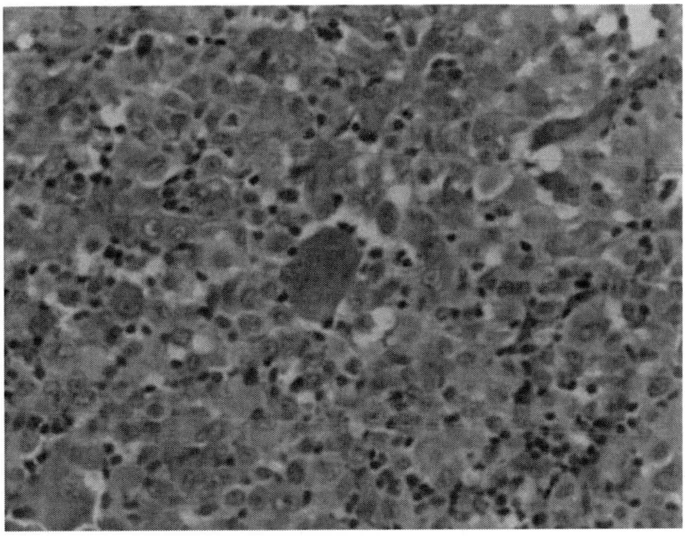

Figure 4. Multinucleated histiocytes (HE 400x).

We also performed immunostaining to support the diagnosis. The immunostaining was positive for CD1a, S100 protein, Langerin (performed by Prof TSY, SGH), and CD68, and negative for LCA, BCL6, CD10 (Figure 5, 6). The immunostaining confirmed the diagnosis of Langerhans cell histiocytosis and the patient received chemotherapy and was given Vinblastin, Etoposide, 6–MP, and Prednisone. At the time of study, the patient was still under control and showing recent signs of improvement.

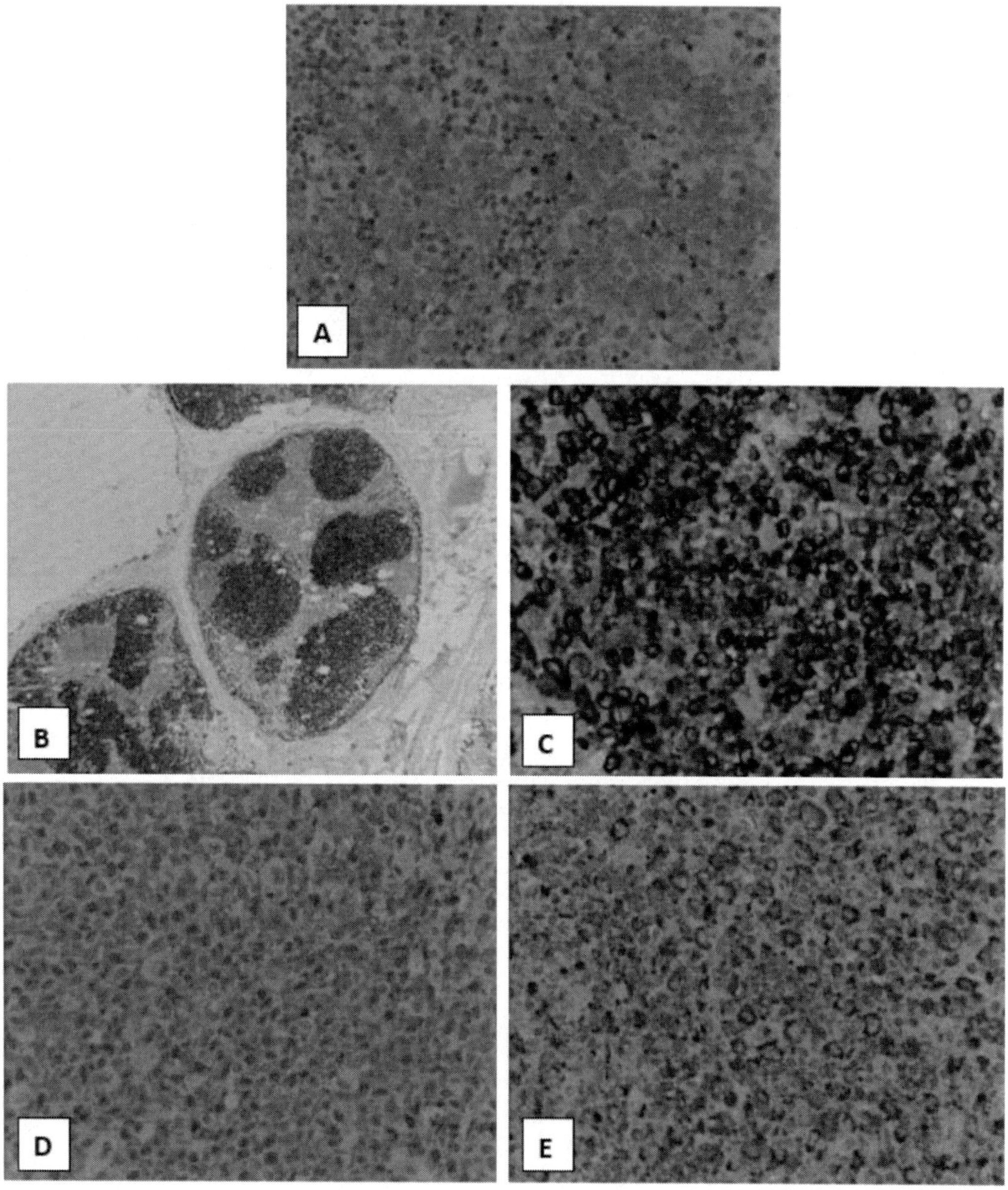

Figure 5. Immunostaining (a) CD1a (IHC 100x), (b) Langerin (IHC 40x), (c) Langerin (IHC 100x), (d) S100 (IHC 100x), and (e) CD68 (IHC 100x).

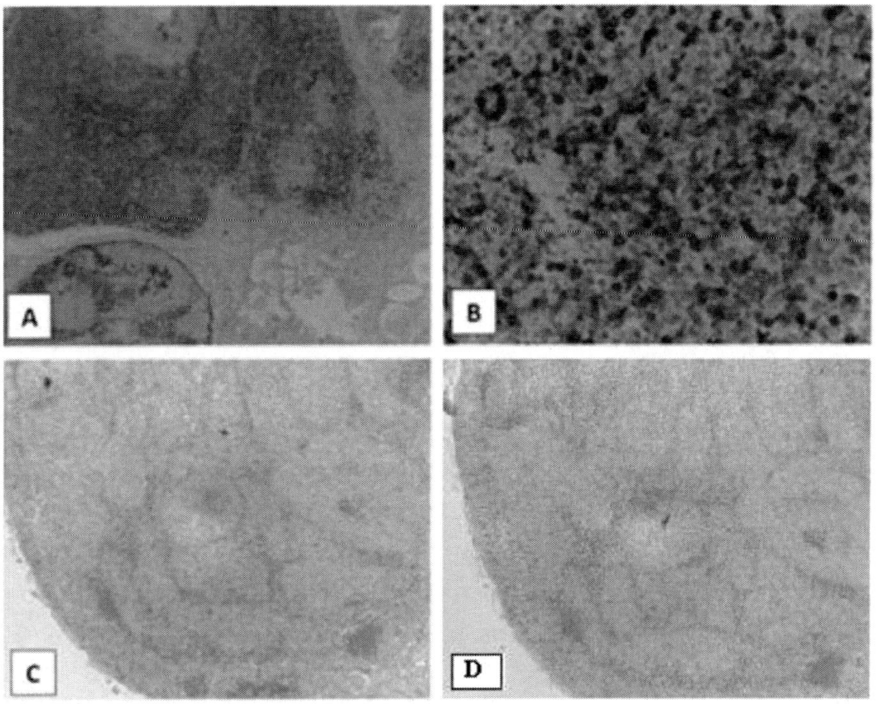

Figure 6. Negative immunostaining (a) LCA (IHC 40x), (b). LCA (IHC 100x), (c) BCL6 (IHC 40x), and (d) CD10 (IHC 40x).

DISCUSSION

LCH is characterized by the proliferation of pathologic cells with the phenotype of Langerhans cells (LCs) [5]. The Langerhans cell is a dendritic cell or antigen that originates from bone marrow and migrates through the blood to regional lymph nodes via the afferent lymphatics. Silberberg-Sinakin et al. in their study demonstrated the migration of Langerhans cell with an attached antigen to the afferent lymphatics and their appearance in the paracortical zone of regional lymph nodes, where they could present antigen to T-lymphocytes. This process is mediated by a local cytokine response. In regional lymph nodes, LCs interact with antigen-specific T-cells that are activated and proliferate to form effector and memory T-cells. LCH cells are derived from mature LCs that have been transformed. Yu et al. in their study demonstrated that LCH cells have little or no alloantigen presenting capacity because of suppressor cytokines that inhibit the function of the LCH cell. LCH cells will produce a wide variety of cytokines. The cytokines include IL-2, IL-3, IL-4, IL-5, IL-7, TNF-α, IL-1α, GM-CSF, IFN-γ and cause decreased apoptosis resulting in the accumulation of LCH cells. Circulating cytokines may be responsible for organ damage and responsible for systemic disease symptoms particularly fever, which may be related to the production of IL-1β and failure to thrive, which may be due to TNF-α production. Little is known about the molecules involved or about the routes taken by homing cells to find their way into the lymph nodes. Chemokines such as CCR1, CCR2, CCR5, CCR6, and CXCR1 are also important for the migration of LCs [5].

The etiology and pathogenesis of LCH are still unclear and whether this is a reactive process or a neoplasm has long been debated. Evidence of clonality in LCH was reported to support LCH as a neoplastic process [1,11]. A mutation of the BRAF proto-oncogene typically occurs in 38%–69% of LCH patients and supports the neoplastic origin. The BRAF mutation activates the RAS-RAF-MEK-ERK pathway that is involved in many neoplastic diseases. Activation of the BRAF gene leads to the production of a BRAF V600E mutant protein and was found in more than half of all LCH cases, suggesting that this is a genuine driver mutation in this disease [12,13].

Patients with LCH can be of any age, but it is most common in children aged one to three years old [7,14]. Males are affected more frequently with the ratio ranging from 1.2:1 to over 2:1. Singh T et al. in their study reported that the incidence of LCH is 0.5–5.4 million/year with children under 15 years old affected more than 50% [13]. There are 40 cases of LCH reported from the Anatomical Pathology Department Faculty of Medicine Cipto Mangunkusumo Hospital from 2005 until 2015. Twenty-one cases were males and 19 cases were females. In our case, the patient was an eleven-month-old boy.

Many organs can be involved in LCH including bone, lung, lymph node, skin, liver, spleen, and bone marrow. The organs have been classified into low and high-risk organs. The low-risk organs include skin, bone, lungs, and lymph nodes. The high-risk organs include liver, spleen, and bone marrow. However, a small subset of LCH patients present with isolated lymphadenopathy and with no other systemic signs or symptoms. Cervical lymph nodes are most frequently affected but supraclavicular, axillary, and inguinal lymph nodes can also be involved [7]. In our case, the patient had a single system and low-risk organ involvement that was neck and inguinal lymph nodes.

The clinical symptoms of LCH are varied and depend on the site of involvement. If affected, the lymph nodes will be enlarged. In our case, the patient had a lump on his neck and inguinal region.

The diagnosis of LCH is based on morphological and immunostaining analysis [10,14]. In our patient, the definitive diagnosis was made based on the morphological and immunostaining analysis of the lymph node biopsy specimens. In most cases of LCH, the morphology shows polymorphous cells arranged in diffuse sheets. There was no report published that showed LCH in nodular patterns. The mechanism by which LCH cells proliferate and accumulate as a nodular aggregate remains unknown. In our case, we found that cells were arranged in nodular features with Langerhans cell characteristics. This is the first case of LCH with nodular features that we have treated at the Cipto Mangunkusumo Hospital. When we first saw this pattern, we thought that it mimics follicular lymphoma. The morphological diagnosis rests on the characteristic morphology of the Langerhans cells. Langerhans cells have moderate to abundant amounts of eosinophilic cytoplasm and the presence of classical nuclear grooves and folds ("twisted towel" nuclei). The background is characteristically rich in eosinophils with varying amounts of macrophages and small lymphocytes, and neutrophils and plasma cells are absent or rare.

Multinucleated histiocytes are more numerous in bone lesions than in skin, lung, or lymph nodes. Immunostaining characteristics for LCH include positivity for CD1a, Langerin, and S100 protein. Additionally, the cells are positive for vimentin, CD68, and HLA-DR. CD45 expression is low. Ki67 is highly variable. We found the features above in the present case. The follicular lymphoma was excluded by immunostaining because it was negative for BCL6 and CD10. Electron microscopy searching for cytoplasmic granules, called Birbeck granules, wasn't done for this patient. Birbeck granules are specific for Langerhans cell and have a tennis racket-like appearance, are 200–400 nm long and 33 nm wide, and contain the protein Langerin [3,10].

The differential diagnosis of LCH includes Langerhans cell sarcoma, Rosai–Dorfman disease, and Dermatopathic lymphadenopathy [1,9]. Langerhans cell sarcoma can be distinguished from LCH by the presence of high-grade nuclear atypia and high mitotic rate. Rosai–Dorfman disease is sinus histiocytosis with massive lymphadenopathy, and the sinuses are distended by distinctive histiocytes that have round nuclei, central nucleoli, and abundant cytoplasm with well-defined cytoplasmic membranes and common emperipolesis. Langerhans cell sarcoma is most common in children. The immunostainings are positive for the S100 protein and CD68, but negative for CD1a. Dermatopathic lymphadenopathy is composed of interdigitating dendritic cells and Langerhans cells that expand to the paracortical area of the lymph node. Dermatopathic lymphadenopathy has a nodular growth pattern, pigment-laden histiocytes, and absence of necrosis or eosinophil background [9].

Patient prognosis is based at the age of first diagnosis, on whether there is a low or high risk of organ involvement, and on responses to the initial round of therapy. Single system LCH has a good prognosis with more than 80% remaining disease-free after initial therapy. In our case, the patient was 11 months old at first diagnosis, had a single organ LCH that involved the lymph nodes, and responded well to the initial treatment [1,6].

A wide spectrum of treatment modalities has been adopted to deal with LCH, including surgical excision combined with radiotherapy. Other treatment strategies have been suggested and include chemotherapy, isolated radiotherapy, and the use of corticosteroids [15]. In the present case, the patient underwent open surgical biopsy, chemotherapy and was given corticosteroids. He has now completed chemotherapy and is due for follow-up at the clinic once every six months.

Conclusion

LCH is a rare disease that can impact any age group but is most commonly seen in young children. In most cases, the morphological features showed polymorphous cells that arrange in diffuse sheets, but the pathologist must be aware that there is another different feature of LCH that was nodular. This pattern mimics follicular lymphoma but was excluded by immunostaining that was negative for BCL6 and CD10. The immunostaining was positive for CD1a, Langerin, S100, and CD68. Whether or not there is different pathogenesis or biological behavior in nodular LCH remains unclear. Treatment options include surgery, radiotherapy, chemotherapy, and corticosteroids. Our patient received Vinblastin, Etoposide, 6-MP, and Prednisone and responded well to the treatments.

References

[1] Harmon, C. M., Brown, N. (2015). Langerhans cell histiocytosis: a clinicopathologic review and molecular pathogenetic update. *Archives of Pathology and Laboratory Medicine,* 139: 1211-1214.

[2] Burns, P., Foster, A., Moran, T., Blayne, A. (2010). Multifocal Langerhans cell histiocytosis: a case report. *Irish Journal of Medical Science,* 179: 611-613.

[3] Jaffe, R., Weiss, L. M., Facchetti, F. (2008). Tumours derived from Langerhans cells. In: Swerdlow, S. H., Campo, E., Harris, N. L., editors. *WHO classification of tumours of haematopoietic and lymphoid tissues.* (4th ed.pp.358-360). Lyon: IARC.

[4] Ioachim, H. L., Medeiros, L. J. (2009). Granulocytic, histiocytic, and dendritic cell neoplasms. In: Ioachim, H. L., Medeiros, L. J., editors. *Lymph Node Pathology.* (4th ed.pp. 537-542). Philadelphia: Lippincott Williams & Wilkins.

[5] Abla, O., Egeler, R. M., Weitzman, S. (2010). Langerhans cell histiocytosis: current concepts and treatments. *Cancer Treatment Reviews*, 36: 354-359.

[6] Grana, N. (2014). Langerhans cell histiocytosis. *Cancer Control*, 21: 328-334.

[7] Elia, D., Torre, O., Cassandro, R., Caminati, A.; Harari, S. (2015). Pulmonary Langerhans cell histiocytosis: a comprehensive analysis of 40 patients and literature review. *European Journal of Internal Medicine,* 26: 351-356.

[8] Kumar, V., Abbas, A. K., Aster, J. C. (2015). Diseases of the immune system. In: Kumar, V., Abbas, A. K., Aster, J. C., editors. *Robbins and Cotran pathologic basis of disease.* (9th ed.pp. 192). Philadelphia: Saunders Elsevier.

[9] Weiss, L. (2008). Histiocytic and dendritic cell neoplasms. In: *Lymph Nodes.* (1st ed.pp.237-241). New York: Cambridge University.

[10] Agarwal, P., Kaushal, M. (2014). An unusual presentation of Langerhans cell histiocytosis. *Journal of Cytology*, 31: 227-229.

[11] Rizzo, F. M., Cives, M., Simone, V., Silvestris, F. (2014). New insight into the molecular pathogenesis of Langerhans cell histiocytosis. *The Oncologist*, 19: 151-163.

[12] Morimoto, A., Oh, Y., Shioda, Y., Kudo, K., Immamura, T. (2014). Recent advances in Langerhans cell histioctosis. *Pediatrics International,* 56: 451-461.

[13] Egeler, R. M., Katewa, S., Leenen, P., Beverley, P., Collin, M., Ginhoux, F. et al. (2016). Langerhans cell histiocytosis is a neoplasm and consequently its recurrence is a relapse. *Pediatric Blood and Cancer*, 63: 1704-1712.

[14] Singh, T., Sateesh, C. T., Appaji, L., Aruna, K., Mamatha, H. S., Giri, G. V. et al. (2010). Langerhan's cell histiocytosis: a single institutional experience. *Indian Journal of Medical and Paediatric Oncology*, 31: 51-53.

[15] Allen, C. E., Li, L., Peters, T. L., Leung, H., Yu, A., Man, T. et al. (2010). Cell-specific gene expression in Langerhans cell histiocytosis lesions reveals a distinct profile compared with epidermal Langerhans cells. *Journal of Immunology*, 184: 4557-4567.

In: Case Reports in Surgery
Editors: Ahmad Jabir Rahyussalim et al.
ISBN: 978-1-53616-582-1

Chapter 33

PITFALLS IN THE HISTOPATHOLOGICAL DIAGNOSIS OF SCLEROSING RHABDOMYOSARCOMA

***Fetisari Kurniawan*[1], *Nurjati Chairani Siregar*[1,*], *Ludi Dhyani Rahmartani*[2], *Marcel Prasetyo*[3] *and Kshetra Rinaldhy*[4]**

[1]Department of Anatomical Pathology, Faculty of Medicine, Universitas Indonesia, Cipto Mangunkusumo Hospital, Jakarta, Indonesia
[2]Department of Pediatrics, Faculty of Medicine, Universitas Indonesia, Cipto Mangunkusumo Hospital, Jakarta, Indonesia
[3]Department of Radiology, Faculty of Medicine, Universitas Indonesia, Cipto Mangunkusumo Hospital, Jakarta, Indonesia
[4]Department of Pediatric Surgery, Faculty of Medicine, Universitas Indonesia, Cipto Mangunkusumo Hospital, Jakarta, Indonesia

ABSTRACT

Rhabdomyosarcoma (RMS) is the most common soft tissue malignancy occurring in childhood and adolescence. RMS was previously classified into the following three main subtypes: embryonal, alveolar, and pleomorphic. In the latest classification, a new variant of RMS, spindle/sclerosing RMS, has been included. This variant is rare, occurring in 5%–10% of all cases of RMS. It is characterized by prominent hyaline and sclerosis stroma that mimics an osteoid or chondroid with a pseudovascular, microalveolar, or cord growth pattern. Therefore, it might be easily mistaken during initial evaluation as osteosarcoma, chondrosarcoma, angiosarcoma, infiltrating carcinoma, spindle cell sarcoma, or other RMS types. Awareness of the existence of this entity is important for not only diagnosis but also prognosis and treatment. Here we present the case of a child with sclerosing RMS that was not easily diagnosed. This report aims to discuss the potential diagnostic pitfalls associated with other look-alike sarcomas.

* Corresponding Author's E-mail: nuryati.chairani@ui.ac.id.

Keywords: rhabdomyosarcoma, sclerosing rhabdomyosarcoma

INTRODUCTION

Rhabdomyosarcoma (RMS) is the most common soft tissue malignancy in childhood and adolescence, accounting for 5%–8% of all pediatric malignancies [1, 2]. According to the World Health Organization (WHO) 2013 classification, RMS can be classified into the following four subtypes: embryonal (including botryoides and anaplastic variants), alveolar (including solid and anaplastic variants), pleomorphic, and spindle cell/sclerosing RMS [3].

The latest WHO classification has grouped spindle cell and sclerosing RMSs into a single pathological entity, as both commonly share overlapping histological features. It is considered that spindle cell and sclerosing RMSs are a continuous spectrum [1, 4]. Sclerosing RMS was first reported by Mentzel and Katenkamp in 2000, and since then, additional cases with similar features have been described [5]. This variant is rare and accounts for 5%–10% of all cases of RMS [3, 4, 6]. It occurs over a wide age range (0.3–79 years) and shows male predominance [2, 3, 7, 8]. Its symptoms might vary depending on the location and size. Although spindle cell and sclerosing RMSs are under the same pathological group, their site predilections differ. Spindle cell RMS occurs predominantly in the para-testicular region among pediatric patients and in the head and neck region and at genitourinary sites among adult patients [3, 6]. On the other hand, sclerosing RMS commonly affects the extremities and the head and neck region [2, 6].

Macroscopically, both tumors show a well-demarcated border, with a mean size >5 cm [3, 4, 6]. Additionally, the outer surface appears gray/white. In a cut section, necrosis and hemorrhage might be noted [3]. Histologically, the term spindle cell RMS is used when fascicular or intersecting spindle cell morphology is the prominent feature (>80% of the tumor area), with rare, scattered eosinophilic rhabdomyoblasts [3, 6]. Therefore, it might resemble other spindle cell sarcomas [4]. On the other hand, sclerosing RMS is characterized by abundant production of a hyaline matrix, which imitates a primitive osteoid or chondroid; thus, it might be confused with osteosarcoma or chondrosarcoma at the initial evaluation. The tumor cells are usually arranged in a pseudovascular/microalveolar pattern; thus, the tumor might be mistaken for angiosarcoma or alveolar RMS [3-6]. Most cases show mixed features of spindle and sclerosing patterns. Immunohistochemically, spindle cell RMS shows positivity for desmin (diffuse), myogenin (nuclear expression), smooth muscle actin (SMA), and muscle-specific actin (MSA). On the other hand, sclerosing RMS shows strong positivity for myoD1 [3].

Spindle cell and sclerosing RMSs have distinct genetic abnormalities that differentiate them from other RMS types. They are characterized by the presence of *NCOA2* and *VGLL2*-related fusions in congenital/infantile cases and *MYOD1* mutations co-existing with *PIK3CA* mutations in both pediatric and adult cases [1, 4]. Overall, spindle cell and sclerosing RMSs arising in adult patients have more aggressive behaviors when compared with tumors arising in pediatric patients [4].

Here, we present a child with sclerosing RMS that was not easily diagnosed. This report aims to share the potential diagnostic pitfalls associated with other look-alike sarcomas. Understanding of histopathological features and appropriate use of immunohistochemical analysis are essential to achieve an accurate diagnosis.

CASE REPORT

An 8-year-old girl had an enlarging mass in the left mandibular region since 1 year before admission to our hospital. Initially, she complained about severe toothache at her left jaw. Following tooth extraction, her gum swelled and gradually increased in size, causing difficulty in eating and drinking.

Clinical examination revealed that she was stunted and underweight (both height and weight for age were below −3SD). A large mass measuring 10×5×2.5 cm was noted at the left buccal and mandibular region, and lymphadenopathy measuring 1 cm in diameter was noted at the right colli (Figure 1). Laboratory results indicated hypochromic microcytic anemia (hemoglobin level, 8 g/dL; mean corpuscular volume, 64 fL; mean corpuscular hemoglobin, 19 pg/ml; mean corpuscular hemoglobin concentration, 30 g/dL), leukocytosis (14,500/μL), and thrombocytosis (690,000/μL). She was clinically suspected to have RMS.

Plain radiography and computed tomography showed a multilobulated soft tissue mass extending from the deep maxillary and neck region. Tumoral expansion resulted in bony thinning and deformity of the left zygoma, maxilla, and mandible. The tumor occupied the left oral cavity. There was no significant bone destruction (Figure 2 a-c). Magnetic resonance imaging showed a solid heterogeneous mass with a necrotic component. These findings were consistent with a malignant soft tissue neoplasm (Figure 3 a-d).

Debulking excision surgery was performed, and it resulted in 70% mass reduction. The surgical specimens were sent to the Anatomical Pathology Department. There were 11 resected specimens varying in size from 3×2×0.5 cm to 8×6×3 cm (white to brownish in color), with firm consistency. In a cut section, a yellowish mass was noted without hemorrhage or a necrotic area (Figure 4).

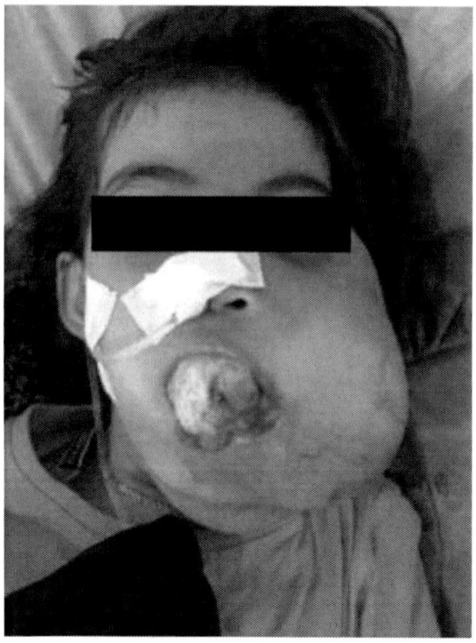

Figure 1. Mass at the left buccal and mandibular region at the initial presentation.

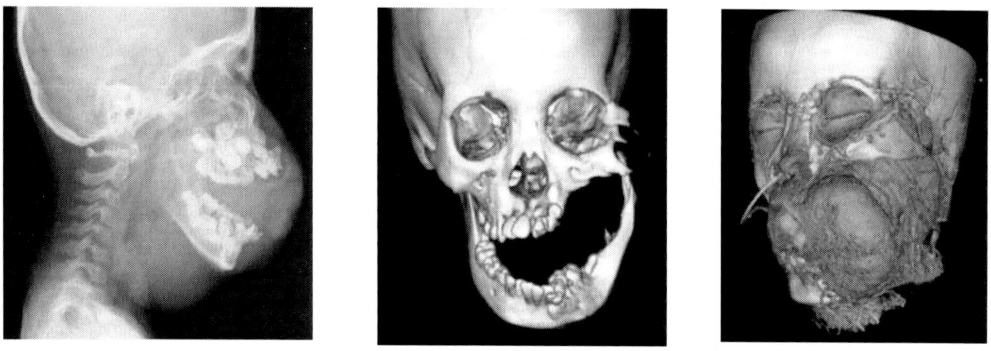

(a) (b) (c)

Figure 2. Radiography and computed tomography. (a) Plain radiography, lateral projection; (b, c) Computed tomography with three-dimensional bone reconstruction.

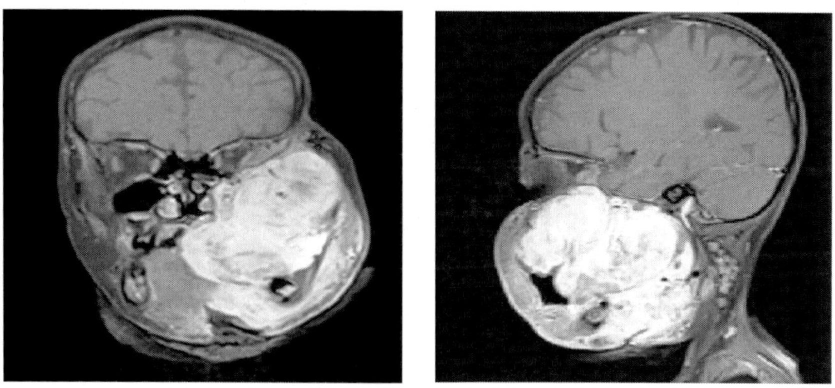

(a) (b)

Figure 3. (Continued).

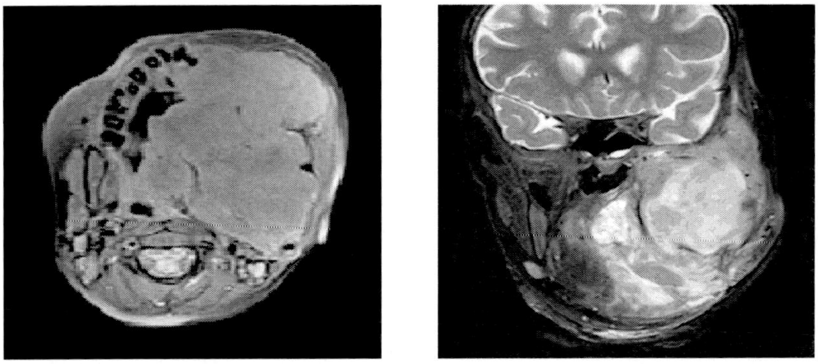

(c) (d)

Figure 3. Magnetic resonance imaging. (a) T1 contrast, coronal; (b) T1 contrast, sagittal; (c) T1, axial; (d) T2, coronal.

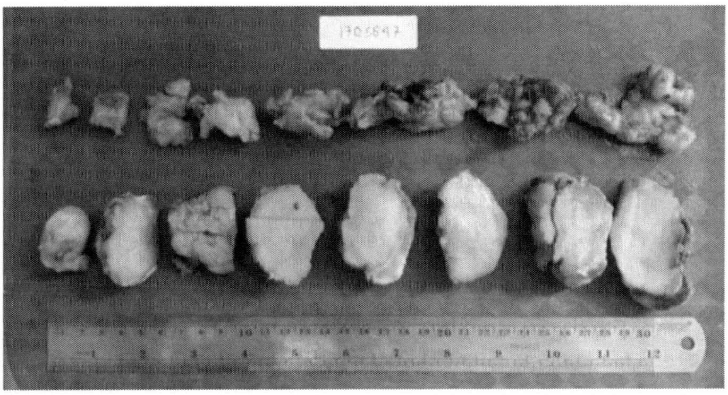

Figure 4. Gross specimens. Firm tumors varying in size (white to brownish in color) without hemorrhage or a necrotic area.

Histopathological examination showed mesenchymal tumor cells arranged in diverse patterns, including solid, microalveolar, and linear patterns (Figure 5a-c). Some areas showed alternating hypercellular and hypocellular zones (Figure 5d) with a myxoid stromal background (Figure 5e). The tumor cells appeared round/oval and spindle shaped with marked nuclear pleomorphism and bizarre, hyperchromatic, or vesicular nuclei, and some cells showed conspicuous nucleoli and eosinophilic cytoplasm (Figure 5f). Typical mitosis and atypical mitosis were easily found. A lace-like osteoid matrix mimicking that in osteosarcoma was seen interspersed between tumor cells (Figure 5g). Additionally, there was prominent hyaline stroma (Figure 5h). No rhabdomyoblasts were noted. These microscopic findings initially concluded as conventional osteosarcoma.

A tumor board meeting was held owing to the discrepancy between the clinical diagnosis and histopathological results. Immunohistochemical analysis was then performed (Figure 6a-d). The neoplastic cells were immunopositive for desmin (cytoplasmic positive, diffuse), myoD1 (nuclear strong positive, diffuse), myogenin (nuclear positive, focal), and SMA (cytoplasmic positive, focal). Thus, the diagnosis of sclerosing RMS (WHO grade 3) was confirmed.

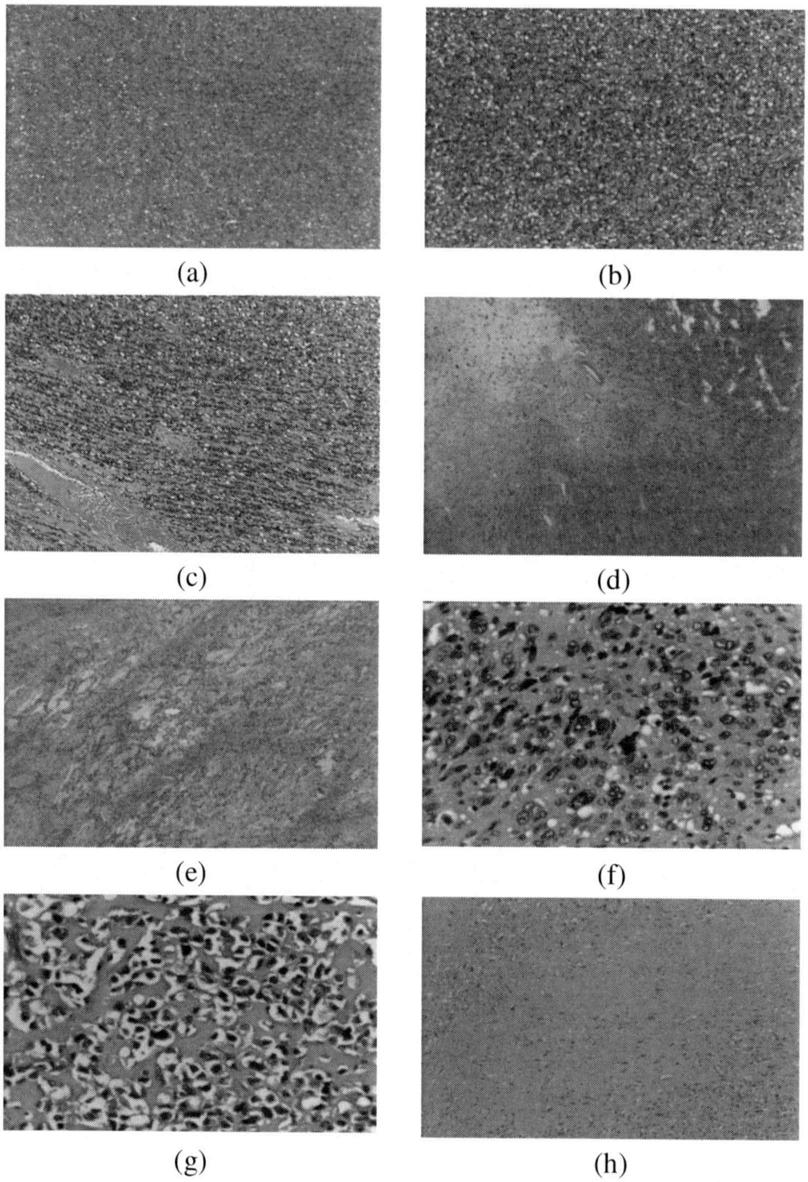

Figure 5. Histological analysis. (a) Solid pattern (hematoxylin and eosin [H&E], magnification 100×); (b) Microalveolar pattern (H&E, 40×); (c) Linear pattern (H&E, 40×); (d) Alternating hypercellular and hypocellular zones (H&E, 40×); (e) Myxoid stromal background (H&E, 40×); (f) Tumor cells and mitosis (H&E, 400×); (g) Osteoid-mimicking matrix (H&E, 400×). (h) Prominent hyaline and sclerosis matrix (H&E, 100×).

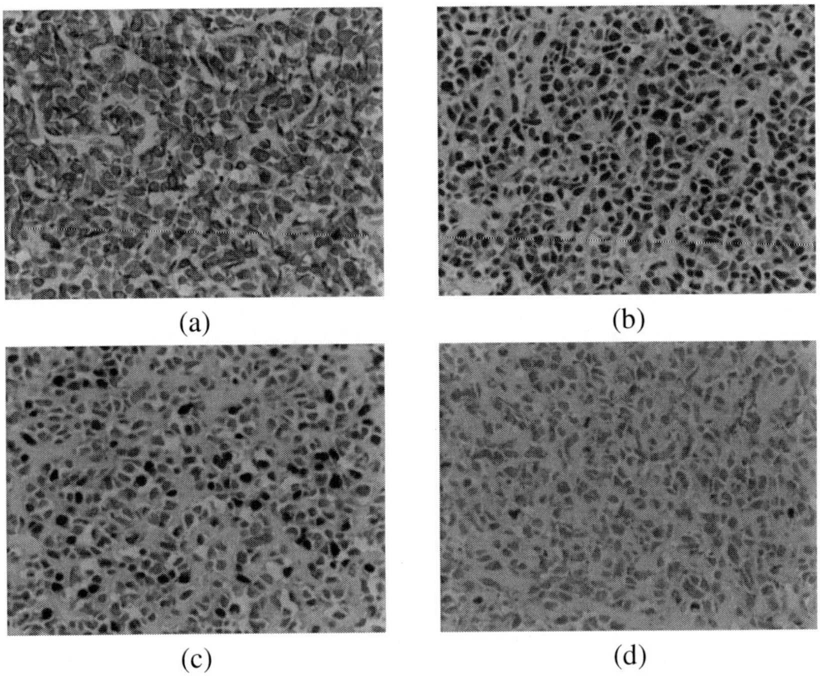

Figure 6. Immunohistochemical analysis. (a) Desmin (cytoplasmic positive, diffuse; magnification 400×); (b) MyoD1 (nuclear strong positive, diffuse; 400×); (c) Myogenin (nuclear positive, focal; 400×); (d) SMA (cytoplasmic positive, focal; 400×).

Discussion

Sclerosing RMS has been reported to occur over a wide age range, including in pediatric patients, and males are six times more frequently affected than females [2, 3, 7, 8]. The two most common sites of involvement are the extremities and head and neck region [2, 6, 9]. Lesions usually form a large bulky mass with a median size >5 cm [3, 4, 6]. Our present 8-year-old female patient had an enlarging mass measuring 10×5×2.5 cm in her left mandibular region. Our findings are similar to the findings of these previous reports in terms of onset age, predilection site, and tumor size at presentation.

Microscopic examination revealed that the tumor produced abundant hyaline stroma mimicking a primitive osteoid in conventional osteosarcoma. The tumor cells were round/spindle shaped with pleomorphic nuclear and brisk mitotic figures arranged in various patterns. The presence of solid and microalveolar patterns might resemble the appearance of alveolar RMS, alternating cellular zones with myxoid background stroma might resemble the appearance of embryonal RMS, and a linear pattern might resemble the appearance of metastatic breast carcinoma.

Classically, conventional osteosarcoma has a bimodal age distribution (10–14 years of age and >40 years of age) with long bone predilection sites, especially the femur [3, 10]. It is composed of pleomorphic or anaplastic tumor cells in a permeative pattern with an osteoid lace-like matrix in between cells (Figure 7a) [3, 10]. It genetically exhibits complex abnormalities [3], and there are no specific immunohistochemical studies to confirm a diagnosis of osteosarcoma [10]. The tumor in our case also showed nuclear pleomorphism with a mimicking osteoid lace-like matrix in between cells (Figure 7b). It can be very difficult to subjectively distinguish between an osteoid and eosinophilic extracellular matrix [3]. Immunohistochemical analysis confirmed that the origin of the tumor cells was skeletal muscle.

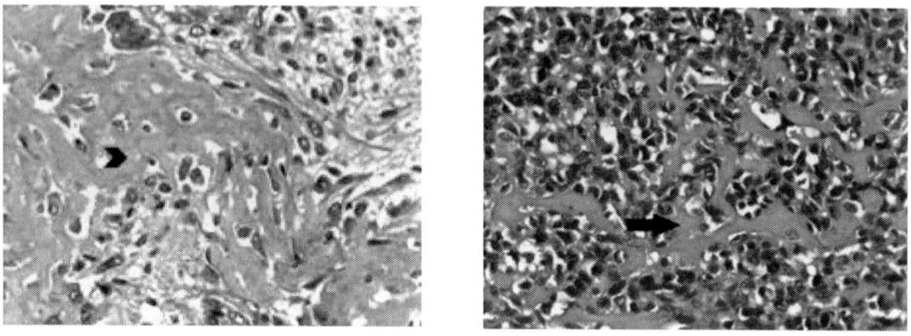

(a) (b)

Figure 7. Comparison between conventional osteosarcoma case and the tumor in the present case. (a) Conventional osteosarcoma with osteoid lace-like matrix (H&E, 400×) (arrow head); (b) Prominent hyaline stroma in sclerosing rhabdomyosarcoma mimicking an osteoid matrix (H&E, 400×) (arrow).

Classically, alveolar RMS arises in adolescents and young adults, with soft tissue extremities as the predilection site [3, 8, 11]. It is composed of nests containing primitive round cell tumors separated by thin fibrous septa creating a pseudoalveolar pattern (Figure 8 a) [3, 11]. The nests usually show central loss of cohesion and are peripherally arranged in a picket fence-like arrangement [3, 12]. Wreath cells with rhabdomyoblastic differentiation might also be noticeable [3]. The solid variant of alveolar RMS lacks fibrous septa and forms a tumor sheet [3]. It genetically exhibits either *PAX3-FOXO1* or *PAX7-FOXO1* fusion genes [3, 13].

Immunohistochemical analysis shows diffusely positive staining for myogenin [3, 12]. On the other hand, in our case, there was a microalveolar pattern formed by hyaline stroma that entrapped a smaller cluster of cells with thicker septa and lack of central loss of cohesion and picket fence-like arrays instead of the classic pseudoalveolar pattern (Figure 8 b) [12]. No rhabdomyoblastic differentiation was seen in our case. In contrast to the alveolar RMS predilection site, the tumor in our case arose in the head and neck region. Moreover, in contrast to the immunohistochemical findings of alveolar RMS, the tumor in our case showed prominent staining for myoD1, with only focal reactivity for myogenin. Unfortunately, molecular testing data were not available to exclude the presence of *PAX-FOXO* fusion genes.

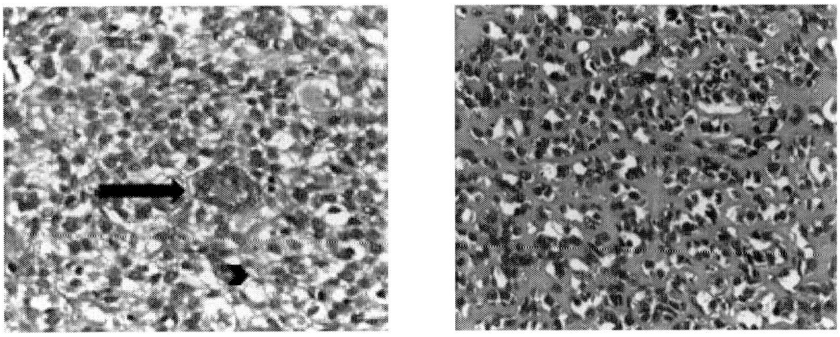

(a) (b)

Figure 8. Comparison between alveolar rhabdomyosarcoma (RMS) case and the tumor in the present case. (a) Alveolar RMS with wreath cell (arrow) and thin fibrovascular septa (arrowhead) (H&E, 400×); (b) Sclerosing RMS with a microalveolar structure (H&E, 400×).

Classically, embryonal RMS affects patients of younger age (typically <5 years) with head and neck region and genitourinary predilections, and only few cases involve the extremities [3]. It involves patternless primitive mesenchymal tumors in various stages of myogenesis with variable cellularity and myxoid stroma (Figure 9 a) [3, 11]. Scattered rhabdomyoblasts are often conspicuous (Figure 9 b) [11, 14]. It genetically exhibits 11p15.5 anomaly [7, 9]. Immunohistochemical analysis shows nuclear positive staining for myoD1 [3]. The tumor in our case also occurred in the head and neck region and showed a prominent profile of myoD1 over myogenin immunohistochemically. Although it histologically exhibited an alternating cellular zone, it lacked rhabdomyoblast differentiation and occurred at an older age compared with typical embryonal RMS (Figure 9 c). Unfortunately, molecular testing data were not available to exclude the presence of 11p15.5 anomaly.

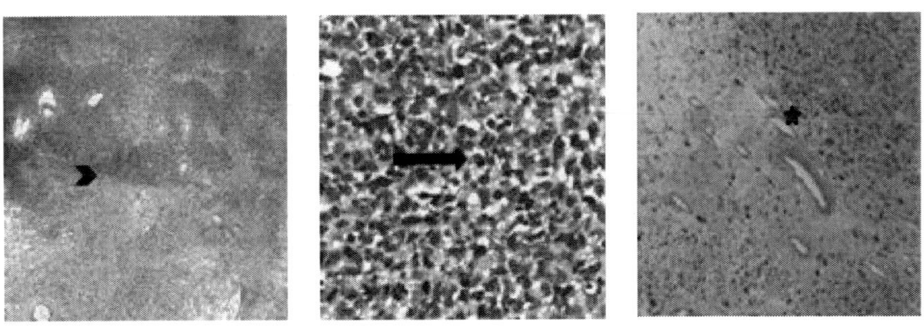

(a) (b) (c)

Figure 9. Comparison between embryonal rhabdomyosarcoma (RMS) case and the tumor in the present case. (a) Embryonal RMS with a marbled appearance (H&E,25×) (arrow head); (b) Rhabdomyoblastic differentiation in embryonal RMS (H&E,400×) (arrow); (c) Sclerosing RMS with alternating cellularity zones (H&E,400×) (star).

Classically, invasive lobular carcinoma of the breast shows discohesive cells arranged in a single-file linear pattern invading the fibrous stroma (Figure 10a) [15, 16]. Immunohistochemical analysis shows loss of E-cadherin expression [15]. On the other hand, in our case, the tumor cells lacked discohesiveness (Figure 10b). Invasive lobular carcinoma of the breast is rarely found in children, and it rarely metastasizes to the head and neck region [3].

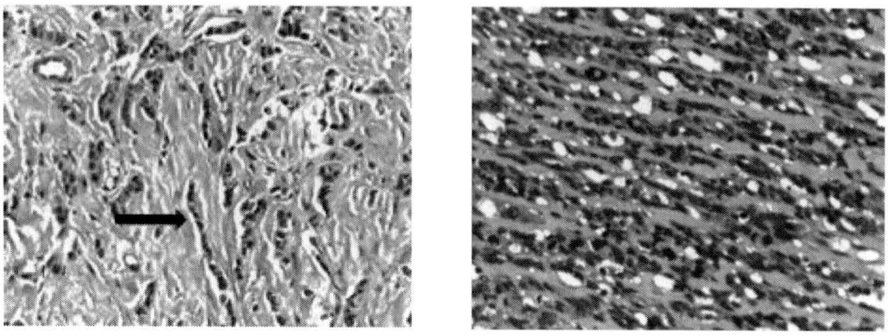

(a) (b)

Figure 10. Comparison between classical invasive lobular carcinoma of the breast case and the tumor in the present case. (a) Classical invasive lobular carcinoma of the breast shows single-file arrangement (H&E, 400×) (arrow); (b) Sclerosing rhabdomyosarcoma shows a linear pattern (H&E, 400×).

CONCLUSION

Spindle cell/sclerosing RMS is a new variant included in the latest WHO classification. Histopathologically, the tumor might show various growth patterns with abundant hyalinized stroma mimicking other look-alike sarcomas. In this report, several differential diagnoses have been presented, including conventional osteosarcoma, alveolar RMS, embryonal RMS, and invasive lobular carcinoma of the breast. The use of immunohistochemical analysis, especially for myoD1 is important in the confirmation of the diagnosis. Recognition and awareness of the existence of this entity and appropriate use of immunohistochemical analysis are essential to achieve an accurate diagnosis.

REFERENCES

[1] Alaggio, R., Zhang, L., Sung, Y. S., Huang, A. C., Chen, C. L., Bisogno, G., Zin, A., Agaram, N. P., LaQuaglia, M. P, Wexler, L. H. & Antonescu, C. R. (2016). A molecular study of pediatric spindle and sclerosing rhabdomyosarcoma identification of novel and recurrent VGLL2-related fusions in infantile cases. *Am. J. Surg. Pathol.*, 40(2), 224-235.

[2] Wang, J., Tu, X. & Sheng, W. (2008). Sclerosing rhabdomyosarcoma: a clinicopathologic and immunohistochemical study of five cases. *Am. J. Clin. Pathol.*, 129, 410-415.

[3] Fletcher, C. D. M., Bridge, J. A., Hogendoorn, P. C. W. & Mertens, F. (2013). *WHO classification of tumours of soft tissue and bone* (4th ed). Lyon: IARC.

[4] Owosho, A. A., Chen, S., Kashikar, S., Zhang, L., Chen, C. L., Wexler, L. H., Estilo, C. L., Huryn, J. M. & Antonescu, C. R. (2016). Clinical and molecular heterogenity of head and neck spindle cell and sclerosing rhabdomyosarcoma. *Oral. Oncol.*, 58, e6-11.

[5] Mentzel, T. & Katenkamp, D. (2000). Sclerosing, pseudovascular rhabdomyosarcoma in adults clinicopathological and immunohistochemical analysis of three cases. *Virchows Arch.*, 436, 305-311.

[6] Yasui, N., Yoshida, A., Kawamoto, H., Yonemori, K., Hosono, A. & Kawai, A. (2015). Clinicopathologic analysis of spindle cell/sclerosing rhabdomyosarcoma. *Pediatr. Blood. Cancer.*, 62, 1011-1016.

[7] Lin, X. Y., Wang, Y., Yu, J. H., Liu, Y., Wang, L., Li, Q. C. & Wang, E. H. (2013). Sclerosing rhabdomyosarcoma presenting in the masseter muscle: a case report. *Diagn. Pathol.*, 8, 18.

[8] Robinson, J. C., Richardson, M. S., Neville, B. W., Day, T. A. & Chi, A. C. (2013). Sclerosing rhabdomyosarcoma: report of a case arising in the head and neck of an adult and review of the literature. *Head Neck Pathol.*, 7, 193-202.

[9] Kumar, A., Singh, M., Sharma, M. C., Bakshi, S. & Sharma, B. S. (2014). Review article pediatric sclerosing rhabdomyosarcomas: a review. *ISRN Oncol.*, 9.

[10] Nielsen, G. P., Rosenberg, A. E., Deshpande, V., Hornicek, F. J., Kattapuram, S. V. & Rosenthal, D. I. (2017). *Diagnostic pathology bone* (2nd ed). Philadelphia: Elsevier.

[11] Linberg, M. R., Lucas, D., Cassarino, D. S., Gardner, J. M. & Stalling-Archer, K. (2016). *Diagnostic pathology soft tissue tumors* (2nd ed). Philadelphia: Elsevier.

[12] Chiles, M. C., Parham, D. M., Qualman, S. J., Teot, L. A., Bridge, J. A., Ullrich, F., Barr, F. G. & Meyer, W. H. (2004). Sclerosing rhabdomyosarcomas in children and adolescents: a clinicopathologic review of 13 cases from the Intergroup Rhabdomyosarcoma Study Group and Children's Oncology Group. *Pediatr. Dev. Pathol.*, 7, 583-594.

[13] Vadgama, B., Sebire, N. J., Malone, M. & Ramsay, A. D. (2004). Sclerosing rhabdomyosarcoma in childhood: case report and review of the literature. *Pediatr. Dev. Pathol.*, 7, 391-396.

[14] El-Naggar, A., Chan, J. K. C., Grandis, J. R., Takata, T. & Slootweg, P. J. (2017). *WHO classification of head and neck tumours* (4th ed). Lyon: IARC.

[15] Lakhani, S. R., Ellis, I. O., Schnitt, S. J., Tan, P. H. & Vijver, M. J. V. (2012). *WHO classification of tumours of the breast* (4th ed). Lyon: IARC.

[16] Hicks, D. G. & Lester, S. C. (2016). *Diagnostic pathology breast* (2nd ed). Philadelphia: Elsevier.

In: Case Reports in Surgery
Editors: Ahmad Jabir Rahyussalim et al.
ISBN: 978-1-53616-582-1

Chapter 34

PRIMARY MALIGNANT GIANT CELL TUMOR OF PROXIMAL RIGHT TIBIA: A RARE CASE REPORT

Mirna Albertina Wijaja[1], Nurjati Chairani Siregar[1,*], Evelina Kodrat[1], Yogi Prabowo[2] and Thariqah Salamah[3]

[1]Department of Anatomical Pathology, Universitas Indonesia, Jakarta, Indonesia
[2]Department of Orthopaedics and Traumatology, Universitas Indonesia, Jakarta, Indonesia
[3]Department of Radiology, Universitas Indonesia, Jakarta, Indonesia

ABSTRACT

Primary malignant giant cell tumor of bone (PMGCTB) refers to a high-grade sarcoma arising from adjacent to benign giant cell tumor located in bone tissue. This type of sarcoma is rare and accounts for approximately 7% of all giant cell tumors. This report shares our experience of diagnosing a rare case. A 53-year-old man presented with a mass on the upper end of his tibia that appeared 6 years before he was admitted to the hospital and had no previous history of radiation therapy or surgery. A radiograph showed an aggressive bone tumor at the metadiaphysis with a suspicious femorotibial joint involvement. Histopathology showed mononuclear cell proliferation, multinucleated giant cells with abundant nuclei, identical with mononuclear cells in the stroma, and a high-grade sarcoma area juxtaposition to the benign giant cell tumor. PMGCTBs arise *de novo* and are extremely rare. From these findings, we concluded this case as PMGCTB. Malignant giant

* Corresponding Author's E-mail: nuryati.chairani@ui.ac.id.

cell tumor of bone (MGCTB) prognosis is poor with a 5-year survival of 50%, and PMGCTB has a better prognosis than secondary MGCTB.

Keywords: Primary malignant giant cell tumor, high-grade sarcoma, tibia

INTRODUCTION

Jaffe et al., identified giant cell tumor of bone (GCTB) as an entity many years ago and classified it into a primary benign bone tumor that may evolve into a malignant lesion.The etiology of malignant transformation of benign GCTB remains unknown [1-3]. Malignant GCTB (MGCTB) is rare and encompasses 2%–9% of all GCTB. There are only a small number of MGCTB cases published in the literature [4, 5]. In the Cipto Mangunkusumo Hospital, there were two cases reported from 2013 to 2017.

MGCTBs are divided into primary (PMGCTB) and secondary (SMGCTB). PMGCTB is a high-grade sarcoma that presents a *de novo* juxtaposition with conventional giant cell areas. SMGCTB is a high-grade sarcoma that arises at the area previously treated as a conventional GCTB with surgery or radiation. MGCTB diagnosis is challenging because of the variety of malignant tumors containing giant cells. Effective treatment is tough because of the limited existing studies that distinguish PMGCTB, SMGCTB, or post-radiation cancer [4, 5].

The incidence of MGCTB occurs in a wide range of ages, but typically in those 30–55 years of age and more frequently in men with a ratio of 3:1 [6-8]. According to Bertoni F et al., PMGCTB impacts those between 20 and 68 years, whereas SMGCTB impacts those 30–77 years. Both cancers frequently occur in the long bones near the knee joint with 90% of cases located in the meta-epiphyseal segments of the long bones [6, 7].

PMGCTB is extremely unusual and occurs less frequently than SMGCTB. Nascimento et al., reported eight cases, and five cases had been reported by the Mayo Clinic. The most common symptoms of PMGCT are a pain (80%) and swelling (40%) [4, 6]. The radiographic pattern may be identical to conventional GCTB. Most cases are poorly circumscribed. Cortical destruction and soft tissue invasion may occur because of a large area of sarcomatous tissue [9, 10].

Histopathological findings of PMGCTB showed high-grade sarcoma juxtaposed with conventional GCTB areas that are identifiable at the time of the initial presentation. The transition between both components varies considerably. A high-grade sarcoma component includes fibrosarcoma, osteosarcoma, and undifferentiated high-grade pleomorphic sarcoma (UPS) [4-6]. There is a high mitotic activity of both stromal and tumor giant cells, with multiple atypical mitosis present. The prognosis of PMGCTB is still indefinite because of its rareness and short follow-up. Most reports consider the prognosis poor [5, 6].

Here, we report a case of PMGCTB that had a history before the initial presentation and was defined as high-grade sarcomas originating from a giant cell tumor (GCT). The aim of this case report is to define the clinicopathologic and histologic features of malignancy in GCTs.

CASE REPORT

A 53-year-old male presented with a mass on the upper end of his right tibia without a prior history of radiation therapy or surgery. Seven years ago, the patient was in a motorcycle accident that caused a lump on the upper end of his right tibia, but he decided not to go to the hospital. Five years after the accident, the size of the lump remained the same.

One year later, the lump began to grow as large as an egg without pain and made it difficult to walk, but he did not go to the doctor and instead went to a traditional masseur. Five months later, he went to an orthopedic surgeon in Ambon because the lump was getting bigger and was accompanied by pain. He underwent x-ray examination, and the orthopedic surgeon said that there was a benign tumor. He was then referred to the Cipto Mangunkusumo Hospital.

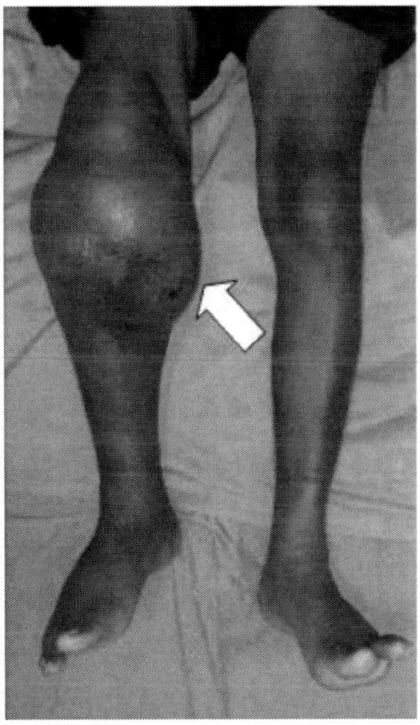

Figure 1. Mass on the upper end of the right tibia.

One month later, he went to the Cipto Mangunkusumo Hospital and met the orthopedic surgeon. It was determined that there was a mass on the area below the right knee, which produced serious hemorrhage from the ulcers of the mass, redness, and distal edema. The mass on the right leg was 55 cm in diameter, solid, fixed, and felt warmer than the surrounding tissue (Figure 1). The patient underwent a second x-ray examination and a magnetic resonance image (MRI) while at Cipto Mangunkusumo Hospital (Figures 2 and 3). He also underwent several chest x-rays that showed multiple nodules in both lungs with infiltrates, suggestive of metastasis (Figure 4).

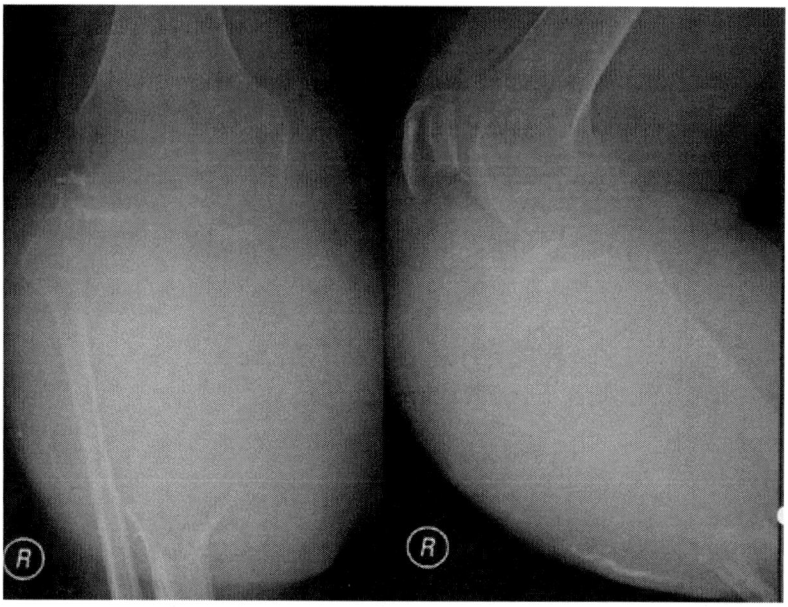

Figure 2. Plain x-ray of the right knee shows an aggressive tumor at metadiaphysis of the upper end of the right tibia. There is a suspicion that the tumor is also present at femorotibial joint (arrow).

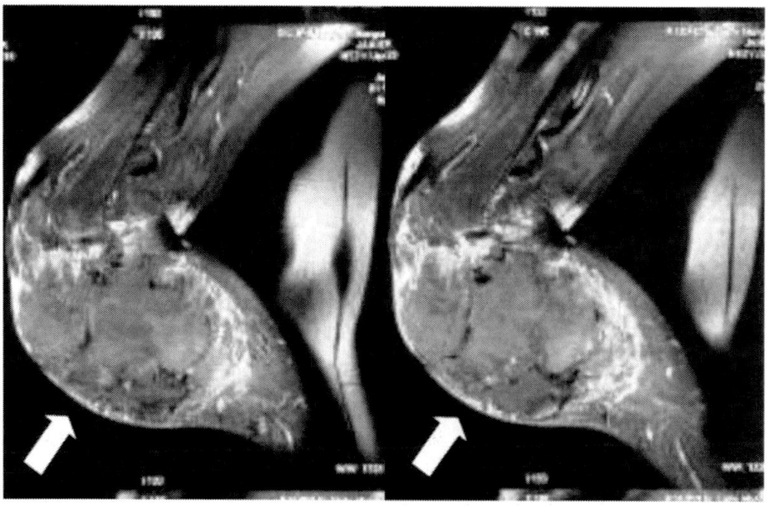

Figure 3. MRI of the right knee shows a mass of solid aggressive tumor, covering epimetadiaphysis of the proximal tibia, femorotibial joint, fibula, and neurovascular anterior tibia (arrow).

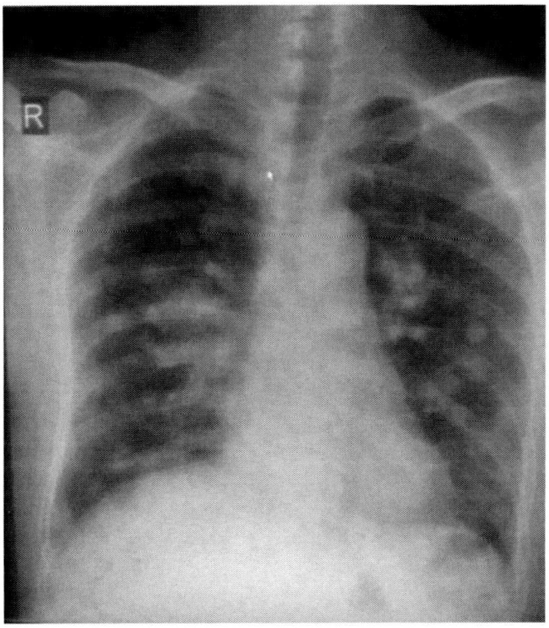

Figure 4. The second chest x-ray showed multiple nodules in both lungs with infiltrates suggestive of metastasis.

Fine-needle aspiration was performed, and cytology showed a predominantly necrotic area with fibrous tissue, a few round or spindle cells occurring in clusters, coarse chromatin, and multiple giant cells. From the cytology, we concluded the mass was a bone lesion containing giant cells that cannot be determined to be either benign or malignant (Figure 5). Nine days later, the patient underwent transfemoral amputation of the lower end of the femur. The specimen was sent to the anatomical pathology laboratory. Dissection revealed a solid mass measuring 17 × 16 × 11 cm, white-brown, and firm. The cut section was yellowish, uncircumscribed, and contained areas of hemorrhage and necrotic tissue. Representative sections were submitted in 22 blocks (Figure 6).

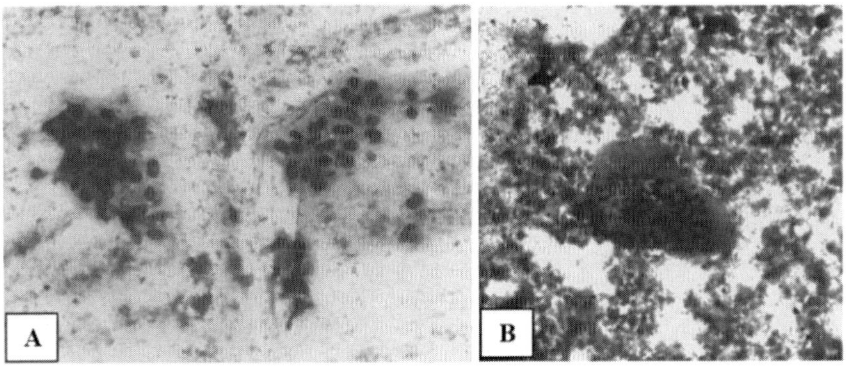

Figure 5. A. Cytology specimen showed round or spindle cells in clusters (Giemsa 100×). B. Multinucleated giant cell (Giemsa 100×).

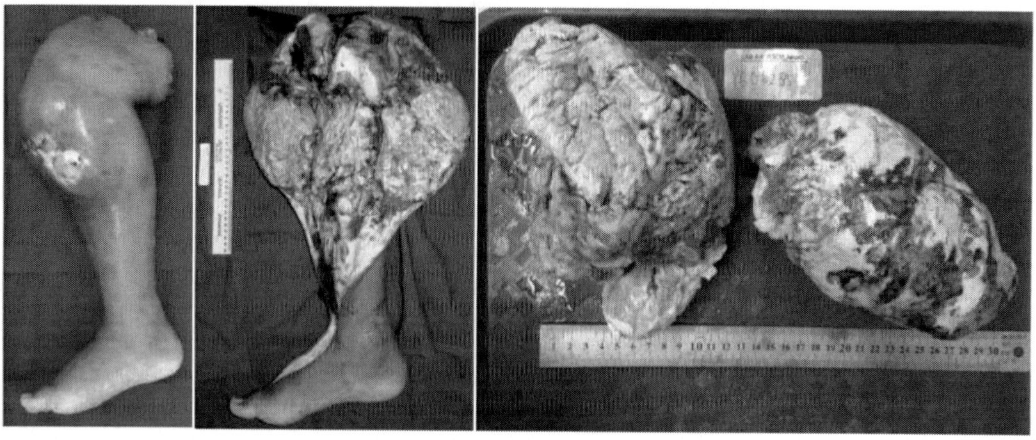

Figure 6. Mass from the right leg. Note the uncircumscribed yellowish mass with areas of hemorrhage and necrosis.

The histopathological findings showed an area of benign GCT that consisted of mononuclear cell proliferation, and multinucleated giant cells were sparsely spread in the stromal cells. The stromal cells had round, oval, or some spindle-shaped nuclei, with vesicular chromatin and variably prominent nucleoli. There were abundant nuclei of giant cells, which was identical to the mononuclear cells observed in the stroma. There was also a high-grade sarcoma area juxtaposed to the benign GCT. The sarcomatous area consisted of cells with the spindle, pleomorphic, bizarre nuclear, vesicular chromatin, and prominent nucleoli. The cytoplasms were eosinophilic. Mitotic activity was 9–12/10 HPF, and some had atypical features (Figures 7 and 8). Focal reactive bone formations, intravascular invasion, hemorrhage, and necrotic areas were also found (Figure 9). Histological findings were compatible with PMGCTB.

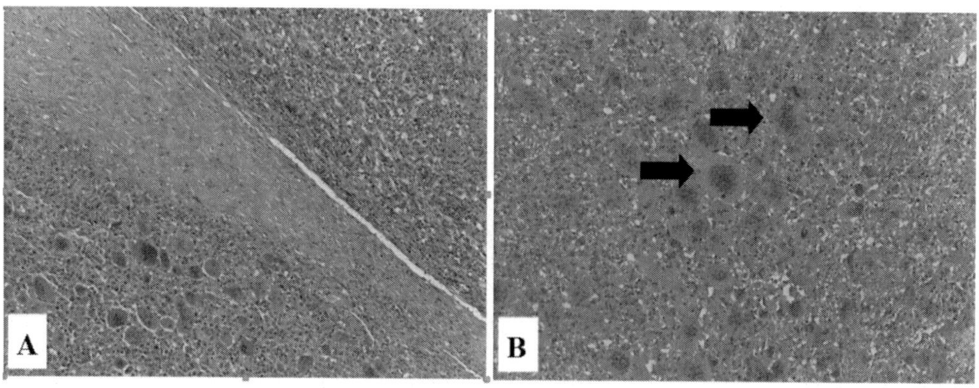

Figure 7. A. The juxtaposition between GCT (on the bottom left) and sarcomatous area (on the upper right, HE 100×). B. Conventional giant cell tumor with scattered multinucleated giant cells (arrow, HE 100×).

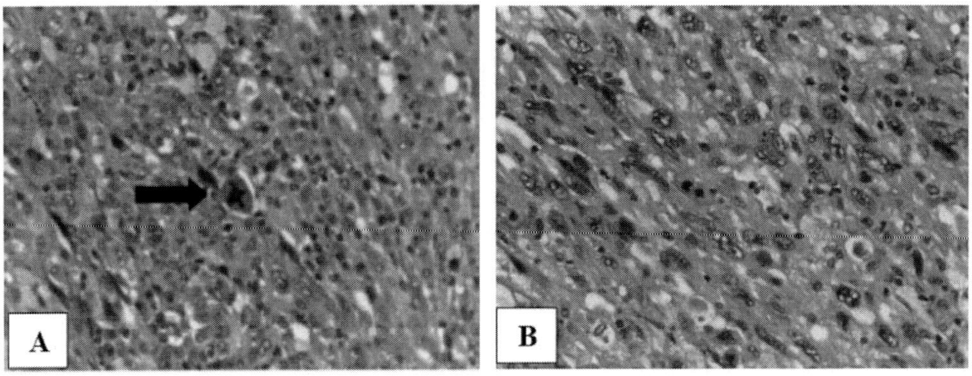

Figure 8. A. Atypical mitotic of high-grade sarcoma (HE 400×). B. High-grade sarcoma (HE 400×).

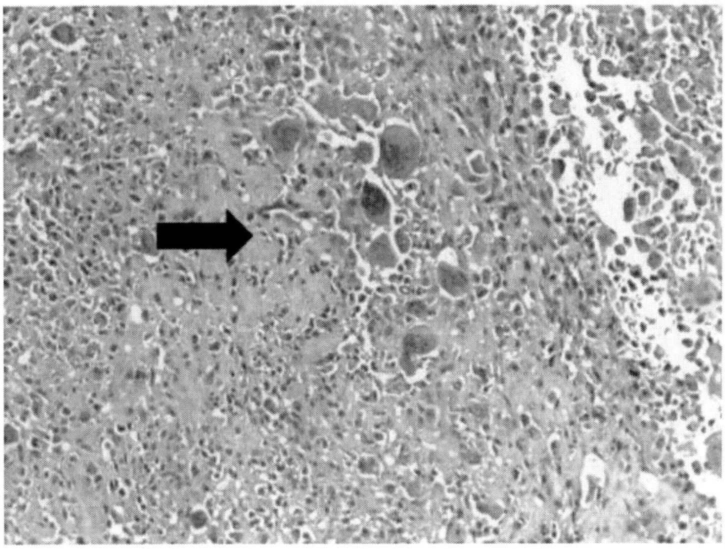

Figure 9. Focal reactive bone formation (arrow) (HE 100×).

After surgery, the patient experienced worsening dyspnea. Cytopathological testing of the sputum was performed and showed a negative result. Three months later, the patient did not receive any chemotherapy due to the long queue, and based on his family, he died because of lung metastasis.

DISCUSSION

In this case, the patient was a 53-year-old male with a mass on the upper end of his right tibia and no history of previous GCT, radiation therapy, or surgery. According to the literature, PMGCTB is a high-grade sarcoma diagnosed during the first treatment for GCTB [4]. PMGCTB typically occurs during the sixth decade of life and more frequently in men [8, 11]. The common sites are at the distal ulna, proximal and distal femur, and proximal tibia (Figure 10) [6], which is consistent with our case.

The x-ray and MRI showed an aggressive bone tumor at the metadiaphysis involving adjacent soft tissue. According to the literature, the radiographic pattern of a PMGCTB may be similar to conventional GCTB. A well-defined lytic lesion involves both the epiphysis and metaphysis. Although well-circumscribed, at least one has a thin cortex and may also be extended or destroyed [9, 11]. Aggressive radiological features such as large soft tissue component or cortical breakthrough may be seen in PMGCTB as well as in SMGCTB and benign recurrences of GCTB. The degree of overlap of the radiological findings in benign and MGCTB makes a histological analysis of tissue critical for diagnosis [8, 12].

FNAB findings, in this case, showed a predominantly necrotic area and fibrous tissue with a small number of round or spindle cells occurring in clusters, coarse chromatin, and multiple giant cells. From the cytology, we conclude that it was a bone lesion containing giant cells that cannot be determined to be either benign or malignant. Giant cell-rich lesions of bone have overlapping cytological features.

Therefore, clinical evaluation and radiological findings can help to distinguish these entities and to aid in an accurate diagnosis [13]. In smears showing giant cells and mononuclear cells, it is wise not to make a definitive diagnosis of GCTB even if suggested by radiological imaging. With regard to the differential diagnosis of other benign tumors with numerous giant cells, full knowledge of clinical and radiographic data is essential for a correct type-specific diagnosis [14].

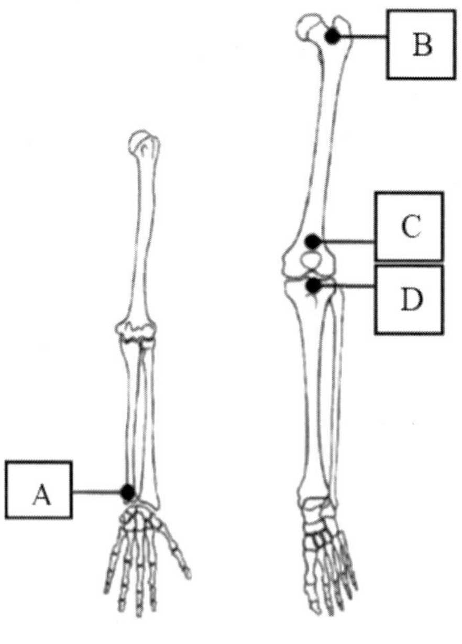

Figure 10. Common sites of PMGCTB. A. Distal ulna. B. Proximal femur. C. Distal femur. D. Proximal tibia [6].

Gross evaluation, in this case, showed a solid mass that was white-brown and firm. The cut surface was poorly circumscribed and showed a yellowish mass with areas of hemorrhage and necrotic tissue. Macroscopically, PMGCTB usually does not differ from those of GCTB. However, cut sections of PMGCTB typically appear to be soft, and the tumor tissue was focally gray-white and firm, intermixed with hemorrhagic, brownish-red, or a yellowish area of necrosis [4, 11].

Histopathology, this case showed proliferation of mononuclear cells and multinucleated giant cells with abundant nuclei, which was identical to the mononuclear cells in the stromal and a high-grade sarcoma area adjacent to the benign GCT. There were atypical mitoses, some focal reactive bone formation, and intravascular invasion. In the literature, there were distinct areas of typical GCT juxtaposed with a high-grade sarcoma. The high-grade sarcoma included fibrosarcoma, osteosarcoma, and UPS, whereas in this case, the sarcomatous component was UPS. Mitotic activity is always present, and atypical mitosis is also found [4, 6, 11]. Reactive bone can be present focally and should be appropriately identified as not being an integral part of the lesion [15]. It has been previously hypothesized that permeation of GCTB cells into vessels causes some emboli to escape and be lodged in the pulmonary parenchyma and remain viable [16].

The differential diagnosis of PMGCTB is giant cell-rich osteosarcoma, malignant fibrous histiocytoma (MFH) and SMGCTB. The diagnosis of giant cell-rich osteosarcoma requires a component of malignant bone-forming tumor [15]. In MFH, benign GCT areas are not present, and there are multinucleated giant cells with large and pleomorphic nuclei [11]. In SMGCTB, there is a history of GCTB, the recurrence information and remnants of conventional GCTB are visible microscopically [4].

Low incidence of MGCTB made it difficult to determine an appropriate therapy for this case, and the resulting prognosis was poor. Treatment typically includes surgery combined with chemotherapy and radiotherapy. Unfortunately, chemotherapy results are inconsistent but may increase the 5 year survival rate, yet the benefit disappears when most patients reach 5 years post-surgery [5]. The prognosis is poor and many patients die rapidly [4]. In this case, the patient had surgery and had planned chemotherapy, but he never received the latter. He later died within 3 months of the operation.

The limitations of this case report include the lack of concrete evidence that the patient did die. According to several chest x-rays that showed multiple nodules in both lungs with infiltrates, we anticipate that this information was true due to the suggestive metastasis. There was also no histopathological examination of multiple nodules of both lungs, and the sputum smear was negative.

REFERENCES

[1] Marui, T., Yamamoto, T., Yoshihara, H., Kurosaka, M., Mizuno, K., Akamatsu, T., (2001). De novo malignant transformation of giant cell tumor of bone. *Skeletal Radiol*, 30: 104-108.

[2] Campanacci, M., Baldini, N., Boriani, S., Sudanese, A., (1987). Giant-cell tumor of bone. *JBJS,* 69: 106-114.

[3] Knochentumoren, A., Becker, W.T., Dohle, J., Bernd, L., Braun, A., Cserhati, M., Enderle, A., Hovy, L., Matejovsky, Z., Szendroi, M., Trieb, K., Tunn, PU., (2008). Local recurrence of giant cell tumor of bone after intralesional treatment with and without adjuvant therapy. *J. Bone Joint Surg. Am.* American volume, 90: 1060-1067.

[4] Gong, L., Liu, W., Sun, X., Sajdik, C., Tian, X., Niu, X., Huang, X., (2012). Histological and clinical characteristics of malignant giant cell tumor of bone. *Virchows Archiv*, 460: 327-334.

[5] Domovitov, S.V., Healey, J.H., (2010). Primary malignant giant-cell tumor of bone has high survival rate. *Ann. Surg.* Oncol, 17: 694-701.

[6] Bertoni, F., Bacchini, P., Staals, E.L., (2003). Malignancy in giant cell tumor of bone. *Cancer*, 97: 2520-2529.

[7] Renard, A.J., Veth, R.P., Pruszczynski, M., Wobbes, T., Lemmens, J.A., Van-Horn, J.R., (1994). Giant cell tumor of bone: oncologic and functional results. *J. Surg.* Onco, 57: 243-251.

[8] Heffernan, E.J., O'Sullivan, P.J., Adibeig, M., Louis, L.J., Ryan, A.G., Neilsen, T.O., Munk, P.L., (2007). Primary malignant transformation of giant cell tumor of bone. *Eur. J.* Radiol, 62: 89-93.

[9] Khurana, J.S, McCarthy, E.F. (2010). Giant cell lesions: Giant cell tumor. In: Khurana, J.S., McCarthy, E.F., Zhang, P.J. editors. *Essentials in bone and soft tissue pathology (*pp.134-137). New York: Springer; 2010.

[10] Athanasou, N.A., Bansai, M., Forsyth, R., Reid, R.P., Sapi, Z. (2013). Giant cell tumour of bone. In: Fletcher CDM, Bridge JA, Hogendoorn P, Mertens F, editors. *WHO classification of tumours of soft tissue and bone* (4th ed.pp.321-324). Lyon: IARC.

[11] Nascimento, A.G., Huvos, A.G., Marcove, R.C., (1979). Primary malignant giant cell tumor of bone. A study of eight cases and review of the literature. *Cancer*, 44: 1393-1402.

[12] Bacchini, P., Bertoni, F. (2010). Giant cell tumour of bone. In: Folpe AL, Inwards CY, editors. *Bone and soft tissue pathology: a volume in the series foundations in diagnostic pathology* (1st ed.pp.400-407). Philadelphia: Saunders Elsevier.

[13] Gupta, K., Dey, P., Goldsmith, R., Vasishta, R.K., (2004). Comparison of cytologic features of giant-cell tumor and giant-cell tumor of tendon sheath. *Diagn. Cytopathol*, 30: 14-18.

[14] Jain, M., Aiyer, H.M., Singh, M., Narula, M., (2002). Fine-needle aspiration diagnosis of giant cell tumour of bone presenting at unusual sites. *Diagn.Cytopathol*, 27: 375-378.

[15] Czerniak, B. (2016). Giant cell lesion. In: Czerniak B, editor. *Dorfman and czerniak's bone tumors* (2nd ed. pp. 692-742). Philadelphia: Saunders.

[16] Okubo, T., Saito, T., Mitomi, H., Takagi, T., Torigoe, T., Suehara, Y., Kaneko, K., Yao, T., (2013). p53 mutations may be involved in malignant transformation of giant cell tumor of bone through interaction with GPX1. *Virchows Archiv*, 463: 67-77.

In: Case Reports in Surgery
Editors: Ahmad Jabir Rahyussalim et al.
ISBN: 978-1-53616-582-1

Chapter 35

SECONDARY MALIGNANT GIANT CELL TUMOR OF THE BONE: A CASE REPORT AND RARE EXPERIENCE

Fadhlina Muharmi Harahap[1], Nurjati Chairani Siregar[1,*], Yogi Prabowo[2] and Thariqah Salamah[3]

[1]Department of Anatomical Pathology, Faculty of Medicine, Universitas Indonesia, Cipto Mangunkusumo Hospital, Jakarta, Indonesia
[2]Department of Orthopaedic and Traumatology, Faculty of Medicine, Universitas Indonesia, Cipto Mangunkusumo Hospital, Jakarta, Indonesia
[3]Department of Radiology, Faculty of Medicine, Universitas Indonesia, Cipto Mangunkusumo Hospital, Jakarta, Indonesia

ABSTRACT

Giant cell tumor of bone (GCTB) is a primary bone neoplasm composed of mononuclear cells proliferating among scattered macrophages and large, osteoclast-like giant cells. Secondary malignant GCTB is a sarcoma arising at a site where a GCTB has been previously documented. This case report is about a 32- year-old female who presented with right knee pain of one year duration. The patient had a history of bone tumor, at the same site, six years ago. Radiographs showed a mass in the epimetaphy seal, extending into the tibiofemoral and patellofemoral junction. Such findings were consistent with a recurrent lesion. Following microscopic investigation, spindle- cell with atypical mitoses and nuclear pleomorphism, admixed with conventional GCTB, were identified. Sarcomatous changes in malignant GCT develop many years, or even decades, following the primary lesion's removal. Radiologic features are represented by large lesions with cortical destruction and prominent invasion into the soft tissue. Microscopically, the

* Corresponding Author's E-mail: fadhlinamuharmi@gmail.com.

conventional GCTB is adjacent to, or intermixed with, the sarcomatous area. Based on such findings, we conclude this case is a secondary malignant GCTB.

Keywords: giant cell tumor of the bone, secondary malignant

INTRODUCTION

Giant cell tumor of bone (GCTB) is a primary bone neoplasm composed of mononuclear cells proliferating among numerous scattered macrophages and large, osteoclast-like giant cells [1]. It represents around 4% – 5% of all primary bone tumors. Its peak incidence is between the ages of 20 and 45, with a slight predominance in females. In terms of localization, GCTB generally arises at the ends of long bones (e.g., distal femur, proximal tibia, distal radius and proximal humerus). The lesion commonly involves epiphysis and adjacent metaphysis [1-3].

Malignant transformation in GCTB is a rare event. It is classified as primary and secondary [4-6]. Primary malignant GCTB is defined as GCTB composed of sarcomatous growth juxtaposed with zones of typical benign GCTB in an individual without a previous history of surgery or radiotherapy [4-7]. It occurs in 1% – 3% of all GCTB cases [6]. Secondary malignant GCTB is described as sarcomatous growth at the site of a previously documented benign GCT [4-7]. It occurs in 5% – 10% of all GCTB cases [6]. Most secondary malignant GCTBs have a history of irradiation treatment for the primary lesion. Therefore, malignant changes occurring after only surgical procedures represent an extremely rare phenomenon [5, 8].

Histologically, tumors are characterized by many osteoclast-like giant cells, uniformly scattered among numerous oval or plump, spindle- shaped mononuclear cells. The nuclei of mononuclear and giant cells are similar; specifically, they both have round or oval nuclei with regular outlines, evenly distributed fine chromatin, prominent nucleoli, and eosinophilic cytoplasm. Occasionally, a subset of giant cells may present with 50 – 100 or even more nuclei. Mitotic figures are typically observed [1, 9]. Sarcomas are identified based on the presence of atypical mitotic figures and cytological anaplasia in the round or spindle-shaped mononuclear cells associated with conventional GCTB [1, 10].

In the present case report, we describe a 32-year-old female patient with a recurrent bone tumor in the right distal femur. She had an earlier history of bone tumor (in 2009). Upon X-Ray examination, an epimetaphyseal mass in the right distal femur was identified. Histologically, the lesion presented as a high grade sarcoma, consistent with secondary malignant of GCTB.

Secondary malignant GCTB's diagnosis is based on several aspects, such as patient history (age, symptoms, and physical examinations), preferred location, radiographs and histopathology. Secondary malignant GCTB is a rare event. This case report aims to share the experience of diagnosing a rare case.

CASE REPORT

A 32-year-old female presented with right knee pain, which started about one year before evaluation. The patient had a medical history of bone tumor and underwent surgery six years ago. A histopathological examination was not performed. Physical examination of the right knee showed deformity, shortening, a 2cm leg length discrepancy, external rotation, and a mass. The mass was 8 x 8 x 2cm in size, firm, tender and warm (Figure 1).

X- ray of the right knee showed a plate and screw internal fixation from distal to mid-diaphysis of the right femur in good condition. There was also swelling of the right distal femur soft tissue (Figure 2). An X- ray of the right femur showed a lytic lesion in distal femoral metadiaphysis with thickening of the surrounding soft tissues (Figure 3).

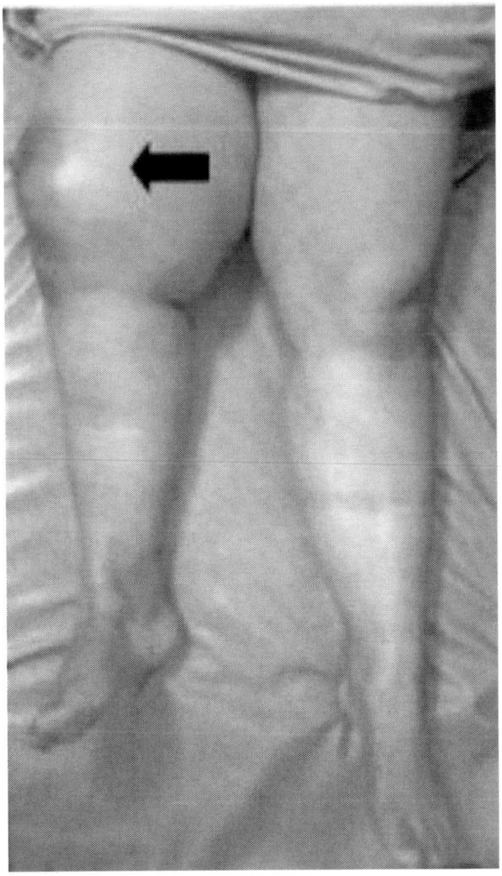

Figure 1. Tumor mass in the right femur (arrow).

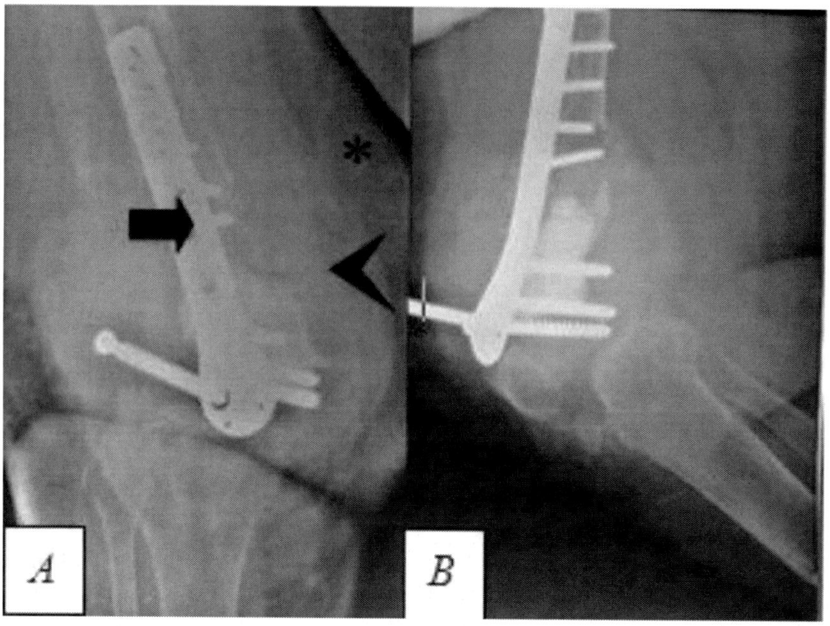

Figure 2. An X- ray of the right knee in (a) anteroposterior and (b) lateral views. Plate and screw internal fixation (arrow) and GCT (arrow head) with right distal femur soft tissue swelling (asterisk) are shown.

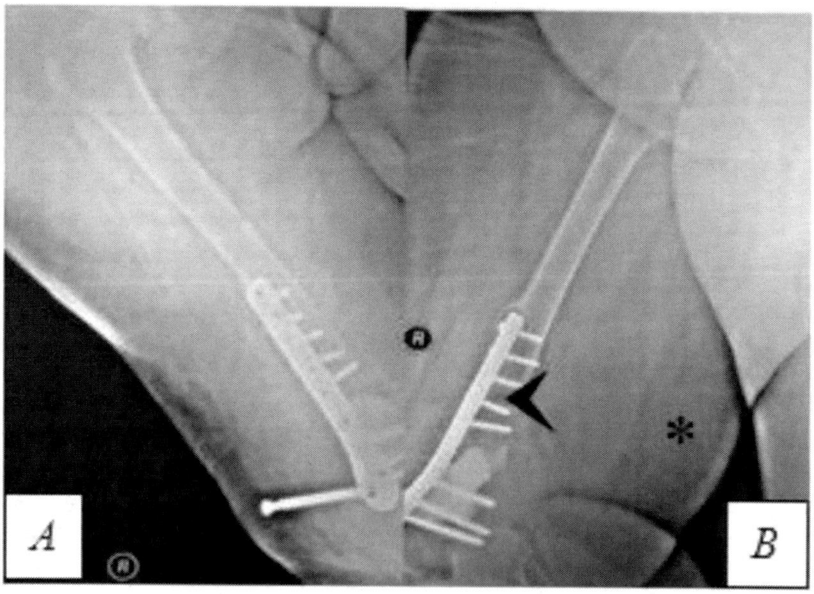

Figure 3. X- ray of the right femur in (a) anteroposterior and (b) lateral views. Lytic lesion (arrow head) with thickening of surrounding soft tissues (asterisk) are shown.

A CT scan of the right knee showed a right distal femur epimetaphyseal (6.1 × 10.2 × 11cm in size), extending into the tibiofemoral and patellofemoral junction, consistent with a recurrent lesion (Figure 4).

Core biopsy sample revealed tissues contained giant cells with >20 nuclei resembling stroma cell nuclei. The nuclei were round/oval, mild pleomorphic, hyperchromatic, and often vesicular with conspicuous nucleoli. Histological findings were compatible with a giant cell containing lesion, which can be identified in GCTB (Figure 5).

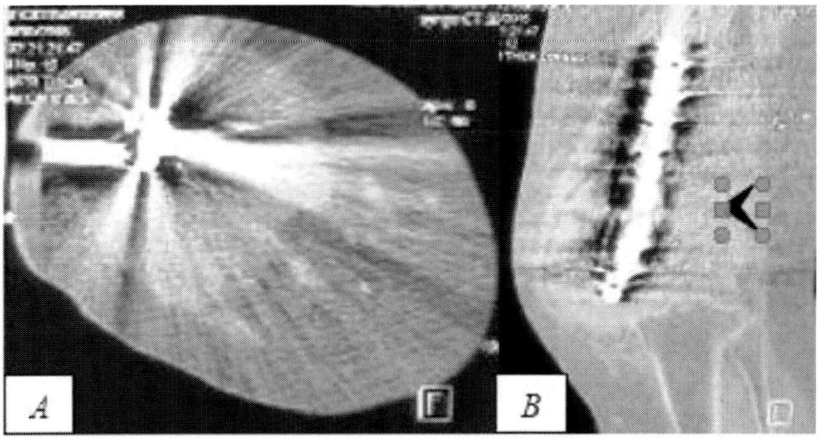

Figure 4. A CT scan of the right knee in (a) axial plane and (b) sagittal plane views. The right distal femur epimetaphyseal mass (arrow head), extending into the tibiofemoral and patellofemoral junction, are shown.

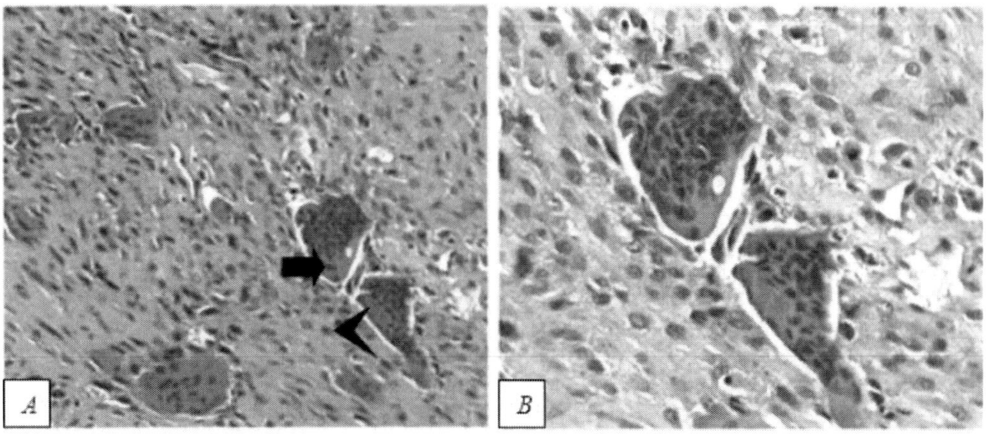

Figure 5. Core biopsy of the right distal femur. (a) Giant cells with >20 nuclei (arrow) resemble the stroma cell nuclei (arrow head) (HE 100X). (b) Round/oval nuclei, mild pleomorphic, hyperchromatic and often vesicular with conspicuous nucleoli (HE 400X).

The patient underwent a second surgery one month later. A surgical specimen sized 21 x 14 x 9cm was collected. The cut surface presented as well-circumscribed white mass with solid consistency (Figure 6).

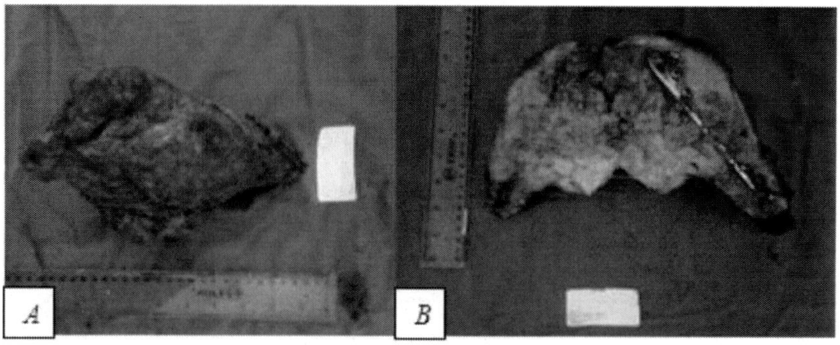

Figure 6. (a) Mass removed from the right knee. (b) The well-circumscribed white mass with solid consistency.

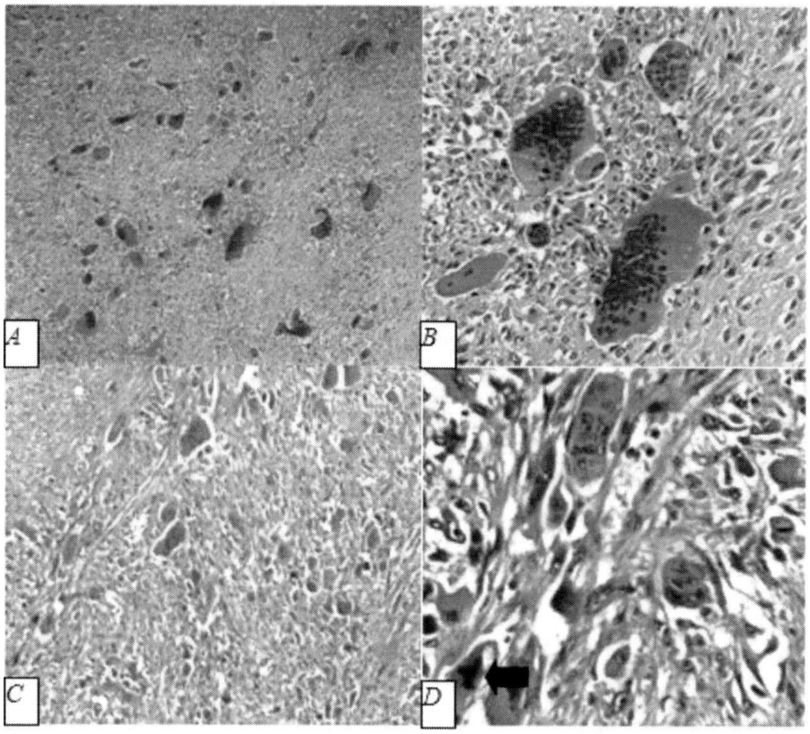

Figure 7. Histological sections of a surgery specimen. (A&B) Conventional GCT area (HE 40X & 400X). (C&D) Sarcomatous area with atypical mitosis (arrow) (HE 40X & 400X).

Representative sections were submitted in 11 cassettes. Histological evaluation revealed tumor tissues contained giant cells with >20 nuclei. There was a similarity among subsets of giant cells and stromal cells nuclei. Nuclei were round/oval, mild pleomorphic, vesicular, eosinio philic cytoplasm. High cellular stroma were found and arranged in storiform pattern, sarcomatous with oval/spindle nuclei, pleomorphic to bizarre, hyperchromatic, eosinophilic cytoplasm. The mitotic count was 2/10 HPF. Giant cells with bizarre nuclei, lymphovascular invasion, and areas of necrosis were also identified (Figure

7). Histological findings were compatible with high grade sarcoma, which can be found in secondary malignant GCTB.

Discussion

About 70% of GCTB cases are diagnosed in patients 20 – 40 years old, with a peak incidence in the third decade of life [9]. Women are affected about 1.5 times more frequently than men [1, 2, 9]. In line with current reports, the present case involved a 32-year-old female patient.

GCTB is commonly located in the epiphyseal ends of long tubular bones, usually in the distal end of the femur, the proximal end of the tibia, and the distal end of the radius. In the present case, the tumor was at the end of the long bone (right distal femur). Such a location was where the GCTB was previously diagnosed.

GCTB tends to progress to a high grade malignancy. Sarcomatous changes in malignant giant cell tumors can also develop for several years, or even decades, following removal of the primary lesion. Transformation to high grade sarcoma rarely occurs spontaneously. Specifically, it takes place with higher- frequency, post-irradiation therapy [8]. Alternatively, it can occur following a single local recurrence or multiple recurrences. [9] A histological or radiological differentiation between the two is impossible [6]. Clinically, the recurrence of pain and swelling many years post-GCT treatment is a clue of malignant transformation [1, 7]. In the present case, the patient was diagnosed with a bone tumor and underwent the first surgery six years ago, with no histopathological examination. The histopathologic findings from the second surgery, performed one year later, were consistent with high grade sarcoma, corresponding to secondary malignant GCTB. The patient did not have history of irradiation.

GCTB typically occurs as an eccentric, purely lytic lesion involving the end of the bone. It usually extends up to the subchondral bone plate. As a consequence of the tumor growth, the cortex is frequently destroyed. The lesion expands to soft tissues, where it is covered with a thin shell of reactive new bone [2]. Radiologically, a giant cell tumor with malignant change has the features of a large destructive lesion with cortical destruction and prominent invasion into soft tissues.

Plain X-rays of primary malignant GCTB demonstrate the presence of a lytic process extending to the end of the long bone. Imaging rarely shows typical GCT features and sclerotic destructive tumors juxtaposed with it. Plain X-rays of secondary malignant GCTB are characterized by a destructive process, with poor margination, situated at the site of a previously diagnosed GCTB [1]. In the case presented here, an X- ray showed lytic lesions in the distal femoral metadiaphysis, with thickening of the surrounding soft tissues. A CT scan showed a right distal femur epimetaphyseal mass 6.1 × 10.2 × 11 cm in size. The lesion appeared to extend into the tibiofemoral and patellofemoral junction, consistent with a recurrent lesion.

The gross appearance of malignancy in GCT is a large, fleshy tumor often with a soft tissue extension that is commonly seen in sarcomas [1, 2]. In the present case, the tumor's cut surface showed a well-circumscribed white mass, of solid consistency, with soft tissue extension.

Secondary malignant GCT are a rare condition, defined as a sarcomatous growth that occurs at the site of a previously documented benign GCT [4-8]. Characterised histologically by atypical mitoses and pleomorphism spindle cell nuclear that is next to or intermixed with conventional GCT [9, 11, 12]. Of note, immunohistochemical studies are not required for the transformation's diagnosis [12]. In the present case, a histopathological examination from the first surgery was not available for our review. A core biopsy performed before the second surgery revealed a giant cell containing lesion consistent with GCTB. The histological sections from the second surgery revealed giant cells with >20 nuclei admixed with round and spindle mononuclear cells. Subsets of the giant cells and mononuclear cells' nuclei were similar. In some areas, the spindle stromal component predominated and proliferated. Cells were arranged in storiform pattern with hyperchromatic and pleomorphic to bizarre nuclei. Atypical mitotic, lymphovascular invasion, and necrotic areas were identified. Based on these findings, we conclude that there was a malignant change characterized by sarcomatous growth that occurred next to, or intermixed with, the conventional GCT.

Malignant changes in GCT may be in the form of fibrosarcoma, malignant fibrous histiocytoma, osteosarcoma, or undifferentiated high- grade pleomorphic sarcoma. In an earlier study, Gong et al. reported malignant components, including osteosarcoma (11 cases), undifferentiated, high grade pleomorphic sarcoma (two cases), and fibrosarcoma (four cases) [13]. Additionally, Rock et al. found three times more fibrosarcomas than osteosarcomas among secondary malignant GCTB cases [14]. Bertoni et al. reported osteosarcomas in primary malignant GCTB (four of five cases), osteosarcomas in secondary malignant GCTB (9 of 12 cases), fibrosarcomas (two postradiation secondary malignant GCTBs) and malignant fibrous histiocytomas (one primary malignant GCTB and one postsurgical secondary malignant GCTB) [15]. In the present case, the malignant change was in the form of an undifferentiated high-grade pleomorphic sarcoma.

Secondary malignant GCTB needs to be differentiated from giant cell-rich osteosarcoma. Osteosarcoma's diagnosis requires the presence of a malignant bone-forming tumor [9]. In the present case, no malignant bone-forming tumor was identified.

The prognosis for patients with secondary malignant GCTB is similar to high grade sarcomas. Reports have shown that, in such patients, the prognosis is worse than in those with primary malignant GCTB [1].

The present case report presents a limitation. Specifically, no histopathological examination was performed at the time of the first surgery. However, from the second surgery's microscopic examination, we identified areas of anaplastic pleomorphic tumor cells and atypical mitoses were intermixed with conventional GCT. Such findings were the key in diagnosing malignant changes in GCT [9, 11, 12].

SUMMARY

Malignancy in GCT is a sarcoma arising within the GCT or at the site where a GCT had been previously documented. Malignant transformation in GCTB is rare. Giant cell tumors with malignant changes have radiologic features of large, destructive lesions with cortical destruction and prominent invasion into soft tissues. Key microscopic features in diagnosing malignant changes in GCT are atypical mitoses and pleomorphism spindle cell nuclear that is next to or intermixed with conventional GCT.

REFERENCES

[1] Athanasou, N. A.; Bansai, M.; Forsyth, R.; Reid, R. P.; Sapi, Z. Giant cell tumour of bone. In: Fletcher, C. D. M.; Bridge, J. A.; Hogendoorn, P.; Mertens, F.; editors. *WHO classification of tumours of soft tissue and bone.* 4th ed. Lyon: IARC. 2013. p. 321 - 324.

[2] Silverberg, S. G. Giant cell tumor. In: Silverberg, S. G.; editor. *AFIP atlas of tumor pathology: Tumors of the bones and joints.* Series 4. Washington: Armed forces institute of pathology. 2005. p. 282 - 295.

[3] Bacchini, P.; Bertoni, F. Giant cell tumor of bone. In: Folpe, A. L.; Inwards, C. Y.; editors. *Bone and soft tissue pathology*, p. 401 - 407.

[4] Saito, T.; Mitomi, H.; Suehara, Y.; Okubo, T.; Torigoe, T.; Takagi, T.; Kaneko, K.; Yao, T. A case of de novo secondary malignant giant- cell tumor of bone with loss of heterozygosity of p53 gene that transformed within a short - term follow- up. *Pathology-Research and Practice,* 2011 207, 664 - 669.

[5] Saito, T.; Mitomi, H.; Izumi, H.; Suehara, Y.; Okubo, T.; Torigoe, T.; Takagi, T.; Kaneko, K.; Sato, K.; Matsumoto, T.; Yao, T. A case of secondary malignant giant-cell tumor of bone with p53 mutation after longterm follow- up. *Human Pathology,* 2011 42, 727 - 733.

[6] Georgiev, G. P.; Slavchev, S.; Dimitrova, I. N.; Landzhov, B. Giant cell tumor of bone: current review of morphological; clinical; radiological; andtherapeutic characteristics. *Journal of Clinical and Experimental Investigations,* 2014 5,475 - 485.

[7] Grote, H. J.; Braun, M.; Kalinski, T.; Pomjanski, N.; Back, W.; Bleyl, U.; Böcking, A.; Roessner, A. Spontaneous malignant transformation of conventional giant cell tumor. *Skeletal Radiology,* 2004 33, 169 - 175.

[8] Oda,Y.; Sakamoto, A.; Saito, T.; Matsuda, S.; Tanaka, K.; Iwamoto, Y.; Tsuneyoshi, M. Secondary malignant giant- cell tumour of bone: molecular abnormalities of p53 and H- ras gene correlated with malignant transformation. *Histopathology*, 2001 39, 629 - 637.

[9] Czerniak, B. *Giant cell lesion*. In: Czerniak, B.; editor. Dorfman and czerniak's bone tumors. 2nd ed. Philadelphia: Saunders. 2016. p. 692 - 742.

[10] Zheng, M. H.; Robbins, P.; Xu, J.; Huang, L.; Wood, D. J.; Papadimitriou, J. M. The histogenesis of giant cell tumour of bone: a model of interaction between neoplastic cells and osteoclasts. *Histology and Histopathology*, 2001 16, 297 - 307.

[11] Bullough, P. G. Benign nonmatrix- producing bone tumors. In: Bullough, P. G.; editor. *Orthopaedic pathology*. 5th ed. Mosby elsevier: Missouri. 2010. p. 466 - 474

[12] Miller, I. J.; Blank, A.; Yin, S. M.; Mcnickle, A.; Gray, R.; Gitelis, S. A case of recurrent giant cell tumor of bone with malignant transformation and benign pulmonary metastases. *Diagnostic Pathology,* 2010 5, 62.

[13] Gong, L.; Liu, W.; Sun, X.; Sajdik, C.; Tian, X.; Niu, X.; Huang X. Histological and clinical characteristics of malignant giant cell tumor of bone. *Virchows Archiv.,* 2012 460, 327 - 334.

[14] Rock, M. G., Sim, F. H., Unni, K. K., et al. Secondary malignant giant-cell tumor of bone. Clinicopathological assessment of nineteen patients. *J. Bone Joint Surg. Am.,* 1986 68, 1073 - 1079.

[15] Bertoni, F.; Bacchini, P.; Staals, E. L. Malignancy in giant cell tumor of bone. *Cancer,* 2003 97, 2520 - 2529.

In: Case Reports in Surgery
Editors: Ahmad Jabir Rahyussalim et al.
ISBN: 978-1-53616-582-1

Chapter 36

SEGMENTAL ABSENCE OF INTESTINAL MUSCULATURE: CASE REPORT OF A RARE CAUSE OF NEONATAL INTESTINAL OBSTRUCTION

Ignasia Andhini Retnowulan[1] and Nur Rahadiani[2,*]
[1]Anatomical Pathology Residency Program, Faculty of Medicine, Universitas Indonesia, Jakarta, Indonesia
[2]Department of Anatomical Pathology, Faculty of Medicine, Universitas Indonesia, Jakarta, Indonesia

ABSTRACT

Segmental absence of intestinal musculature is a distinct histopathological entity with rare occurrence. The condition typically presents in neonates, with the primary manifestation being intestinal obstruction or perforation. Here we present the case of a neonate who initially presented with a high lesion of anal atresia. In the first few days following colostomy, the infant exhibited signs of intestinal obstruction. An exploratory laparotomy revealed ileal stenosis. A resected ileum specimen showed a narrowed segment of the ileum. Histopathological examination showed focal hypoplasia to total absence of muscularis propria with intact mucosal, submucosal, and serosal layers. Histochemical and immunohistochemical studies confirmed the absence and hypoplasia of muscularis propria, presence of ganglion cells, and absence of Cajal cells in the pathological segment. In cases of neonatal intestinal obstruction due to segmental absence of intestinal musculature, the possibility of defects of intestinal musculature should be investigated, particularly in conjunction with other congenital diseases.

* Corresponding Author's E-mail: nur.rahadiani@ui.ac.id.

Keywords: congenital defect, segmental absence of intestinal musculature

INTRODUCTION

Segmental absence of intestinal musculature (SAIM) is a distinct histopathological entity with rare occurrence. The condition was reported for the first time in 1943 [1]. Since then, the number of reported cases has been increasing, reaching approximately 25 cases in the English and Asian relevant literature [2]. However, thus far, there have been no such cases reported in Indonesia.

Typically, the condition presents in the neonatal age group, although several cases have been reported in adults [3]. The main manifestation of the disease is intestinal obstruction or perforation, along with other congenital anomalies, such as intestinal atresia, biliary atresia, patent ductus arteriosus, and ventricular septal defect [2, 4, 5]. Patients are mainly admitted to the hospital with complaints of abdominal distention, hypoactive bowel, ileus, and failure to pass meconium [6]. The majority of SAIM cases are discovered through surgery; however, a definitive diagnosis is based on histopathological findings [6]. Following gross examination, several cases demonstrated a thin-walled resected bowel, consistent with wall atrophy with paper-like consistency. Studies have reported an almost translucent color of the resected bowel [1]. Histological findings showed segmental absence or atrophy of intestinal musculature, with normal remaining intestinal layers. Other less common findings include fibrosis, inflammatory infiltration in the pathologic segment, and an underdeveloped capillary network [1,4,7]. The condition may involve the stomach, small intestine, or colon [1].

The pathogenesis of SAIM remains uncertain. However, several theories have been proposed. Abnormality during embryogenesis is thought to lead to incomplete myogenesis. Other theories described an etiology of an ischemic process during pre- or post-natal life, or as part of the remnant of developmental diverticula [2, 8]. Nevertheless, whether the disease is primarily due to malformation, or an ischemic or inflammation process remains controversial [4].

Currently, the condition is not widely recognized among clinicians and pathologists; hence, it is thought that the disease may be underdiagnosed. The aim of this case report was to familiarize pathologists and clinicians with this rare disease.

Case Report

Clinical Summary

A neonate was admitted to Cipto Mangunkusumo General Hospital 20h after birth due to congenital absence of the anal opening. The full-term infant was born through a spontaneous midwife-assisted labor from a mother who underwent irregular prenatal care. There was no record of the Appearance, Pulse, Grimace, Activity, Respiration (APGAR) score; however, the mother stated that the infant cried immediately after birth. The weight of the infant at birth was 3,000g. There were no other congenital anomalies identified at birth. In addition, there was no maternal illness or pregnancy complications reported. The 27-year-old mother denied consuming any medication or herbal drinks during pregnancy other than vitamins prescribed by the midwife. However, the mother revealed a history of untreated leukorrhea during pregnancy. Both parents did not report a family history of congenital anomalies. The older sibling of the patient was aged 5 years and born without any congenital anomalies or complications during pregnancy and labor.

At the time of hospital admission, physical examination showed normal vital signs with pale acral. It was observed that the abdominal distention with an abdominal circumference of 34cm, exceeded the normal limit (Figure 1) [9]. Laboratory testing showed a slight increase in leucocyte count (24,400/μL) and prolonged prothrombin time/activated partial thromboplastin time (1.46×/1.57×). Abdominal X-ray and babygram examination confirmed the diagnosis of a highlesion of anal atresia.

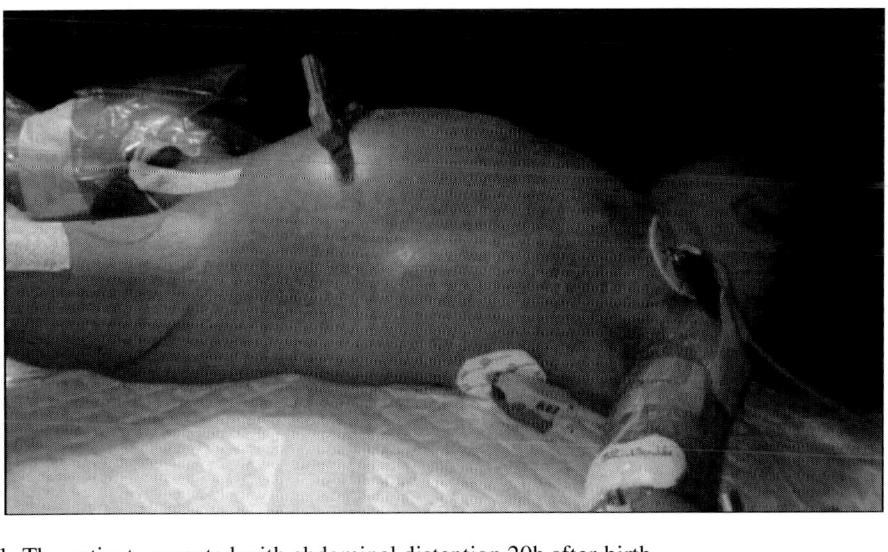

Figure 1. The patient presented with abdominal distention 20h after birth.

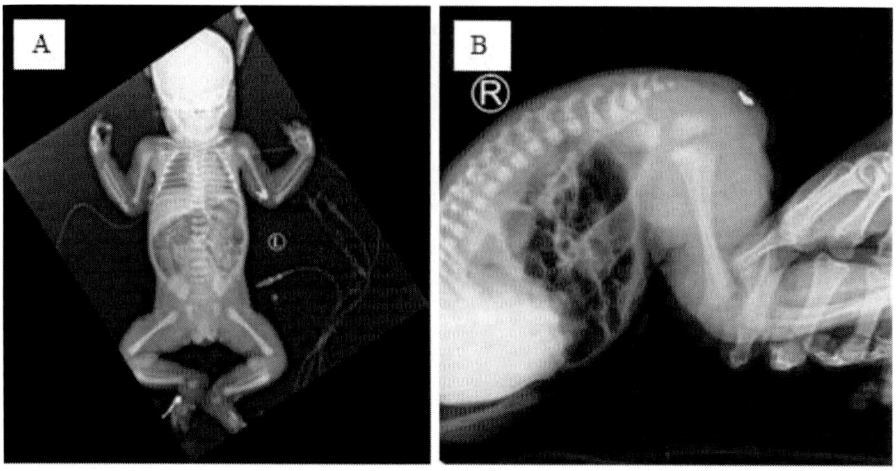

Figure 2. Radiological examination performed at the time of hospital admission. (a) Babygram imaging. (b) Abdominal X-ray examination in the knee-chest position.

The colon and small bowel were distended and filled with fecal mass (Figure 2a, 2b). The early babygram did not reveal ileal atresia. The initial diagnosis was anal atresia with suspicion of late-onset neonatal sepsis.

At the age of 2 days, the patient underwent colostomy. In the first few days following surgery, the patient developed signs and symptoms of intestinal obstruction, such as vomiting, abdominal distention, and decreased production of stoma. The intestinal obstruction became apparent on day 8. The patient was lethargic and serum markers of inflammation increased. The levels of C-reactive protein and procalcitonin were 16.4 and 0.44, respectively. Repeated abdominal X-ray examinations showed intestinal dilatation, indicating the presence of high intestinal obstruction. Subsequently, an exploratory re-laparotomy was performed. Intraoperative findings revealed ileal stenosis, located 120cm from the Treitz ligament.

Evaluation of the colostomy stoma did not demonstrate obstruction or presence of pus. Adhesion between the ileum and sigmoid was found. A 2.5-cm specimen of the ileal stenosis was resected, and an ileo-ileal anastomosis and adhesiolysis were performed. Post-operative abdominal X-ray examination did not show signs of intestinal obstruction. Post-operative laboratory testing showed a decrease in the level of C-reactive protein from 16.4 to 10.9; however, the level of procalcitonin was slightly increased from 0.44 to 0.54. There was no vomiting reported, and the production of colostomy stoma was within normal limits. Several days following the surgery, an enteral diet was initiated. The patient was discharged from the hospital 19 days after surgery. During subsequent outpatient visits, the patient did not show signs of recurring intestinal obstruction. Moreover, the stoma output was within normal limits. Unfortunately, the patient was lost to follow-up after a few months.

Pathological Findings

Histopathological examinationwas performed using a resected specimen of the ileum (2.5cm in length and 1cm in diameter). The specimen revealed a narrowing segment of the ileum (Figure 3). Histopathological examination showed intact mucosa with a normal to shortened ileal villous. The lamina propria to serosal layers were mildly infiltrated with chronic inflammatory cells, neutrophils and eosinophils of 5–10 per high-power field. Muscularis propria showed focal hypoplasia to total absence of smooth muscle fibers.

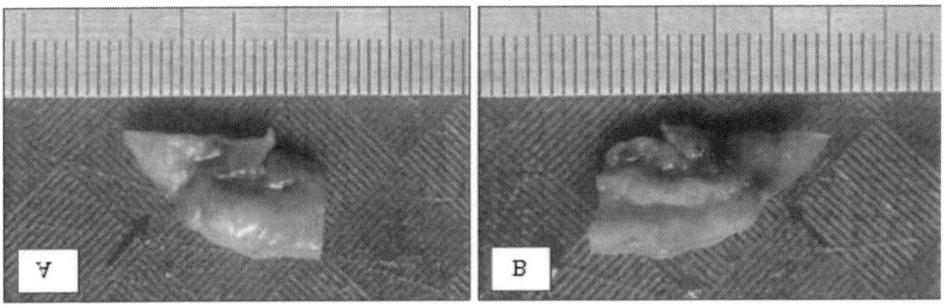

Figure 3. Gross examination showed a narrowing segment (red arrow) of the resected ileum.(a) Serosal surface and (b) Luminal surface.

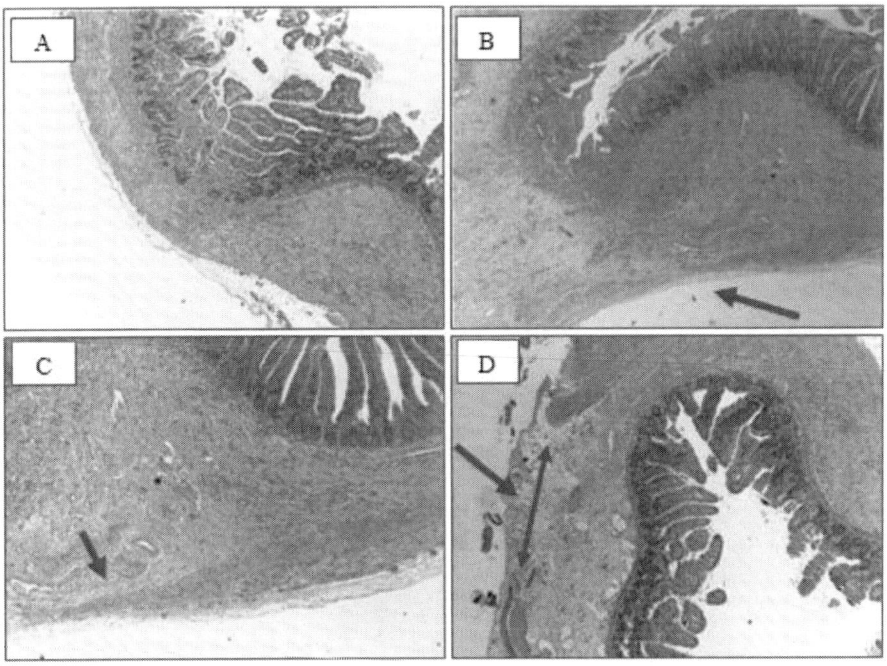

Figure 4. Histopathological examination. (a) Relatively normal segment of the ileum (HE, 40×). (b) Focal hypoplasia of the muscularis propria (hematoxylin & eosin [HE], 40×). (c) Focal hypoplasia of the muscularis propria (HE, 100×). (d) Total absence of the muscularis propria (HE, 40×). b-d. Intact mucosal, submucosal, and serosal layers.

There were no vascular network abnormalities, vasculitis, or ischemic changes present (Figure 4).

Histochemical and immunohistochemical staining was performed for further assessment of both the muscle fibers and innervation of the ileum. Gomori trichrome staining showed normal connective tissue fibers in both the normal and stenotic segments of the bowel. Smooth muscle actin showed positivity in the smooth muscle, in terms of normal thickness and hypoplastic muscle. CD117 immunostaining was non-reactive, thus revealing the absence of Cajal cells in both segments where the muscularis propia were hypoplastic and absent. Calretinin, which was positive in normal ganglion cells, showed normal submucosal and myenteric ganglion cells in the narrowed segment and revealed slightly hyperplastic ganglion cells in the normal segment (Figure 5, 6).

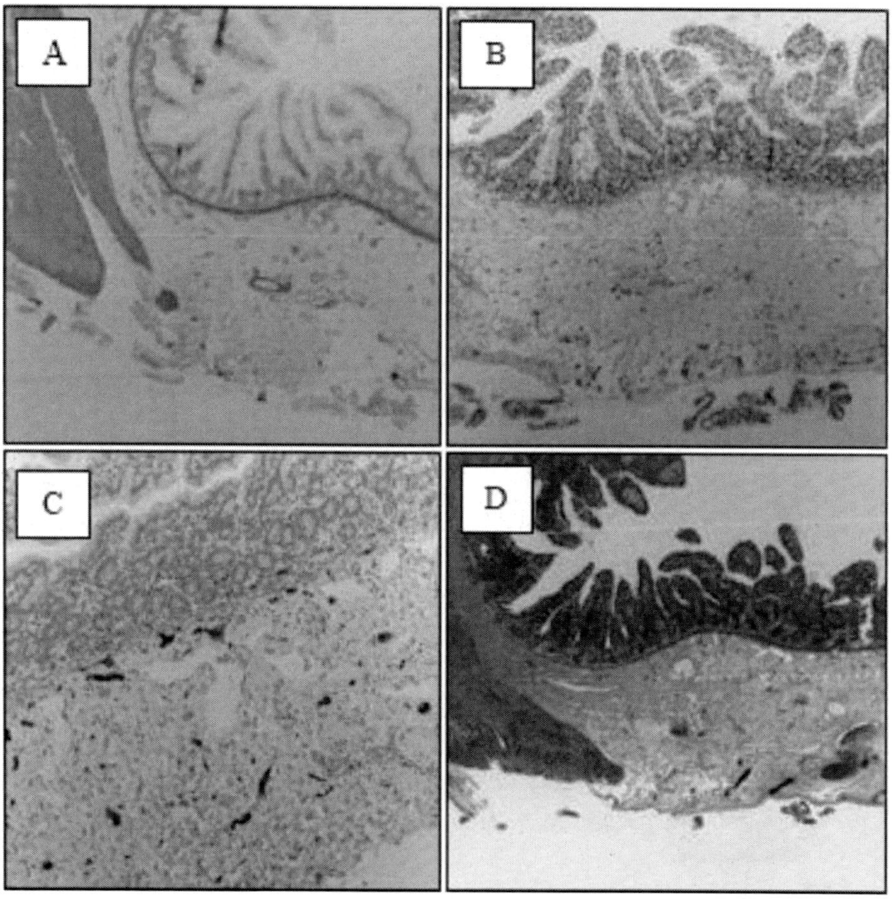

Figure 5. Histochemical and immunohistochemical staining in the total absence of muscularis propria. (a) SMA, 40×; (b) CD117, 40×; (c) Calretinin, 100× and (d) Gomori trichrome, 40×.

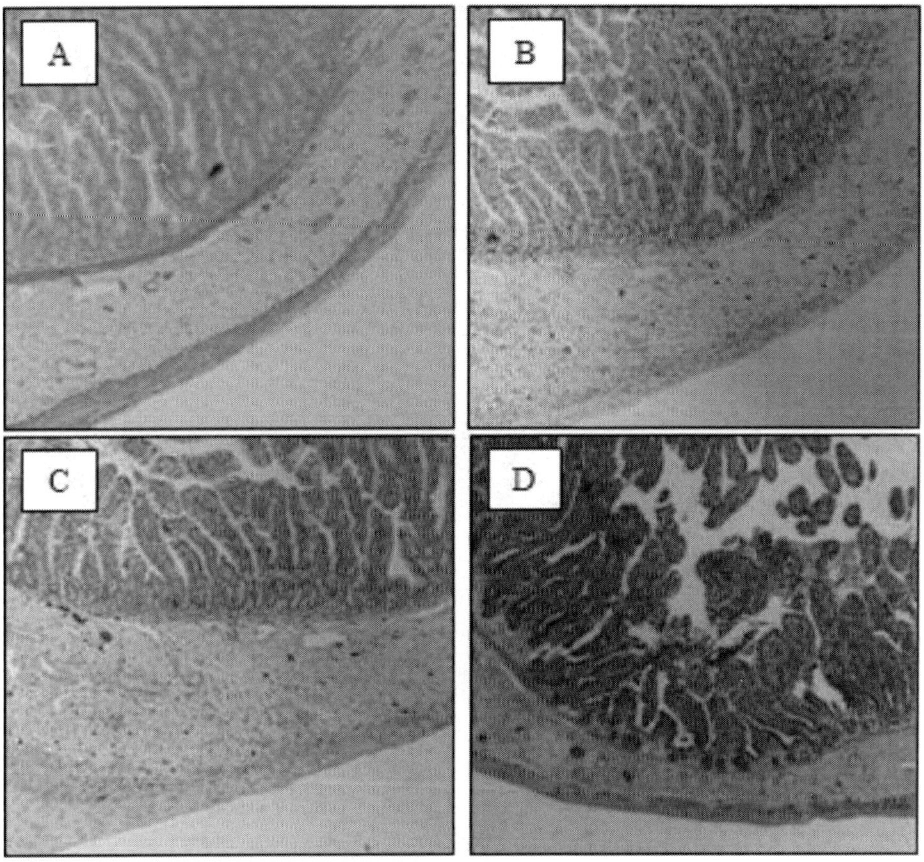

Figure 6. Histochemical and immunohistochemical staining of the hypoplastic muscularis propria. (a) SMA, 40×; (b) CD117, 40×; (c) Calretinin, 100× and (d) Gomori trichrome, 40×.

DISCUSSION

Neonatal intestinal obstruction commonly results in admission to the Neonatal Intensive Care Unit. The incidence rate is approximately 1 in 2,000 live births [10]. The cardinal signs of this condition are polyhydramnion, bilious emesis, failure to pass meconium in the first 24–48 hours of life, and abdominal distention [10, 11]. The blockage along the gastrointestinal tract may be structural or functional [11, 12]. Structural obstruction includes atresia, stenosis, intussusception, volvulus, intussusception, hernias, bands, and presence of masses [11]. In contrast, functional obstruction can be caused by Hirschsprung's disease, sepsis, electrolyte imbalance, meconium plug syndrome, and other secondary conditions that lead to loss of peristaltic activity [11, 13]. The most common cause of intestinal obstruction in newborns is intussusception (20.8%), followed by intestinal atresia (11.8%) [14]. Among intestinal atresias, jejunoileal and anal atresia are the most common conditions, with an incidence rate of 1 in 5,000 live births [10]. Initial treatment involves nasogastric decompression, fluid resuscitation, and administration of broad-spectrum antibiotics. Most cases usually require non-emergent operative repair, except for malrotation and volvulus. However, surgical management should proceed promptly [10].

On the other hand, gastrointestinal perforation in newborns exhibits a slightly higher incidence rate of approximately 0.6% in the neonatal intensive care unit [15]. However, the exact incidence rate is yet to be determined. The mortality rate remains high (30–50%), despite the development of antibiotics and surgical procedures [15, 16]. The leading cause of gastrointestinal perforation in newborns is necrotizing enterocolitis (NEC), which occurs in approximately 1–3 per 1,000 live births [12]. Other causes of perforations are sepsis, intestinal obstruction, iatrogenic trauma, Hirschsprung's disease, and spontaneous intestinal perforations [15].

SAIM is a rare condition that mainly occurs in neonates and presents with other congenital anomalies, such as patent ductus arteriosus, ventricular septal defect, intestinal atresia, and biliary atresia [1, 2, 4]. The main manifestation of this disease is a progressively acute abdomen due to bowel obstruction or perforation. Patients are admitted to the hospital with complaints of moderate-to-severe abdominal distention, diminished bowel sounds, failure to pass meconium, and bilious vomiting [17]. The incidence of SAIM is difficult to determine due to its rarity. In the neonatal age group, the age of onset ranges from 1 to 99 days. Davis *et al.* reported five cases of SAIM, all of whom were born preterm through cesarean section, with very low-birth-weight ranging from 490g to 1166g [17]. The majority of preterm neonates with SAIM also present with respiratory distress syndrome [4]. Although typically present in neonates, studies have also reported the occurrence of SAIM in adults. There is no sex predilection of this defect in adults. The age of onset ranges from 26 to 64 years, with a higher incidence reported in the older age group [3]. Two studies reported a family history of congenital anomalies, such as congenital megacolon and osteogenesis imperfect [3, 18].

In the present case, the clinical presentation was similar to that observed in other reported cases, with regards to chief complaints, age of onset, and correlation with other congenital anomalies. The patient was admitted to the hospital primarily due to anal atresia. Abdominal distention was also reported at the time of admission. An initial diagnosis of bowel obstruction was considered due to the anal atresia. However, abdominal distention, vomiting, and the absence of stoma production persisted after colostomy. These signs and symptoms led to the diagnosis of intestinal obstruction, which was located proximally to the stoma. According to the history of pregnancy, the patient was born full term, with a birth weight within normal limits (3,000g). This may raise awareness among clinicians, as most reported neonatal cases occur in preterm, low-birth-weight infants. This case shows that full-term infants with a normal birth weight may also harbor a congenital defect.

Following gross examination, the resected SAIM showed a thin-walled bowel, with paper-like consistency [3]. Investigators have reported several cases exhibiting segments of intestine with an almost translucent color [1]. Therefore, intraoperative transillumination is recommended as part of the diagnostic process [1, 17]. In this case, intraoperative findings and gross examination of the resected small intestine showed a narrowing segment of the ileum that manifested as an intestinal obstruction. Macroscopically, the observed atrophic intestinal wall was consistent with findings reported in previous studies. Unfortunately, transillumination was not performed during surgery.

Nawar and Sawyer stated that all the cases they reviewed showed a gradual or abrupt loss of the muscularis propria of both the longitudinal and circular layers. Inflammation and mesenteric vessel thrombosis are uncommon findings. Approximately half of the cases demonstrated loss of nerve plexuses in affected segments [3, 19]. Our histopathological findings showed segmental hypoplasia to total absence of the muscularis propria, with remaining intact mucosal, submucosal, and serosal layers. There were mild inflammatory cell infiltrations within the lamina propria. However, vasculitis, thrombosis, or signs of vascular anomaly were not identified. Moreover, there was no fibrosis found in the area of the defect. Innervation was found to be normal. Submucosal and myenteric plexuses were observed in both normal and pathological segments. These findings are consistent with previous results reported in the literature. The diagnosis of SAIM was reached solely based on pathological evaluation.

SAIM may mimic other conditions that manifest as obstruction or perforation. In the presence of obstruction, the closest differential diagnoses are Hirschsprung's disease and intestinal atresia. In the presence of perforation, SAIM may also mimic NEC and intestinal ischemia. Both Hirschsprung's disease and SAIM may cause delay in passing meconium and colonic dilatation. Hirschsprung's disease is diagnosed by the absence of ganglion cells and hypertrophied nerve fibers [12]. SAIM, on the other hand, involves the presence of ganglion cells and absence of muscularis propria. Intestinal atresia varies from a septum obstructing the bowel (i.e., membranous atresia) to a complete gap between the bowel ends with a mesenteric defect and apple-peel atresia [12,14]. However, SAIM may cause dilatation or stenosis of the bowel, while maintaining the continuity of the bowel. However, several articles reported cases of SAIM, which were found in close proximity to intestinal atresia [14, 20]. Therefore, it is possible that both entities share a similar etiology. NEC accounts for the majority of intestinal obstructions occurring in newborns. Therefore, it is the closest differential diagnosis for SAIM, which manifests as perforation. However, NEC shows signs of inflammation, bacterial overgrowth, epithelial regeneration, mucosal edema, and ischemic transmural necrosis [21]. Notably, SAIM shows limited signs of inflammation. The pathology of intestinal ischemia involves mucosal damage, neutrophil infiltration, neuronal damage, and degeneration of muscle, which includes clear cytoplasm, pyknotic nuclei, and apoptotic bodies [22]. In the present case, there was no mucosal damage or acute inflammatory cells identified. The remaining muscularis propria in the hypoplastic segment was normal.

Considering that the clinical presentation of SAIM may mimic other conditions, exploratory laparotomy is the gold standard, and the diagnosis is mainly dependent on histopathological findings. Resection of the affected intestines, ileostomy, and end-to-end anastomosis have been linked to favorable outcomes. Of note, most patients are not in good general condition at the time of diagnosis due to the presence of peritonitis. Therefore, they usually require initial enterostomy [17]. The incidence of SAIM is currently unknown; thus, determining the prognosis of this disease is challenging. Davis *et al.* did not report progression or secondary perforation in five cases of neonatal SAIM [17]. Additionally, Nawar and Sawyer did not report the recurrence of intestinal perforation in adults with SAIM [3]. However, Oyachi *et al.* reported the occurrence of multiple perforations after resection. This condition is caused by unstable mesenteric circulation, which leads to ischemic process and infarction at previously unresected SAIM lesions [5]. Considering that the diagnosis of SAIM lesions during surgery is occasionally challenging, a frozen section procedure may be a useful diagnostic modality to avoid misdiagnosis. Surgeons should ensure that the resection margins are free of lesions prior to performing an end-to-end anastomosis. Preoperative diagnosis of SAIM is not possible; therefore, it is important for surgeons to understand this condition in order to recognize the lesions during surgery and prevent secondary destruction of the muscle layer.

Conclusion

In cases of neonatal intestinal obstruction or perforation, the possibility of defects of intestinal musculature due to SAIM should be investigated, especially in conjunction with other congenital diseases.

Conflict of Interest

None declared.

References

[1] Pereira, S., Tortosa, F., Gonçalves, M. (2014). Segmental absence of intestinal musculature concerning a child with acute appendicitis. *J. Pediatr. Surg.*,3(5), 207-210.

[2] Nandedkar, S.S., Malukani, K., Patidar, E., Nayak, R. (2015). Segmental absence of intestinal musculature: A rare case report. *Int. J. Appl. Basic Med. Res.*, 5(3), 222-224.

[3] Nawar, N.A., Sawyer, P.R. (2016). Segmental absence of intestinal musculature in a 64-year-old female: Case report and literature review. *Am. J. Case Rep.,* 17, 749-54.

[4] Oretti, C., Bussani, R., Janes, A., Demarini, S. (2010). Multiple segmental absence of intestinal musculature presenting as spontaneous isolated perforation in an extremely low-birth-weight infant. *J. Pediatr. Surg.,* 45(8), E25-27.

[5] Oyachi, N., Suzuki, T., Emura, T., Obana, K., Nemoto, A., Naito, A., Oyama, T. (2017). Segmental absence of intestinal musculature with metachronous bowel perforations in an infant. *J. Pediatr. Surg. Case Rep.,* 30, 1-3.

[6] Tawfik, O., Newell, B., Lee, K.R. (1998). Segmental absence of intestinal musculature in an adult. *Dig. Dis. Sci.,* 43(2), 397-399.

[7] Ozguner, I.F., Savas, C., Ozguner, M., Candir, O. (2005). Intestinal atresia with segmental musculature and neural defect. *J. Pediatr. Surg.,* 40(8), 1232-1237.

[8] McCarthy, D., Qualman, S., Besner, G. (1994). Absent intestinal musculature: Anatomic evidence of an embryonic origin of the lesion. *J. Pediatr. Surg.,* 29(11), 1476-1478.

[9] Meldere, I., Urtans, V., Kruze, D., Petersons, A., Abola, Z. (2013). Neonatal anthropometry: Measurement of the abdominal circumference in newborns. *Acta Chir. Latviensis,* 1, 47-50.

[10] Juang, D., Snyder, C.L. (2012). Neonatal bowel obstruction. *Surg. Clin. North Am.,* 92(3), 685-711.

[11] de Silva, N.T., Young, J.A., Wales, P.W. (2006). Understanding neonatal bowel obstruction: Building knowledge to advance practice. *Neonatal Netw.,* 25(5), 303-318.

[12] de la Hunt, M.N. (2006). The acute abdomen in the newborn. *Semin. Fetal Neonat. Med.,* 11(3), 191-197.

[13] Kiho, T., L., Scheimberg, I., Phelps, S., Misra, D., Ward, H., Colmenero, I. (2011). Neonatal functional intestinal obstruction and the presence of severely immature ganglion cells on rectal biopsy: 6 year experience. *Pediatr. Surg. Int.,* 27(5), 487-490.

[14] Subbarayan, D., Singh, M., Khurana, N., Sathish, A. (2015). Histomorphological features of intestinal atresia and its clinical correlation. *J. Clin. Diagn. Res.,* 9(11), EC26-29.

[15] Sarac, M., Bakal, U., Aydin, M., Tartar, T., Orman, A., Taskin, E., Canpolat, Ş., Kazez, A. (2017). Neonatal gastrointestinal perforations: the 10-year experience of a reference hospital. *Indian J. Surg.,* 79(5), 431-436.

[16] Hakan, N., Aydin, M., Erdogan, D., Cavusoglu, Y.H., Dursun, A., Zenciroglu, A., Okumus, N., Ozguner, I.F., Karaman, A., Karaman, I. (2013). Neonatal gastrointestinal perforations: a 7-year single center experience at a tertiary neonatal intensive care unit in Turkey. *CIB. Tech. J. Surg.,* 3, 1-7.

[17] Davis, J.S., Ryan, M.L., Shields, J.M., Sola, J.E., Perez, E.A., Neville, H.L., Rodriguez, M.M. (2012). Segmental absence of intestinal musculature: an increasingly reported pathology. *J. Pediatr. Surg.,* 47(8), 1566-1571.

[18] Steiner, D.H., Maxwell, J.G., Rasmussen, B.L., Jones, R. (1969). Segmental absence of intestinal musculature. An unusual cause of intestinal obstruction in the neonate. *Am. J. Surg.,* 118(6), 964-967.

[19] Dzieniecka, M., Grzelak-Krzymianowska, A., Kulig, A.(2010). Segmental congenital defect of the intestinal musculature. *Pol. J.Pathol.*, 61(2), 94-96.

[20] Budhiraja, S., Jaiswal, T.S., Sen, R. (2004). Ileal atresia with segmental defect of intestinal musculature. *Indian J. Pediatr.,* 71(2), 177-179.

[21] Tanner, S.M., Berryhill, T.F., Ellenburg, J.L., Jilling, T., Cleveland, D.S., Lorenz, R.G., Martin, C.A. (2015). Pathogenesis of necrotizing enterocolitis: modeling the innate immune response. *Am. J. Pathol.*, 185(1), 4-16.

[22] Pontell, L., Sharma, P., Rivera, L.R., Thacker, M., Tan, Y.H., Brock, J.A., Furness, J.B. (2011). Damaging effects of ischemia/reperfusion on intestinal muscle. *Cell Tissue Res.,* 343,411-419.

In: Case Reports in Surgery
Editors: Ahmad Jabir Rahyussalim et al.
ISBN: 978-1-53616-582-1

Chapter 37

Hemangioma-Like Vessels in the Resection Margin of Giant Hemangiomas of the Liver as a Possible Cause of Recurrence: A Case Series and Literature Review

Marini Stephanie**, *Ening Krisnuhoni, Diah Rini Handjari and Nur Rahadiani
Department of Anatomical Pathology,
Universitas Indonesia/Cipto Mangunkusumo Hospital,
Jakarta-Indonesia

Abstract

Most liver hemangiomas are small and asymptomatic, but large, or giant, hemangiomas may be symptomatic and can occur with hemangioma-like vessels (HLVs) distant from the primary tumor. We report three cases of giant cavernous hemangioma of the liver in adults, with the hemangioma recurring in one of the three patients 8 months after surgical resection. All cases had clusters of HLVs located far from the primary tumor and in the resection margin.

Keywords: giant hemangioma, liver, recurrence, hemangioma-like vessels

*Corresponding Author's E-mail: marini2sh@gmail.com.

INTRODUCTION

Cavernous hemangioma of the liver is the most common benign liver tumor with an estimated incidence ranging from <1% to 20%. It can occur at any age but is most frequently found in young adult women. Increased size may be related with sex hormones. Liver hemangiomas are generally solitary, with only about 10% being multiple. Cavernous hemangiomas can vary in size from a few millimeters to so large that they can replace most of the liver. However, the majority are <4 cm and are usually asymptomatic. Gross sections have a spongy appearance with a lot of blood. Cavernous hemangiomas rarely become malignant, and usually, surgical resection is indicated for large tumors or those that progress. Hemangiomas can have irregular margins that extend between liver cells at the edge of tumor. The presence of small clusters of hemangioma-like vessels (HLVs), located distant from the tumor mass associated with giant hemangioma may be the reason for post-resection recurrence. We report three cases of giant cavernous hemangioma of the liver in adults, one of which recurred after surgical resection [1, 2].

CASE REPORT

Case 1

A 46-year-old man came to the Cipto Mangunkusumo Hospital complaining of intermittent stomach pain for 3 weeks before admission. The patient had a 6-year history of stomach discomfort; however, he noted an enlargement of the stomach accompanied by nausea and fatigue 1 year ago. Enlargement of the abdomen without jaundice was found on physical examination. Abdominal computed tomography (CT) scan showed a hypodense 14 × 16 × 20-cm lesion involved segments V, VI, VII, and VIII, with enhancement in the arterial phase that increased in the venous and delayed phases, consistent with a hemangioma.

Gross examination following hepatectomy revealed a well-demarcated 15 × 14 × 8-cm tumor (Figure 1). The cut surface had a spongy appearance, and tissue sections contained a lot of dark blood, with some areas appearing yellow-white. Microscopic examination showed spaces and vascular channels of varying sizes that were separated by a fibrous matrix, lined by flattened endothelial cells. Organizing thrombi and wide fibrotic areas were observed. The interface between the lesion and the adjacent liver parenchyma was irregular, and many hemangioma-like vessels (HLVs) were seen in the resection margin.

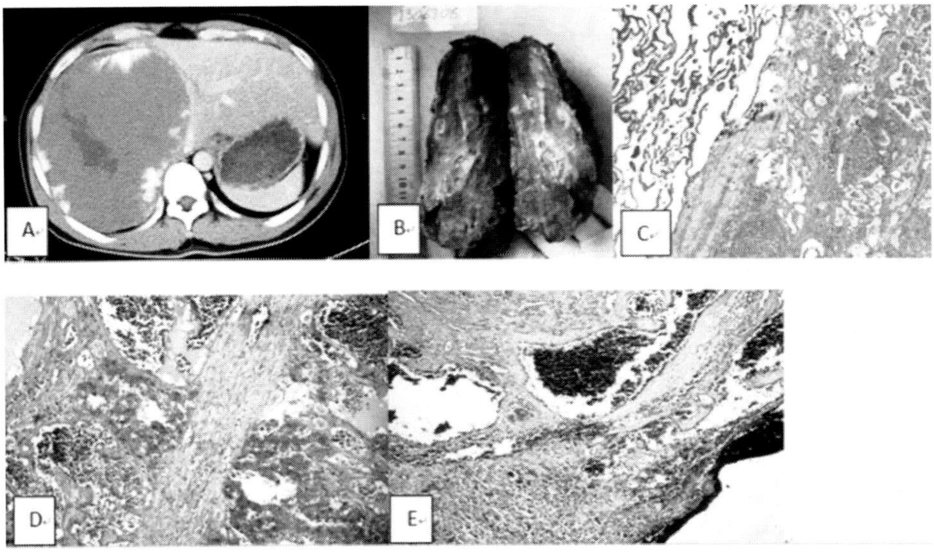

Figure 1. A. Abdominal CT scan, venous phase. B. Macroscopic appearance of the right lobe resection of case one. C. Microscopic appearance of the cavernous hemangioma of case one (HE, ×40); D. Irregular, spongy interface (Trichrome ×100); E. Resection margins with hemangioma-like vessels (HLVs) (Trichrome ×100).

A follow up abdominal CT scan performed 8 months after resection revealed a 5.4 × 5 × 5-cm nodule in the posteromedial right lobe segment VIII. Afterwards the second surgical resection was done to the patient. In intraoperation, a new growth was noted in the post-resection site, and gross examination revealed a 6 × 4 × 3-cm tumor with microscopic features similar to those of the previous tumor with hemangioma-like vessels (HLVs) in the resection margin. Trichrome staining of the interface border revealed a tumor margin with an irregular, spongy interface. Immunohistochemistry was negative for Ki-67.

Case 2

A 53-year-old woman came to the Cipto Mangunkusumo Hospital complaining of enlargement of the abdomen for 1 year before admission, accompanied by nausea, vomiting, and weight loss over the previous 6 months. Physical examination found no jaundice and a palpable mass with indistinct edges in the right hypochondria. An abdominal CT showed a 15.8 × 12.8 × 15.3-cm hypodense mass in the right lobe of the liver, segments IV, V, VII, and VIII with enhancement in the arterial, venous, and delayed phases, consistent with hemangioma. A follow-up CT scan 6 months after transarterial embolization found necrosis with no significant change in the size of the mass. Following hepatectomy, gross examination revealed a 20 × 13 × 9 cm tumor (Figure 2). The cut surface had a spongy appearance and tissue sections contained a lot of dark blood and some areas that were yellow-white in color. Microscopic examination showed spaces and vascular channels of varying sizes lined by flattened endothelial cells and separated by a fibrous network including dispersed thrombi. The interface between the lesion and adjacent live parenchyma was irregular and hemangioma-like vessels (HLVs) were seen in the resection margin. Trichrome staining of the interface border revealed a tumor margin with a predominantly irregular and spongy interface and an interdigitating pattern. Immunohistochemistry was negative for Ki 67.

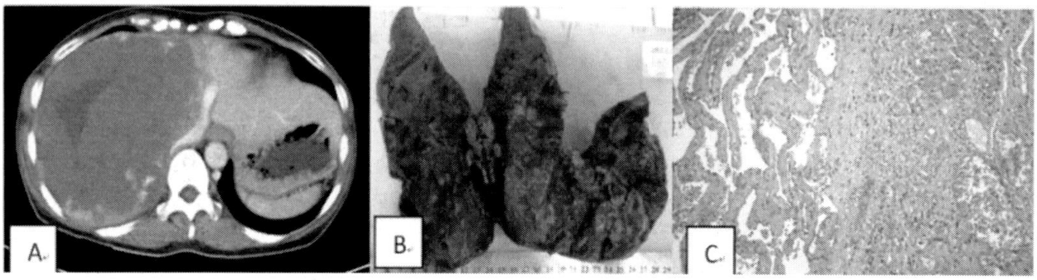

Figure 2. A. Abdominal CT scan, venous phase; B. Macroscopic appearance of right lobe resection of case two; C. Microscopic appearance of the cavernous hemangioma of case two (HE, ×100).

Case 3

A 41-year-old woman came to the Cipto Mangunkusumo Hospital complaining of stomach bloating for 2 months before admission. Physical examination found no jaundice and a solitary palpable mass with indistinct edges in the right hypochondria. An abdominal CT showed a 10.16 × 9.3 × 26.67-cm multilobulated mass with irregular edges involved liver segments V, VI, VII, and VIII that displaced the intestine medially. There was contrast enhancement in the arterial and venous phases and patchy areas of enhancement within the mass, consistent with liver neoplasm and a differential diagnosis of hemangioma and hepatocellular carcinoma. The gross appearance of the hepatectomy specimen revealed a 22 × 16 × 9-cm tumor (Figure 3). The cut surface had a spongy appearance and tissue sections contained a lot of dark blood and some areas that were cystic or yellow-white in color.

Microscopic examination showed spaces and vascular channels of varying sizes lined by flattened endothelial cells and separated by a fibrous network including dispersed thrombi. The interface between the lesion and adjacent live parenchyma was irregular and hemangioma-like vessels (HLVs) were seen in the resection margin. Trichrome staining of the interface border revealed an interdigitating pattern. Immunohistochemistry was negative for Ki 67.

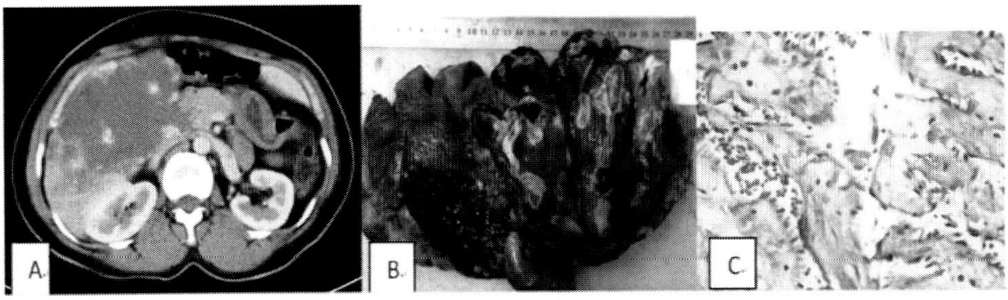

Figure 3. A. Abdominal CT scan, venous phase; B. Macroscopic appearance of right lobe resection of case three; C. Microscopic appearance of cavernous hemangioma of case three (HE, ×400).

DISCUSSION

The ages of these three patients with cavernous hemangiomas of the liver ranged from 41 to 53 yers old. Patients came in a state of advanced may have contributed to the large size of the tumors [2]. All three were found in the right lobe of the liver, and a size of more than 10 cm surpassed the 5 cm needed consideration as a giant hemangioma [1-3]. The ages of a series of 198 cases of hepatic hemangioma reported by Etemadi et al. ranged from 27–84 years. Most were located in the right lobe, and only 18,2% were from 5 to 25 cm in size. Of the 129 who could be followed-up, 7% were treated by surgical resection because of abdominal pain, large size, rupture, or bleeding [4]. The lack of response to arterial embolization in case two is consistent with a report by Koszka et al. that arterial embolization to restrict the growth of a 40 cm giant liver hemangioma was not effective and was followed by a worsening of symptoms [5].

The gross and microscopic appearance of the resected tumor was similar in all three cases and in line with a previous report of the pathological characteristics of the interface border of the tumor and liver parenchyma by Zimmermann et al. [6].

In a previous report, Zimmermann et al. have described four distinct interface patterns that were seen in cavernous liver hemangiomas [6]. Pattern A was characterized by a capsule-like fibrous lamella(fibrous interfaces). In pattern B, the peripheral component of the hemangioma interdigitated with the liver parenchyma, dilated vascular channels were associated with remnants of the portal tract, and a fibrous lamella was absent(interdigitating interfaces). Pattern C included a compressed interface with a thin, vascular tissue layer that separated the tumor and liver parenchyma without the presence of a fibrous lamella or interdigitating vascular channels. Pattern D was a, irregular, spongy interface with a highly irregular border characterized by the presence of liver parenchyma located between dilated vascular channels. Of the 10 cases in their report, 7 showed predominantly pattern A, and with 5 of the 10 exhibiting a single pattern and the remaining 5 a mixed pattern. Only two hemangiomas had a predominant pattern D. Trichrome staining of tissue from our patients revealed that the interface border in case one and two had a predominant pattern D with a highly irregular border and lack of a clear separated of tumor and non tumor tissue. Case three had a pattern B interdigitating interface. Immunohistochemistry was done to exclude a diagnosis of low-grade angiosarcoma, with Ki67 staining of low- and high-grade angiosarcomas as controls.

Case one had the longest follow-up, with recurrence detected on CT at 8 months after hepatectomy. Previously, Conter et al. have reported four cases of recurrence of hepatic hemangiomas, with two of them recurring years after surgery in patients with histories of long-term hormonal therapy [7]. Romano et al. have described a case with three hepatic hemangioma recurrences in the years after surgery in a patient with no history of hormonal therapy [8]. The pathological evaluation of the resection margins or hemangioma-like vessels (HLVs) was not reported in either of those cases. Zhu et al. reported two cases of giant hepatic hemangiomas that recurred 4 and 5 years after resection. Both had irregular interfaces because of the presence of hemangioma-like vessels (HLVs). No hormonal therapy data were reported [9]. Etemadi et al. have reported post-surgical recurrences in three of 198 patients with hepatic hemangioma, but the time of recurrence, pathology data on the resection margin, and the presence of hemangioma-like vessels (HLVs) were not reported [4]. Our case had a short recurrence time, and the tumor, which occurred in the area of the original hepatectomy, had hemangioma-like vessels (HLVs) in the resection margin. The patient did not have a history of hormonal therapy. However, whether HLV in the resection margin or hormonal therapy contributed to the recurrence remained unclear. All three of our patients had hemangioma-like vessels (HLVs) in the margin but only one experienced a recurrence.

Conclusion

Three cases of giant liver hemangiomas had hemangioma-like vessels (HLVs) in the resection margin, two had highly irregular interfacesbut onlyone had a short recurrence time.. However, whether hemangioma-like vessels (HLVs) at the resection margins, an irregular interface, or hormonal therapy contribute to recurrence is not clear.

References

[1] Goodman, ZD, Terracciano, LM, Wee A. Tumours and tumour-like lesions of the liver. In: Burt AD, Ferrel LD, Portmann BC, editors. *MacSween'spathology of the liver*. 7th ed. London: Churchill Livingstone, 2018, 835-37.

[2] Miettinen, M, Fletcher, CDM, Kindblom, LG, Zimmermann, A, Tsui, WMS. Mesenchymaltumours of the liver. In: Bosman FT, Carneiro F, Hruban RH, Theise

ND, editors. *WHO classification of tumours of the digestive system*. 4th ed. Lyon: IARC, 2010, 243-4.

[3] Suriawinata, AA. Miscellaneous tumors and tumor-like lesions. In: Saxena R, editor. *Practical hepatic pathology*. 2nd ed. Philadelphia: Elsevier Saunders, 2011, 583-84.

[4] Etemadi, A, Golozar, A, Ghassabian, A, Zarei, M, HashemiTaheri, AP, Dawsey, SM, Malekzadeh, R. Cavernous hemangioma of the liver: factors affecting disease progression in general hepatology practice. *Eur J Gastroenterol Hepatol*, 2011 23, 354-8.

[5] Koszka, AJM, Ferreira, FG, de Aquino, CG, Ribeiro, MA, Gallo, AS, Aranzana, EMC, Szutan, LA. Resection of a rapid-growing 40-cm giant liver hemangioma. *World J Hepatol*, 2010 27, 292-94.

[6] Zimmermann, A, Baer, HA. Fibroustumor-liver interface in large hepaticneoplasms: its significance for tumor resection and enucleation. *LiverTransplSurg*, 1996 2, 192-9.

[7] Conter, RL, Longmire, WP. Recurrent hepatichemangiomas. Possible association with estrogen therapy. *Ann Surg*, 1988 207, 115-19.

[8] Romano, F, Messinesi, G, Tana, F, Uggeri F. Recurrent giant hemangioma causing severe respiratory distress. *Dig Dis Sci*, 2007 52, 3526-9.

[9] Zhu, H, Obeidat, K, Ouyang, J, Roayaie, S, Schwartz, M, Thung, SN. Recurrent giant hemangiomas of liver: report of two rare cases with literature review. *World J GastrointestSurg*, 2012 4, 262-66.

In: Case Reports in Surgery
Editors: Ahmad Jabir Rahyussalim et al.
ISBN: 978-1-53616-582-1

Chapter 38

46, XX Ovotesticular Disorder of Sex Development, Histopathological View: Report of a Rare Case

Intan Nevita Oktamiya Bernanthos and Budiana Tanurahardja [*]
Department of Anatomical Pathology, Faculty of Medicine,
Universtas Indonesia/Dr. Cipto Mangunkusumo Hospital,
Jakarta, Indonesia

Abstract

Ovotesticular disorder of sexual development (OT-DSD) is a rare congenital anomaly characterized by the simultaneous presence of ovarian tissue with mature ovarian follicles and testicular tissue with distinct seminiferous tubules in the same individual. The most common karyotype of OT-DSD is 46, XX. A 12-year-old boy was brought by his parents to our hospital because of a mass in his right groin area that had enlarged over the past 2 weeks. The patient's medical history included multiple surgeries due to hypospadias and unilateral right-side cryptorchidism. Histopathological analysis revealed the presence of ovarian tissue containing multilocular cysts and uterine tissue with an endometrium component, but no testicular component. Hormone analysis showed elevated levels of luteinizing hormone and follicle-stimulating hormone, with normal levels of testosterone and anti-Müllerian hormones. The patient was diagnosed with 46, XX OT-DSD and assigned as a male.

[*] Corresponding Author's E-mail: budiana.t@gmail.com.

Keywords: ovotesticular disorder of sexual development, 46, XX DSD

INTRODUCTION

Disorder of sex development (DSD) is a rare congenital condition associated with a disagreement between chromosomal, gonadal, and phenotypic sex [1]. Generally, DSD is divided into disorders of the sex chromosomes (such as Klinefelter and Turner syndrome), hormone synthesis or action (such as congenital adrenal hyperplasia), and gonadal development (such as XY gonadal dysgenesis, XX testicular DSD, and ovotesticular DSD (OT-DSD)) [2]. The incidence of DSD is reportedly 1:4500 in newborns with ovotesticular disorders accounting for less than 10% of cases [3]. Disorders of gonadal development with the 46 XX karyotype include testicular DSD, ovotesticular DSD, gonadal dysgenesis, and premature ovarian failure [4].

OT-DSD, formerly known as true hermaphroditism, is a rare congenital anomaly characterized by the simultaneous presence of ovarian tissue with mature ovarian follicles and testicular tissue with distinct seminiferous tubules in the same individual, which accounts for 3%-10% of all cases of DSD. The most common karyotype is 46, XX (60%), followed by chromosomal mosaicism/chimerism (33%), and the 46, XY karyotype (7%) [4-7]. OT-DSD most commonly occurs in XX and XX/XY, but rarely XY individuals, and typically presents in infancy as a range of atypical genitalia.

Generally, clinical manifestations of OT-DSD include ambiguous genitalia, isolated clitoromegaly, perineal hypospadias, and cryptorchidism. Phenotypical males complain of breast development, periodical hematuria, or cryptorchidism. Patients with the female phenotype present with menstrual disorders or clitoromegaly, and more rarely with cyclic pain emanating from a descended or undescended gonad [8].

Ovotesticular DSD is usually detected in infancy as underdeveloped genitalia. The etiology of 46, XX ovotesticular DSD is heterogeneous and may be related to mosaicism or genetic mutations. Most cases (65%) are negative for the sex determining region of the Y chromosome (SRY). XX ovotesticular DSD lies in the spectrum of testicular DSDs. Although the genetic etiology of 46, XX testicular and ovotesticular DSD may be the same, it is critical to detect the presence of ovarian tissue for optimal management [6].

Here, we report a rare case of 46, XX ovotesticular DSD with emphasis on its pathological aspects and clinical significance to increase the awareness of this entity.

Case Report

In December 2016, a 12-year-old boy was brought by his parents to our hospital due to the presence of a mass in his right groin area that had enlarged over the past 2 weeks. The mass caused no pain, redness, or itching. The patient's medical history included multiple genital surgeries due to hypospadias (penoscrotal type) and unilateral cryptorchidism in his hometown and in a hospital in Malaysia, as well as repair urethroplasty due to abnormal erections and urine leakage. There was no remarkable family history or parental consanguinity. The patient was fully alert with stable vital signs. The patient's body weight was 33.5 kg, height of 140 cm, and body mass index of 17.09 kg/m^2 ($-1<z$ score<0). A physical examination showed bilateral breast enlargement. An examination of the external genital examination revealed enlargement of the right testicle (6 ×4 cm), while the size of the left testicle was normal.

Laboratory results showed no elevation in either β-human chorionic gonadotropin or alpha-fetoprotein serum levels (0.100 IU/L and 0.8 IU/mL, respectively). A chromosomal examination using Giemsa banding showed that the karyotype of the patients was 46, XX (Figure 1). SRY gene detection was performed for this patient. Testicular ultrasound revealed multiple cystic lesions and septation of the enlarged right scrotum, but not the left (Figure 2).

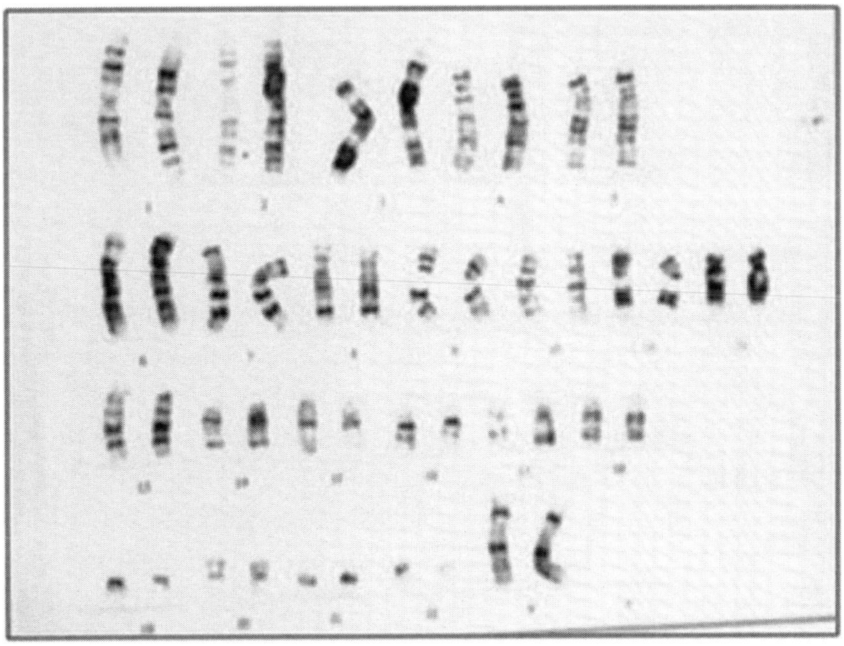

Figure 1. Chromosome analysis results. Giemsa banding of a peripheral blood sample revealed that the karyotype of the patients was 46, XX (46 chromosomes with XX sex chromosomes). There was no major structural abnormality.

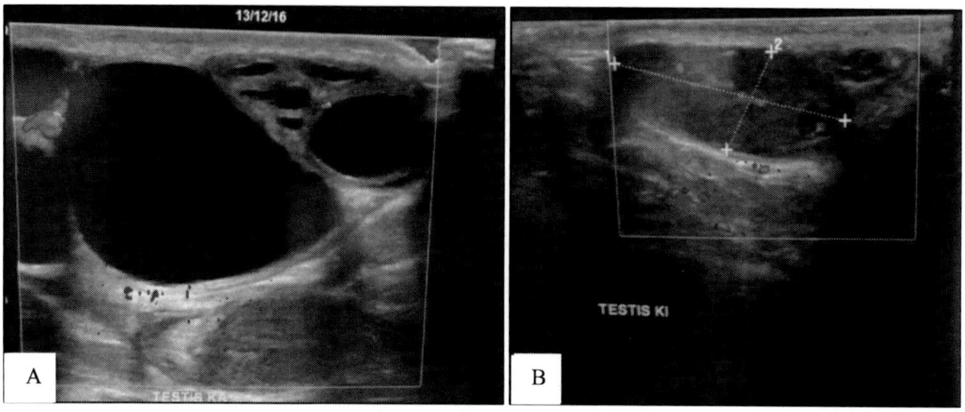

Figure 2. Testicular ultrasound. A. Multiple cystic lesions with septa of the right scrotum. B. The left testis appeared to be solid.

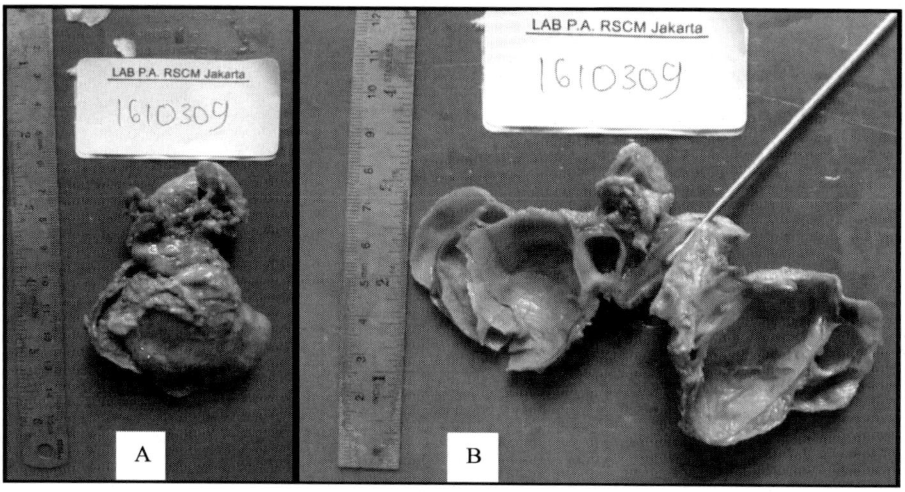

Figure 3. Gross appearance of the right testis. A. Mass with a smooth muscle surface. B. Cut section showing areas with multiple cysts.

The patient was scheduled for explorative surgery. Following identification of the right testicular mass, right orchiectomy was performed. Macroscopically, the tumor was encapsulated with a smooth external surface, measuring 8.5 ×5.0 ×3.5 cm, and gray in color. On a cut section, the tumor appeared to have multiple cysts containing serohemorrhagic fluid with diameters ranging from 0.1 to 4.5 cm. A histopathological examination revealed the presence of ovarian tissue containing multilocular cysts of various sizes, lined by granulosa cells, as well as uterine tissue with the endometrial component lined by ciliated columnar cells, accompanied by endometrial glands arranged in tubular patterns. There was no testicular component of the tissue. The histological findings were consistent with ovarian tissue with follicle cysts and uterine tissue with endometrial cells (Figure 4).

The results of a postoperative hormonal assay showed increased levels of luteinizing hormone (LH), 10,5 mIU/mL (normal 1.7-8.6 mIU/mL) and follicle-stimulating hormone (FSH), 19 mIU/mL (normal 1.5-12.4 mIU/mL), with normal levels of estradiol (5.00 pg/mL; normal range, 5-20 pg/mL), testosterone (159 ng/mL; normal range, 64.9-778 ng/mL), anti-Müllerian hormone (AMH) (26.37 ng/mL; normal range, 3.8-159.8 ng/mL), and dehydroepiandrosterone sulfate (34.7 μg/dL; normal range, 24.4-247 μg/dL). The postoperative serum levels of alpha-fetoprotein and β-human chorionic gonadotropin were within normal limits (0.8 IU/mL and 0.1 IU/L, respectively).

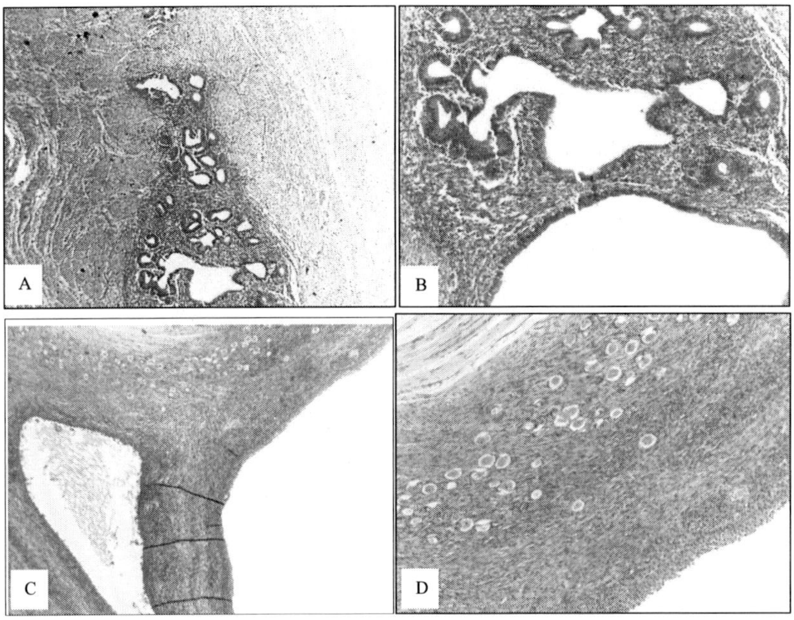

Figure 4. Histopathological examination of ovarian tissue with primary follicles and multilocular cysts, varying in size, lined by granulosa cells and uterine tissue with an endometrial component lined by ciliated columnar cells, with tubuluar ductus. No testicular tissue was observed. (A) Hematoxylin and eosin (H&E) staining, ×40. (B) H&E, ×100. (C) H&E, ×40. (D) H&E, ×100.

Follow-up visits were then scheduled. The urethrocutaneous fistula and webbed peniswere addressed by urethroplasty and penile reconstruction at 6 months after presentation. A tissue sample of the left testicle collected during surgery had a Müllerian duct remnant with extensive squamous metaplasia and ovarian tissue with primary follicles (Figure 5). A repeat urethroplasty was performed within 6 months for repair of recurrent urine leakage. After surgery, erections were normal with no more urine leakage. The patient also underwent breast reduction surgery. Histological analysis of the breast revealed that the tissue was consistent with gynecomastia (florid type) with ductal epithelial hyperplasia, tufting, micropapillary patterns, and increased periductal stromal cellularity (Figure 6).

After psychiatric consultation and evaluation, the patient and his parents decided that the patient was a boy. The patient then continued with hormonal therapy and was scheduled for a routine follow-up.

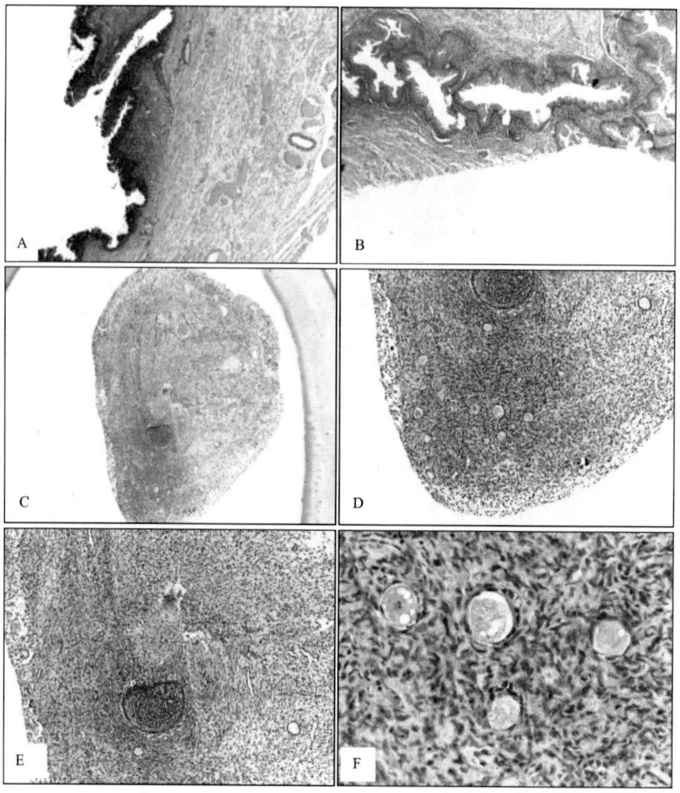

Figure 5. Histopathological features. (A and B) A remnant of a Müllerian duct with extensive squamous metaplasia (H&E, ×100). (C-F) Ovarian tissue with primary follicles (H&E, ×40, ×100, and ×400).

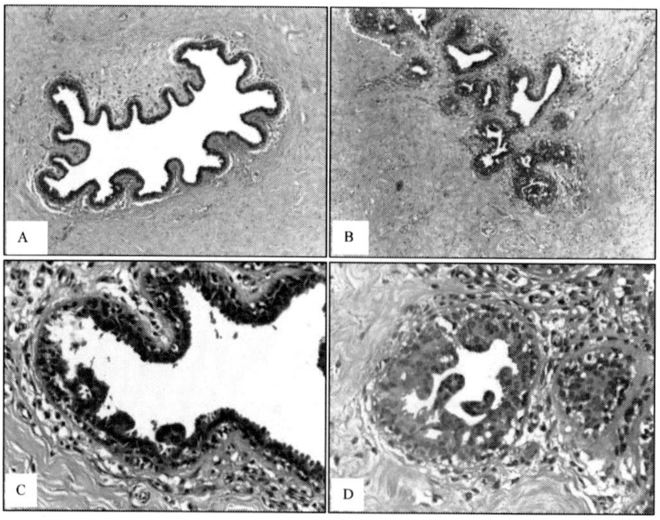

Figure 6. Gynecomastia (florid type). Ductal epithelial hyperplasia with tufting, micropapillary patterns, and increased periductal stromal cellularity (A and B) H&E, ×100. (C and D) H&E, ×400.

DISCUSSION

DSD is rare congenital condition associated with a disagreement between chromosomal, gonadal, and phenotypic sex with an incidence of 1:2000-5.500 live births due to multifactorial etiologies. The Chicago nomenclature divides the condition into six groups (Table 1). The current etiological classification of DSD according to the 2006 consensus of the Lawson Wilkins Pediatric Endocrine Society (LWPES) and the European Society for Pediatric Endocrinology (ESPE) is dependent on adrenal or gonadal involvement and karyotype analysis [1].

Embryologically, the genital and urinary systems have the same origin. The development of the gonads (testes and ovaries) begins at around gestational week (GW) 4 by the formation of urogenital ridges originating from the intermediate mesoderm. From the urogenital ridge cells, two cellular masses evolve successively toward transitional embryonic kidneys (pronephros and mesonephros) and the definitive embryonic kidneys (metanephros). The mesonephros consists of the mesonephric (or Wolffian) ducts and the paramesonephrics (or Müllerian) ducts (Figure 7) [1].

Table 1. DSD classification according to the 2006 LWPES/ESPE consensus

Cases	*Previous nomenclature*	*New nomenclature*
	Intersex	*DSD type*
1.	Congenital adrenal hyperplasia	46, XX DSD
Cases	*Previous nomenclature*	*New nomenclature*
	Intersex	*DSD type*
2.	Male pseudohermaphrodite	46, XY DSD
	Undervirilization of an XY male	
	Undermasculinization of an XY male	
3.	Female pseudohermaphrodite	46, XX DSD
	Overvirilization of an XX female	
	Masculinization of an XX female	
4	True hermaphrodite	Ovotesticular DSD
5.	XX male or XX sex reversal	46, XX testicular DSD
6.	XY sex reversal	46, XY, complete gonadal dysgenesis

Early gonadal differentiation is controlled by various genetic factors (Figure 7). At GW 7, the transcription factor SRY, mapped to Yp11.2 (with only one exon), is activated, while other genes (essentially SF-1, WT1, and CBX2) promote male gonadal development. SRY, also known as testis-determining factor, promotes the transformation of the primary sex cords to testes. Around GW 8, the male-specific hormones testosterone and AMH are produced. Testosterone secreted by Leydig cells promotes the development of the internal genital tract in the male, which consists of the epididymis, vas deferens, seminal vesicles, and ejaculatory ducts. On the other hand, AMH secreted by Sertoli cells induces regression of the paramesonephric ducts and inhibits development of the female internal genitalia [1].

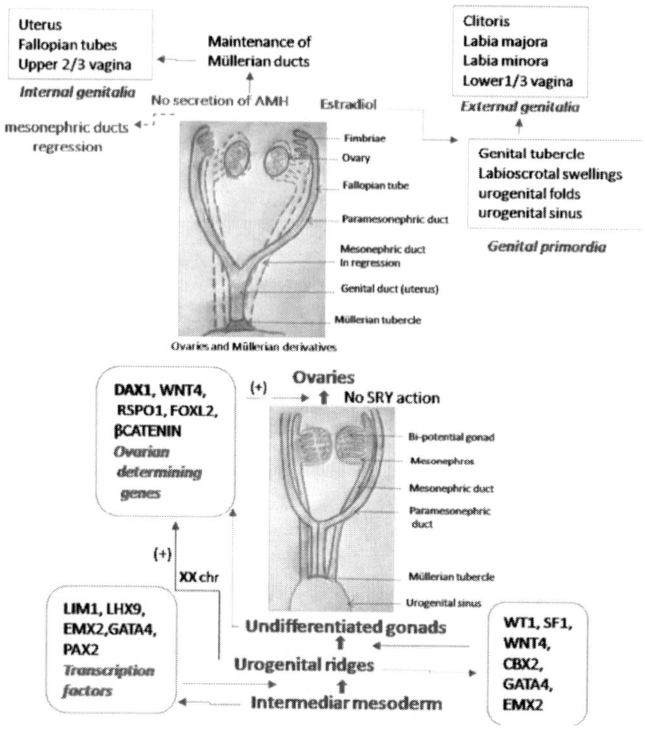

A

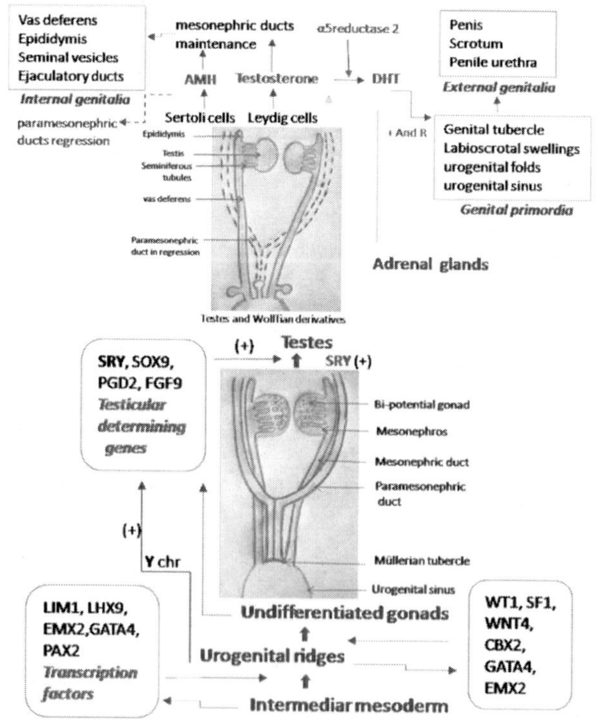

B

Figure 7. Genetic and hormonal factors involved in embryological genital development. (A) Male. (B) Female.

The molecular pathway of sex determination in the 46, XX individual include important genes for the initial formation of the genital ridge, such as Wilms tumor suppressor 1 (*WT1*) and steroidogenic factor 1 (*SF1*). The *WT1* gene is expressed in the urogenital ridge, mesonephros, kidney, gonads, and granulosa cells in females. Mutations to the *WT1* gene occurring in the XY genotype are associated with both gonadal dysgenesis and renal anomalies. *SF1* is also an important gene in early gonadal development. The phenotypic spectrum of genetic defects associated with the *SF1* gene is broad and dependent on the specific mutation. Such genetic defects range from complete testicular dysgenesis with maintenance of Müllerian structures to severe penoscrotal hypospadias with or without adrenal insufficiency. A heterozygous mutation to *SF1* was detected in a 46, XX prepubertal individual presenting with adrenal insufficiency, but apparently normal ovarian differentiation [2].

OT-DSD is a very rare sexual differentiation disorder in infants born with the internal reproductive organs (gonads) of both sexes and is characterized by the presence of ovarian tissue with mature ovarian follicles and testicular tissue with distinct seminiferous tubules in the same gonad (ovotestis) [5, 7, 8]. However, as time passes, the ovarian tissue usually becomes functional and the testicular tissue regresses becoming dysgenetic and showing interstitial fibrosis and lack of spermatogonia [2]. Our patient was diagnosed with suspected OT-DSD as an infant based on a gonadal biopsy that revealed the presence of ovarian tissue, but no testicular tissue. Even though there was no histopathological finding of testicular tissue, the elevated levels of testosterone and AMH supported the presence of functional testicular tissue in this patient.

The types of gonads observed in OT-DSD patients are ovotestis (44%), ovary (33%), and testis (22%). Depending on the type and laterality of the abnormal gonad, OT-DSD is classified into three types: unilateral (ovotestis on one side and a normal gonad on the other side), bilateral (both gonads are ovotestis), and lateral (one gonad is a testis and the other is an ovary) [8].In our patient, both gonads were composed of ovarian tissue.

Various types of chromosomal abnormalities have been described in OT-DSD, including 46, XX; 46, XY; 46, XX/46, XY, and 45, X/46, XY [5, 8-10].Most cases of ovotesticular DSD are sporadic [8]. Genetically, the karyotype of our patient was 46, XX and there was no remarkable family history.

Clinical features of OT-DSD include ambiguous genitalia, isolated clitoromegaly, perineal hypospadias, and cryptorchidism. Phenotypical males complain of breast development, periodical hematuria, or cryptorchidism. Patients with a female phenotype present with menstrual disorders or clitoromegaly, and more rarely with cyclic pain emanating from a descended or undescended gonad [8] (Figure 8), while hormonal levels are typically normal. Patients with OT-DSD have some degree of function and therefore normal levels of FSH, LH, estradiol, and DHT [11]. In the present case, all hormonal levels were normal. The clinical presentations of OT-DSD often go undetected until adolescence when phenotypic males are evaluated for gynecomastia or testicular cysts, which are treated surgically [13].

The diagnosis of OT-DSD is suggested by a mosaic karyotype, but is confirmed by the presence of ovarian and testicular tissue on biopsy [14]. Based on detection of the SRY gene, 46, XX DSD can be clinically classified as SRY-positive or -negative. SRY-positive individuals usually have normal male genitalia, small azoospermic testes, and hypergonadotropic hypogonadism. These characteristics have also been reported in some 46, XX males (testicular DSD). The SRY-negative group includes patients with OT-DSD, which is characterized by the presence of both testicular and ovarian tissues in the gonads of the same individual. Testicular DSD is characterized by the full development of both gonads as testis without any evidence of ovarian tissue [12]. The diagnosis of OT-DSD is based on the exclusion of other DSDs. The differential diagnosis include mixed gonadal dysgenesis, 46, XX testicular DSD, and premature ovarian failure (Table 2).

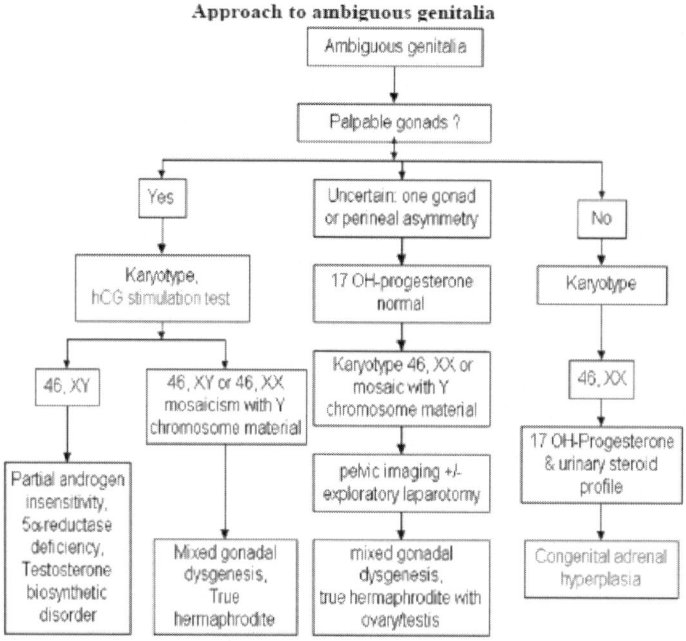

Figure 8. Approach for ambiguous genitalia.

Microscopically, with OT-DSD, the ovary is usually normal (prepubertal ovary with primordial follicles and primary oocytes with a few primary or antral follicles, prepubertal testis with immature seminiferous tubules lined by immature Sertoli cells and primitive germ cells, usually without spermatogonia). Ovotestis is characterized by normal ovarian tissue with atrophic testicular tissue [15] (Figure 9).

Table 2. Differential diagnosis of ovotesticular DSDs [10, 15]

No.	Diagnosis	Common features	Different features	Karyotype	Picture
1.	Mixed gonadal dysgenesis	Cryptorchidism, pubertal masculinization. Asymmetric gonadal differentiation	Ovarian tissue, if present, lacks primordial follicles; internal/external genitalia are not relevant to differentiate these two conditions.Elevated FSH	45, X/46, XY, 45, X/46, XX or 45, X/47, XXY; may also have 46, XX but missing part of one X chromosome	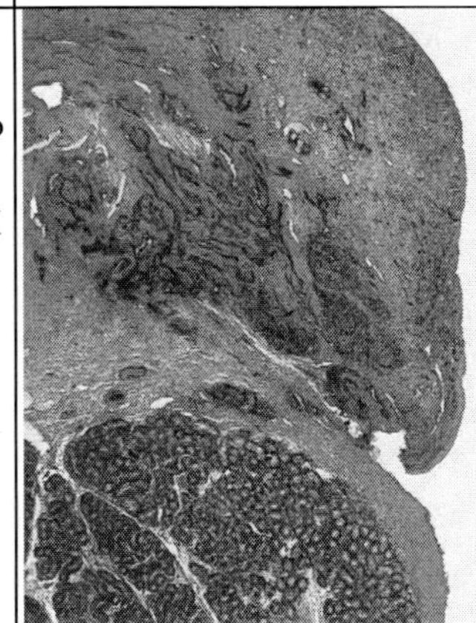 (Top) Streak tissue and rete are separated by the tunica albuginea of the testis. (Bottom) Prepubertal patients develop normal immature testis during puberty with tubules exhibiting mild hypospermatogenesis to total sclerosis. The streak gonad has ovarian stroma without primordial ovarian follicles. The streak ovary has primordial follicles and primitive sex cord-like structures with or without germ cell components within the ovarian type stroma, mimicking gonadoblastoma and tumors composed of granulosa or Sertoli cells.

No.	Diagnosis	Common features	Different features	Karyotype	Picture
2.	46, XX testicular DSD	Gynecomastia, cryptorchidism, hypospadias ambiguous genitalia	No ovarian tissue	46, XX	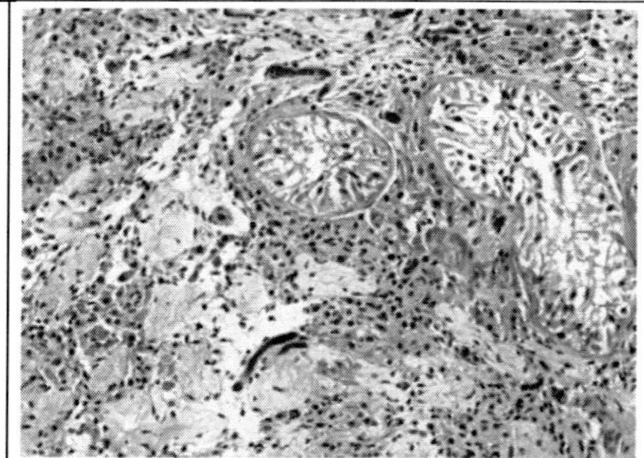 Testicular parenchyma with marked fibrosclerosis of most of the seminiferous tubules, alternating with other tubules lined only with Sertoli cells. Leydig cells are also present.
3.	Premature ovarian failure	46, XX	Sex steroid deficiency and elevated of serum gonadotropins before the age of 40 years [16]	46, XX	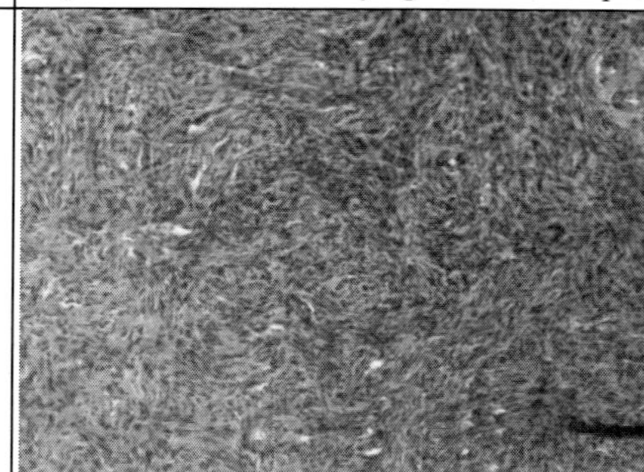 Premature ovarian failure showsdense cortical stroma lacking primordial or developing follicles. This appearance was seen throughout the ovary.

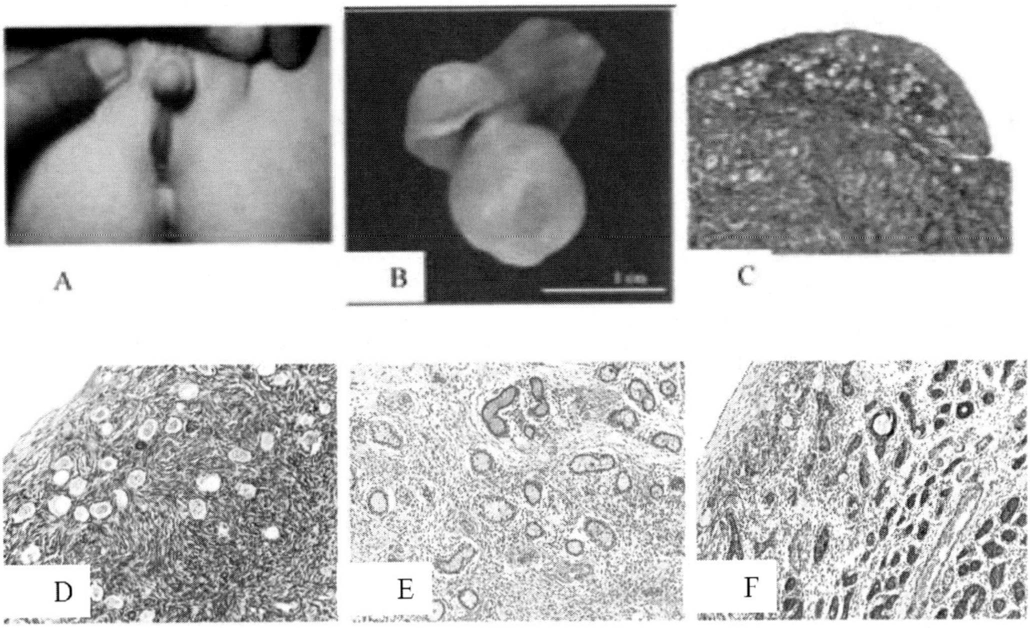

Figure 9. Clinical and pathological aspects of OT-DSD. (A) External male genitalia are hypoplastic with a penile clitoris, hypoplastic labia, and vaginal vestibule. (B) Ovotestis of a child. The ovarian parenchyma forms a cap over the testicle, which is attached by a pedicle. (C) Ovotestis of a child. A gonad with two parts separated by a connective septum. The upper zone shows the ovarian parenchyma overlying the testicular parenchyma. Among some seminiferous tubules, primordial follicles can be identified. (D) Numerous primordial follicles without maturation set in an abundance of spindle cell stroma. (E) Testicular parenchyma rich with cellular stroma similar to ovarian stroma. Some seminiferous tubules are markedly hypoplastic. (F) Epithelial cords with irregular shapes and microliths. Underneath the surface, these cords are embedded in ovarian-like stroma.

The extent of follicular maturation, the corpora lutea, and corpora albicantia varies with OT-DSD. The seminiferous tubules, which rarely contain developing sperm cells, often have Sertoli cells only with a dysgenetic appearance that frequently undergo hyalinization. Sertoli cells are positive for immunostaining of inhibin and maintain the expression of D2-40, which is indicative of immaturity. Many Sertoli cells are negative for the androgen receptor [8] (Figure 10).

Prognostic factors are important to assign gender as soon as possible (before the age of 2-4 years), since there are usually no other developmental anomalies and patients will have a better chance for normal psychological, sexual, and reproductive lives if the gonad inappropriate for gender assignment is removed. Dysplastic gonads are at risk for developing germ cell malignancy and an increased risk for gonadal malignancy if a Y chromosome is present [15].

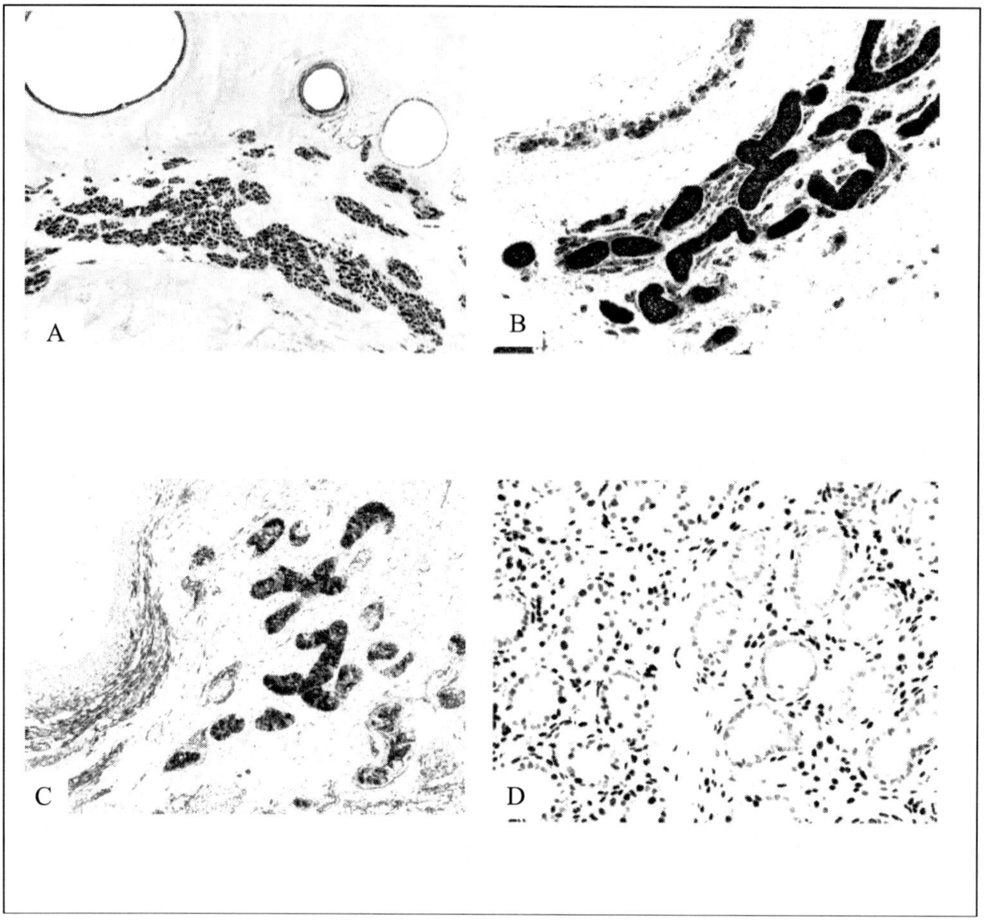

Figure 10. Immunostaining in OT-DSD. (A) Inhibin immunostaining of an ovotestis. Seminiferous tubules are highlighted by inhibin staining, which is also expressed by the immature ovarian follicles. (B) The seminiferous tubules and Leydig cells were positive for inhibin immunostaining. Seminiferous tubules are immature and malformed. (C) Immature and malformed seminiferous tubules as well as the perifollicullar stroma are positive for D240 immunostaining. (D) Androgen receptors are scarcely expressed in Sertoli cells or even absent in some seminiferous tubules, in contrast with the strong expression in peritubular and interstitial cells.

Treatment of OT-DSD is complex because it requires expertise in several subspecialized fields. Also gender assignment should be based on the functional potential of the phenotype. The discordant gonads should be removed as early as possible. In males, the testicular tissue is preserved and orchiopexy is performed. The incidence of testicular tumors in males ranges from 1 to 10%, which are predominantly gonadoblastomas and dysgerminomas, thus long-term surveillance is needed. Hypospadia repair is also required for such males. Males also tend to require hormonal replacement therapy because of progressive testicular fibrosis [14]. The incidence of gonadal tumors is approximately 3% in 46, XY OT-DSD and rare in 46, XX OT-DSD [15].

REFERENCES

[1] Poaty, H. Ondima, I., Moyen, E., Demba Diop, J.P., Moukouma, C., & Ndiaye, R. (2017). Human genetics & embryology disorders of sex development in an infant (46, XX) - A Case Report and Review of Literature. *Hum. Gen. Embryol.*, 7, 3-7.

[2] Barseghyan, H. & Vilain, E. (2014). The genetics of ovotesticular disorders of sex development. *Genet. Steroid Disord.*, 261-263.

[3] Puji, H. T., Julia, M. & Prawirohartono, E. P. (2016). 46 XX ovotesticular disorder of sexual development with detected SRY (Sexdetermining Region Y) gene: A case report. *J. Clin. Case Rep.,* 6, 9-11.

[4] Kousta, E., Papathanasiou, A. & Skordis, N. (2010). Sex determination and disorders of sex development according to the revised nomenclature and classification in 46,XX individuals. *Hormones(Athens)*, 9, 218-231.

[5] Singh, R., Ahluwalia, C. & Mandal, A. K. (2016). Case report ovotesticular disorder of sexual development with rare karyotype. *Ann. Pathol. Lab. Med.*, 3, 69-71.

[6] Vilain, E. (2011). The genetics of ovotesticular disorders of sex development. *Adv. Exp. Med. Biol.*, 707, 105-106.

[7] Scarpa, M.G. (2017). Ovotesticular differences of sex development: Surgery or not sugery? That is the question. *Front. Pediatr.*, 5, 231.

[8] Nistal, M., Paniagua, R., González-Peramato, P. & Reyes-Múgica, M. (2015). Perspectives in pediatric pathology, Chapter 7. Ovotesticular DSD (True Hermaphroditism). *Pediatr. Dev. Pathol.*,18, 345-352.

[9] Pleskacova, J., Hersmus, R., Oosterhuis, J.W., Setyawati, B.A., Faradz, S.M., Cools, M., Wolffenbuttel, K.P., Lebl, J., Drop, S.L., & Looijenga, L.H. (2010). Tumor risk in disorders of sex development. *New Concepts Hum. Disord. Sex Dev.*,5, 259-269.

[10] Nistal, M., Paniagua, R., González-Peramato, P. & Reyes-Múgica, M. (2015). Perspectives in Pediatric Pathology, Chapter 5. Gonadal Dysgenesis. *Pediatr. Dev. Pathol.*,18, 259-278.

[11] Délot, E. C. & Vilain, E. (2018). *Disorders of sex development. in Yen & Jaffe's reproductive endocrinology: physiology, pathophysiology, and clinical management(Eighth Edition).*

[12] Alves, C., Braid, Z., Coeli, F. B. & Mello, M. P. De. (2010). 46,XX Male - Testicular disorder of sexual differentiation (DSD): hormonal, molecular and cytogenetic studies. *Arq. Bras. Endocrinol. Metabol.,* 54, 6-10.

[13] Gatti, J.M. (2014). Ashcraft's Pediatric Surgery: Chapter: Disorders of sexual differentiation. (6th edition, pp. 826-837). Philladelphia. Elsevier.

[14] Al-Hussain, T. True hermaphroditism. PathologyOutlines.com website. Available from: URL: https://www.pathologyoutlines.com/ topic/testistruehermaph.html.

[15] Ebrahimi, M. &AkbariAsbagh, F. (2011). Pathogenesis and causes of premature ovarian failure: an update. *Int. J.Fertil.Steril.*, 5, 54-65.

ABOUT THE EDITORS

Ahmad Jabir Rahyussalim

Editor, Faculty of Medicine Universitas Indonesia

Dr. Rahyussalim, SpOT(K) is an orthopaedic surgeon born in Padang, June 5th 1971. He is currently the Manager of Research and Community Service in Faculty of Medicine, University of Indonesia (FMUI). Dr. Rahyussalim finished his medical doctor degree from FMUI in 1996. He received his orthopaedics and traumatology specialist degre from the same institution in 2008. Later in 2009, Rahyussalim finished his subspecialist degree in spine, and was honored with a Doctorate degree in 2013. He has published 38 papers in several international journals and also is frequently invited as a speaker for national and international scientific programs.

Some of the awards and achievement appreciations given to Rahyussalim include Potential researcher in faculty of medicine Universitas Indonesia based on total articles and impact factor accumulation in SCOPUS ($3 \leq IF \leq 6$) in2013, National publication award on tropical health and infectious disease by Center for Research and Integrated Development of Tropical Health and Infectious Diseases (CRID TROPHID) in 2014, Award on International publication incentive Cipto Mangunkusumo Hospital in2014 and 2015, and Award onIndonesia Innovation and Entrepreneurship Exhibition2016 (IIEE) Universitas Indonesia.

Ismail Hadisoebroto Dilogo

Editor, Faculty of Medicine Universitas Indonesia

Prof. Dr. Ismail, Sp.OT (K) is a professor in orthopedic and traumatology who currently practices at Premier Jatinegara Hospital and Cipto Mangunkusumo Hospital, Jakarta. He completed his specialist education from the Faculty of Medicine, Universitas Indonesia. He has attended several workshops and training related to the orthopedic field, including Current Advances in Orthopedic Trauma, 12th Arthoplasty Simulative Training

Workshop on Total Knee Replacement, The 18th Arthoplasty Simulative Training Workshop on Total Hip Replacement. He is the Secretary of the Orthopedic and Traumatology Study Program in the Trauma and Reconstruction Division at the Faculty of Medicine, Universitas Indonesia. He is also a member of the Association of Indonesian Orthopedic and Traumatology Specialists (PABOI) and the Indonesian Doctors Association (IDI).

Achmad Fauzi Kamal

Editor, Faculty of Medicine Universitas Indonesia

Dr. Achmad Fauzi Kamal, Sp.OT(K) completed his specialist study in orthopedic and traumatology at the University of Indonesia. He also accomplished a Doctorate in the same University in 2012. He is a member of the Indonesian Association of Orthopedic & Traumatology Specialists (PABOI). Dr. dr. Achmad Fauzi Kamal, SpOT(K) practices at Pelni Hospital, Jakarta, RS Kramat 128 Jakarta, and Cipto Mangunkusumo Hospital, Jakarta. He specialty include orthopedic consultation, hemiarthroplasty, elbow replacement surgery, ligament reconstruction, arthroscopy, arthroplasty, leg replacement surgery, shoulder surgery, wrist surgery, hip resurfacing surgery, joint straightening, knee replacement surgery, joint injection, reconstruction of the elbow ligament and shoulder wheel.

Aryadi Kurniawan

Editor, Faculty of Medicine Universitas Indonesia

Dr. Aryadi Kurniawan, Sp.OT(K) finished his general practioner degree in 1995, and then finished his orthopedic and traumatology specialist degree in 2005, studying in University of Indonesia. He was the honored his doctoral degree in the same university in 2016. He is a member of the Association of Indonesian Orthopedic and Traumatology Specialists (PABOI) and Indonesia Surgeon Association (IKABI). Aryadi is currently a medical staff of Orthopedic and Traumatology Department in Cipto Mangunkusumo Hospital and also in Premier Jatinegara Hospital. He is one of the few orthopedic surgeons in Indonesia specializing in pediatric cases, having having studied his pediatric focus in orthopedic after in Fukuoka, Japan and Australia throughout 2006-2008.

Index

B

D

E

F

G

H

I

J

K

L

M

N

O

T

U

V

Related Nova Publications

VASCULAR SURGERY: PROCEDURES, COMPLICATIONS AND RECOVERY

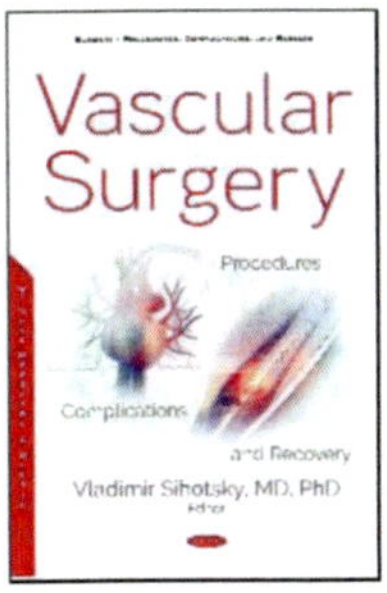

EDITOR: Vladimir Sihotsky, MD, PhD

SERIES: Surgery – Procedures, Complications, and Results

BOOK DESCRIPTION: The book is addressed for students of medicine and also as fundamental principles of vascular surgery for residents of different surgical specializations.

HARDCOVER ISBN: 978-1-53616-454-1
RETAIL PRICE: $230

LIVER STEATOSIS AND BARIATRIC SURGERY

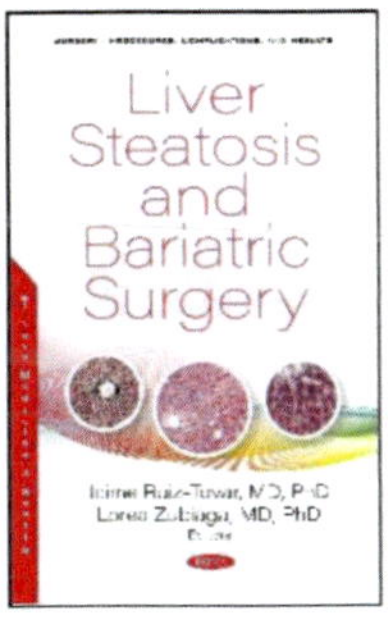

EDITORS: Jaime Ruiz-Tovar, MD, PhD and Lorea Zubiaga, MD, PhD

SERIES: Surgery – Procedures, Complications, and Results

BOOK DESCRIPTION: The aim of this book is to update the actual evidence about liver steatosis, non-alcoholic fatty liver disease and non-alcoholic steatohepatitis in morbidly obese patients, the diagnostic methods and the evolution after the different techniques of bariatric surgery.

HARDCOVER ISBN: 978-1-53616-444-2
RETAIL PRICE: $160

To see a complete list of Nova publications, please visit our website at www.novapublishers.com

Related Nova Publications

Handbook of Surgical Procedures

Editor: Heather Gilbert

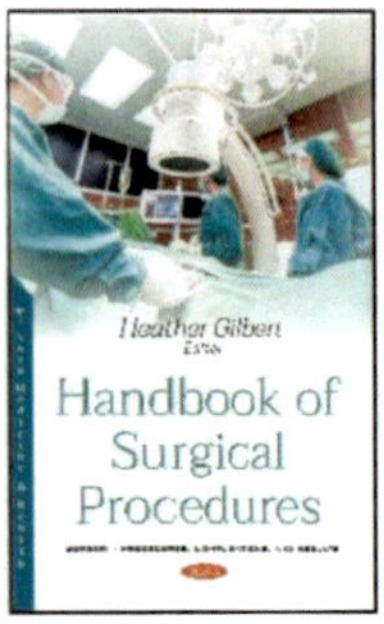

Series: Surgery – Procedures, Complications, and Results

Book Description: In this compilation, the authors begin with a focus on the indications for surgery in hepatocarcinoma and how to perform a liver resection. Long-term outcomes and different theories on the causes of recurrence after resection are also discussed.

Hardcover ISBN: 978-1-53614-580-9
Retail Price: $128

Robotic Surgery: Clinical Perceptions, Approaches and Challenges

Editor: John F. Lazar, M.D.

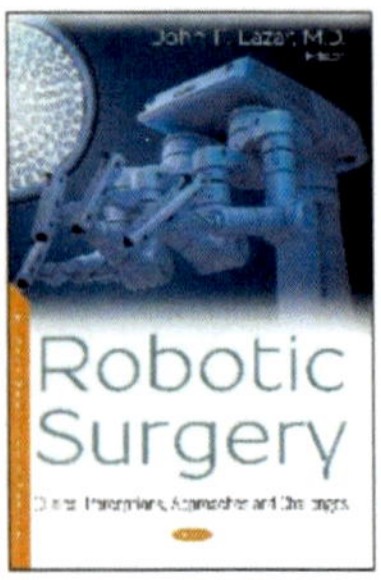

Series: Robotics Research and Technology

Book Description: Robotic surgery is at a significant intersection of technology and the ability to routinely perform high-end minimal invasive surgery. *Robotic Surgery: Clinical Perceptions, Approaches and Challenges* is the robotic surgeon's manual to help achieve the technical and intellectual metrics desired by all surgeons.

Hardcover ISBN: 978-1-53614-325-6
Retail Price: $230

To see a complete list of Nova publications, please visit our website at www.novapublishers.com